CLINICAL AND MOLECULAR ADVANCES IN ANKYLOSING SPONDYLITIS

Edited by **Jacome Bruges-Armas**

Clinical and Molecular Advances in Ankylosing Spondylitis
Edited by Jacome Bruges-Armas

Published by InTech
Janeza Trdine 9, 51000 Rijeka, Croatia

Publishing Process Manager Ivana Zec

Technical Editor Teodora Smiljanic

Cover Designer InTech Design Team

Additional hard copies can be obtained from orders@intechopen.com

Clinical and Molecular Advances in Ankylosing Spondylitis,
Edited by Jacome Bruges-Armas
p. cm.
ISBN 978-953-51-0137-6

For EU product safety concerns:
IN TECH d.o.o., Prolaz Marije Krucifikse Kozulić 3, 51000 Rijeka, Croatia,
info@intechopen.com or visit our website at intechopen.com.

Meet the editor

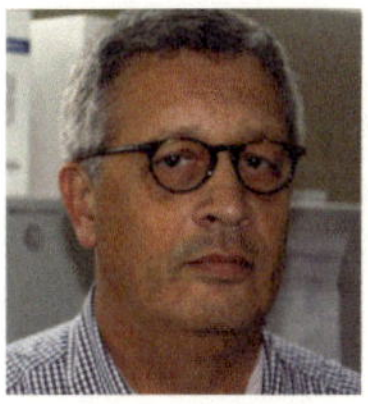

Dr Jácome Bruges Armas is a Senior Specialist in Internal Medicine and is currently the Director of the Genetics and Arthritis Research Group (GARG) at the Institute for Molecular and Cell Biology (IBMC), University of Porto, PortugaL. He is also the Director of the Epidemiology and Molecular Biology Service (SEEBMO) at the Hospital de Santo Espirito de Angra do Heroismo, Terceira Island, The Azores, Portugal. His research interests are mainly the epidemiology and molecular genetics of Spondyloarthritis (SpA), Diffuse Idiopathic Skeletal Hyperostosis (DISH), and Chondrocalcinosis (CC). He is a member of several scientific organizations and a member of the editorial board of several scientific journals.

Contents

Preface

Ankylosing Spondylitis (AS) was first described possibly at the end of the XVII century by Buckley (1931) and Connor, but it was only recognized after the radiologic descriptions of Bechterew, Strumpell and Marie, during the XIX century. In 1964 the American Rheumatism Association classified AS as a distinct disease. About forty years ago (1973), Schlosstein and Brewerton published simultaneously but independently the association of AS with the Class I allele B*27.

Since then, AS has been the target of intense research and an enormous amount of information has been gathered about this disease. Now it is known that AS is one of a group of several diseases known as Spondyloarthritis (SpA): AS, reactive arthritis, unspecified spondyloarthritis, psoriatic arthritis, and entheropathic arthritis.

Also, during the last ten years research has been focused on the understanding of the molecular and cellular processes involved in AS pathogenesis. Genome Wide Association Studies (GWAS) were followed by other studies using candidate genes which allowed the identification of non-HLA genes associated with AS susceptibility.

The more detailed knowledge of the molecular and cellular mechanisms, and the identification of biomarkers and their signaling pathways, contributed to the development of anti-TNFα and anti-IL6 molecules which are highly effective in the treatment of AS. These drugs radically changed the treatment of SpA and improved significantly the quality of life of the patients. With the deeper knowledge of the cellular mechanisms of AS, further therapeutic improvements will follow.

In this book, we have tried through original research and revised chapters, to update the clinical and molecular knowledge of AS and SpA.

The chapters in the first section, *"Clinical Manifestations, Bone Density Measurements and Axial Fractures Treatment"*, cover general and more specific clinical aspects of SpA. Spinal and axial joints are affected in AS, but the hallmark of this disease is the axial aggression, sometimes restricted to the sacroiliac joint, better characterized in the early stages by MRI. Peripheral joints may be involved in 30% of cases, and the earlier involvement of these joints may be an indicator of a more aggressive disease. Extra-articular manifestations are quite common in AS, namely enthesitis, acute anterior uveitis (AUU), cardiac involvement, pulmonary fibrosis, and secondary renal amyloidosis. Psoriatic arthritis has several subgroups and the sub-classification of this disease may be difficult even for the rheumatologist. Up to 50% of AS patients may have gut inflammation when examined by colonoscopy, and SpA may be found in 1-12% of patients with Crohn`s Disease and Ulcerative Colitis, with higher incidence of peripheral arthritis; sacroiliitis may occur asymptomatic or with typical symptoms. Reactive arthritis tends to be more aggressive and as a longer duration in HLA-B*27 positive cases (50%). Asymmetrical acute peripheral arthritis, enthesitis, acute sacroiliitis, urogenital inflammation, and ocular manifestations are common and may last several months to two years. The importance of clinical measurements to evaluate pain, morning stiffness, and functional ability is well evaluated with the BASDAI and BASFI questionnaires. Several measurements may be used by the clinician, to check and control spinal function and flexibility.

The chapter on the incidence, clinical features, pathophysiology, signs, symptoms, and current management of the Temporomandibular Joint (TMJ), reviews how AS affects this joint. TMJ is involved in 4% to 32% of cases, and ranges from mild disease to ankylosis which is exceptional. The non-surgical treatment of TMJ in AS is the most effective way of managing over 80% of patients. Non-pharmacological treatment includes fabrication of intra oral splints, physiotherapy, and patient education. The pharmacological treatment includes NSAIDS, Coxibs, corticosteroids, and anti-TNF agents. The surgical treatment – injection of steroids, joint lavage and total joint replacement -, is indicated in patients with marked trismus, or in cases of the failure of other non-surgical therapies.

The third chapter in this section is dedicated to bone mineral density (BMD) changes in patients with SpA. BMD has been investigated mainly in patients with AS. The authors investigated BMD changes in AS and in other diseases belonging to the SpA group – ReA (Reactive Arthritis), PsA (Psoriatic Arthritis), EnA (Entheropathic Arthritis) - to assess the relationship between changes in BMD and specific disease-related variables like duration, physical disability and immobility, activity of the disease, and medications. The results were also compared with a group of patients with Rheumatoid Arthritis (RA) and healthy people. Several conclusions were obtained but possibly the most relevant are: 1) BMD was identical between patients with SpA and RA; 2) Similar changes were found in patients from the various SpA groups.

The fourth and last chapter in this section is dedicated to surgical treatment in patients with AS. Patients with AS may undergo a fracture with minimal or no history of trauma, and the fracture should be considered as a high-risk injury. New back pain in AS patients should be assumed to be caused by a fracture until proven otherwise. The cervical spine is the most frequent fracture site (75%, C6-C7 and C7-D1) because the anterior and posterior ligaments are more thoroughly ossified and resistant in the thoracic and lumbar spine. Shearing fractures are the most unstable type of fractures and serious complications are: severe neurological symptoms, haemothorax, or the rupture of the aorta. Standard radiographs are inadequate to evaluate shearing fractures due to osteoporosis and the position of the shoulders, and diagnosis may be difficult due to pre-existing spinal alterations. The approach to treatment depends on the type of injury, degree of spinal instability, and neurological status of the patient. The operative treatment of these injuries is effective. Stabilization of fractures is better performed with anterior and posterior support of the spine, but because of frequent associated cardiovascular and pulmonary morbidities, this approach is not always possible.

The second section *"HLA and non-MHC genes, Immune Response, and Gene Expression Studies"* is dedicated to the molecular and immunological processes of AS. HLA-B*27 is a unique HLA Class I molecule: anchoring peptides in the binding grove of B pocket must have an arginine at the P2, and the free thiol Cys67 residue made B*27 easy to form homodimers in the extracellular domain. Twin studies suggest that the HLA-B*27 accounts for more than 50% of AS susceptibility. Until July 2011, 82 subtypes were described based on nucleotide differences. HLA-B*27:05 is the ancestral and most prevalent subtype in the majority of world populations. Several subtypes are clearly disease associated, but B*27:06 and B*27:09 have been reported not to be associated with AS and may have a protective role. According to some authors the level of B27 mRNA may correlate with disease activity and several theories have tried to explain the disease pathogenesis: molecular mimicry and arthritogenic peptides, free heavy chain, and unfolded protein response were considered main streams of hypothesis.

The second chapter in this section deals with the possibility that infectious agents may have an important role as triggering factors for some autoimmune diseases like AS. Previous work reported humoral immune responses to bacteria such as *Klebsiella pneumonia, Salmonella typhimurium, Shigella flexneri, Yersinia enterocolitica,* and *Campylobacter jejuni*. The authors reported that the 30 kDa band (p30) from *S. typhimurium* could be differentially recognized by the immune response in AS patients. In this chapter the authors have investigated whether the p30 antigen recognized by AS patients is specific to *S. typhimurium,* or if it can be found in another serovar of salmonella enterica. Twenty eight AS patients and 28 healthy controls were investigated to analyze the IgG and IgA humoral immune response against Salmonella enterica serovar enteritidis by western-blot. The immune response against *S. typhimurium* appears to be strain specific; patients with AS produce IgG3 antibodies against the p30 of *S. typhimurium* in contrast to healthy controls. The authors also hypothesized that the relationship between the humoral response and the pathogenesis of the disease could be due to Fc◎R polymorphisms of IgG. The authors suggest a link between humoral immune response in a susceptible individual and Fc◎RIII-150-VV.

Other HLA genes have been associated with AS susceptibility, like HLA-B*60 and HLA-DRB1 alleles. A recent publication involving a Spanish/Portuguese cohort reports the association with HLA-DPA1 and HLA-DPB1 alleles and AS. GWAS supported the presence of non-MHC susceptibility genes and further studies narrow down the chromosome areas first identified. ERAP1 (5q15) and IL23R (1p31.3) are the most consistently non-MHC associated genes to AS. ERAP1 is a MHC class I dependent aminopeptidase, and plays a major role in peptide trimming for presentation at the cell surface. Recently it was shown that HLA-B*27 positive and negative AS cases differ in association with ERAP1, suggesting that the mechanism by which B*27 induces AS involves aberrant presentation or handling of peptides. IL23R is a member of the haemopoietin receptor family, and genetic variants of this gene have been reported in association with other autoimmune diseases such as inflammatory bowel disease (IBD), psoriasis, and systemic sclerosis. The association of several IL23R SNPs with AS was first reported by the Consortium WTCCC/TASC in 2007 and, since then, it has been replicated in several populations. The attributable risk for this gene was calculated to be 9%. KIF21B belongs to a family of kinesin motor proteins and was recently found with a strong association to AS in caucasians. Several other genes are suggestively associated with the AS: IL-1 gene cluster, ANTXR2, TNFSF15, TNFRSF1A, and TRADD.

The last chapter of this book explains the recent advances in molecular biology using microarray-based genotyping and expressing assays which are ideal to investigate diseases with underlying complex genetic causes. Microarray expression technology, together with the most recent bioinformatics platforms, can be used for the detection and quantification of differentially expressed genes but, according to the authors, the success of the experiences greatly depends on whether the hypothesis and rationale have been formulated through a clearly delineated question. Although significant inter-individual variations on gene expression may occur, recent studies have been focused on the investigation of gene expression patterns in peripheral blood to identify systemic markers of the disease. Seven papers published since 2007 uncovered pathways and potential biomarkers which may be useful for diagnosis and treatment prediction on SpA. Consistent expression changes in genes such as TLRs, NLRP2 and CLEC4D supports the importance of innate immune mechanisms in AS pathogenesis. Other expression profiles include a pro-inflammatory signature in uSpA and AS, a decreased immune responsiveness and immunosuppressive phenotypes, and two bone remodeling signatures with over-expression of PCSK6, FREMEN1, and catenin alpha-like 1 (CTNNAL1) genes in SpA patients or downregulation of SPOCK2, EP300 and PPP2R1A in AS patients, which are possible mediators in the ossification process. A promising biomarker for early diagnostic of SpA is a member of the family of regulators of G protein signaling (RGS1), although not confirmed in all studies to date. The identification of biomarkers of treatment response to biologic therapies may enable the more appropriate therapy to be chosen, contributing to a patient-specific personalized medicine. LIGHT, RUNX2, and the CX3CL1-CC3CR1 complex may be considered for treatment response in SpA patients.

I am very grateful to all authors for their contribution to this textbook. I sincerely hope that this volume *Clinical and Molecular Advances in Ankylosing Spondylitis* may help to clarify some aspects of the disease contributing to a better understanding of AS pathogenesis.

Dr Jacome Bruges-Armas
Hospital of the Holy Spirit, The Azores,
Portugal

Part 1

Clinical Manifestations, Bone Density Measurements and Axial Fractures Treatment

1

Clinical Features of Ankylosing Spondylitis

Jeanette Wolf
5th Dep. of Inner Medicine
Wilhelminenspital
Vienna
Austria

1. Introduction

Ankylosing spondylitis is an inflammatory rheumatic disease, its cause is yet unknown, a cross-reactivity of antibodies against germs and HLA-B27 is discussed, but not yet proven. Ankylosing spondylitis belongs to the group of seronegative spondyloarthritides (Moll J, Haslock I, Mac Rae IF, Wright V) (Wright V), there is a strong linkage to HLA-B27. Its prevalence lies between 0.1% and 1% with a male predominance of 2-3: 1, the onset of disease lies between 20 and 40 years, very seldom above the age of 45 (Wolf J, Fasching P). So women are less frequently concerned, and the illness tends to take a milder course (Sieper J, Braun J, Rudwaleit M, Boonen A, Zink A) (Gladman DD). On the other hand this puts women to a disadvantage, as the disease is less easily detected, leading to an even longer interval between disease onset and treatment.

General symptoms include morning stiffness of more than 60 minutes, fatigue, sometimes even slightly elevated temperature, but the main initial symptom is low back pain at night and in the morning. All patients with low back pain should be questioned about a positive family history concerning rheumatic diseases, as the risk of developing this illness is higher in patients where family members already have been diagnosed with ankylosing spondylitis. This of course suggests a certain genetic disposition, especially if HLA-B27 is involved (Van der Linden SM, Valkenburg HA, De Jongh BM, Cats A).

As a systemic inflammatory disease it is not restricted to a single organ or part of the body. The following subchapters will deal with the different manifestations of this disease.

2. Spinal manifestations

The first symptoms of this disease are usually a low back pain with its peak at night and in the morning and morning stiffness, which can last for hours. Both symptoms get better with exercise, back pain can worsen with inactivity. Some patients show only a partial involvement of the spine, in others the whole spine is involved. The physician always should examine the patient´s back by patting it gently with one fist, starting at the cervical spine all the way down to the sacrum, asking the patient, if and which part of the spine is painful during this examination.

The disease is caused by chronic inflammation of the spinal joints and entheses, proliferative synovitis and central cartilage fusion, which can lead to total destruction and ankylosis of these joints. Fibroblast proliferation on the other hand leads to increased ossification creating syndesmophytes (Figure 1) between the vertebral bodies and later on bamboo spine (Figure 2). These cause an irreversible loss of spinal flexibility and movement, resulting in the typical habitus still to be seen in older patients with a long disease duration due to significantly enhanced kyphosis of the thoracic part of the spine and loss of lordosis of the lumbal spine, finally making it impossible for the patient to bend any part of his spine.

Inflammation can also be found in the intervertebral disks resulting in discitis and spondylitis, which can be seen as narrowing of the intervertebral space and destruction of the adjacent cover plates. Seldom synovitis and osteitis can be found in the atlantoaxial area leading to erosions and destruction of the lateral atlantoaxial joint. At the worst the joint is destabilized, this may cause cord compression and neurological loss of function.

The costovertebral and costotransverse joints are quite commonly affected, being causal to reduced chest expansion and decreased vital capacity of the lungs.

In some patients ankylosing spondylitis is restricted exclusively to an affection of the sacro-iliac articulation (sacroiliitis), best shown by MRI, as it causes bone marrow edema and cartilage changes. X-ray takes a long time to reveal this arthritis, because there only bone destruction and ankylosis are visible, these are not seen in the early stages of the disease. In the end sacroiliitis can lead to total destruction and ankylosis of the sacroiliacal joint, then of course it is clearly visible in x-ray (Figure 3). Active sacroiliitis can lead to local pressure pain and pain associated with movements of the pelvis.

Finally kyphosis of the thoracic spine, obliteration of the lumbal lordosis and forward stoop of the neck occur, these signs are irreversible. Due to osteoporosis even minor trauma may result in spinal fractures, causing a rapid and significant increase in pain. Fracture fragments can be dislocated and lead to cord compression.

3. Peripheral joints

Almost half of the patients experience arthritis in the hips or the shoulders. Up to 30% of the patients suffer from small joint involvement with swelling, pain and stiffness in the inflamed joints. Often these appear as asymmetrical oligoarthritis. Usually they are non-erosive, but deformity and consequently destruction of the hips have been seen. An early involvement of peripheral joints can be an indicator of a more aggressive progress. Peripheral joint involvement can occur at any stage of the disease (Sieper J, Braun J, Rudwaleit M, Boonen A, Zink A) (Gladman DD).

4. Extra- articular manifestations

Quite common there is an involvement of the enthesis, meaning the insertion of tendons, ligaments and capsules into the bone. These inflammatory changes are referred to as enthesitis (Francois RJ, Braun J, Khan MA). Any enthesis may be concerned, but most frequently an enthesitis of the Achilles tendon is found. Enthesitis causes pain, swelling and thickening as well as loss of function, it can occur all of a sudden, but is found quite often as a chronic inflammation, which can finally lead to rupture of the tendon. Arthritis of the adjacent joint has also been described, enthesitis is presumed to be the starting point of joint inflammation (McGonagle D, Gibbon W, Emery P)

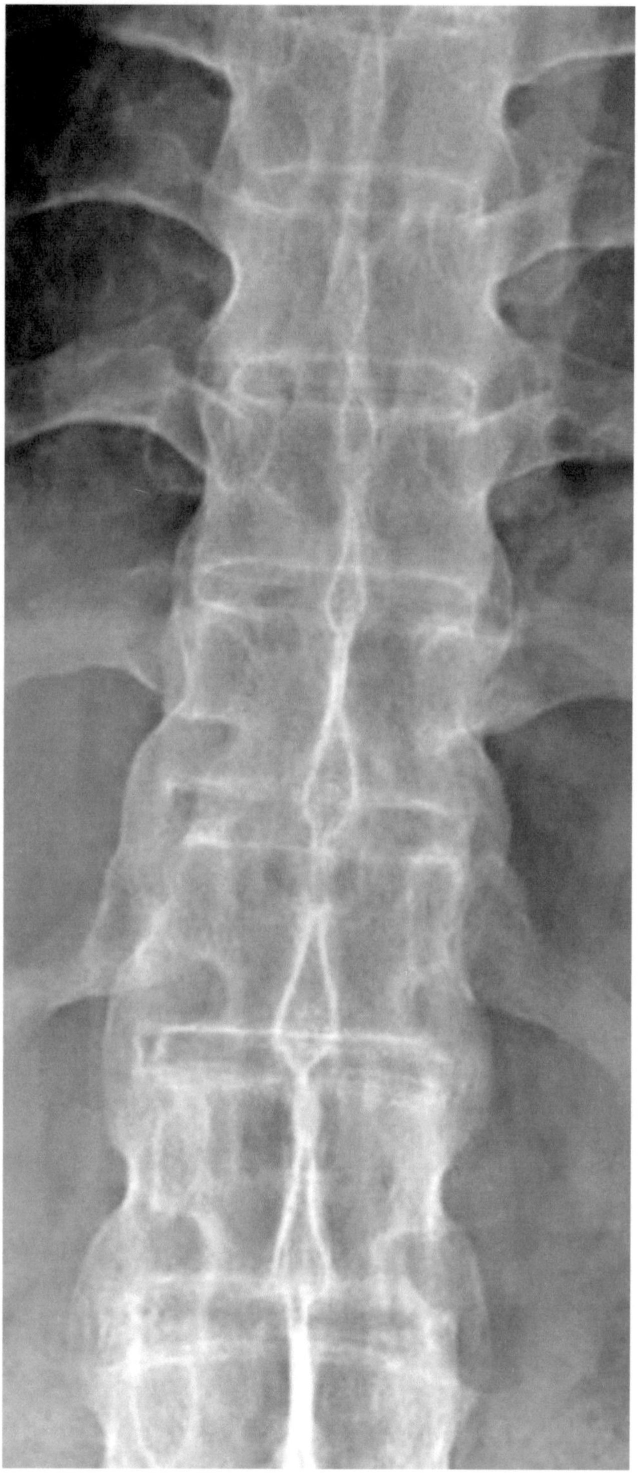

Fig. 1. Syndesmophytes.

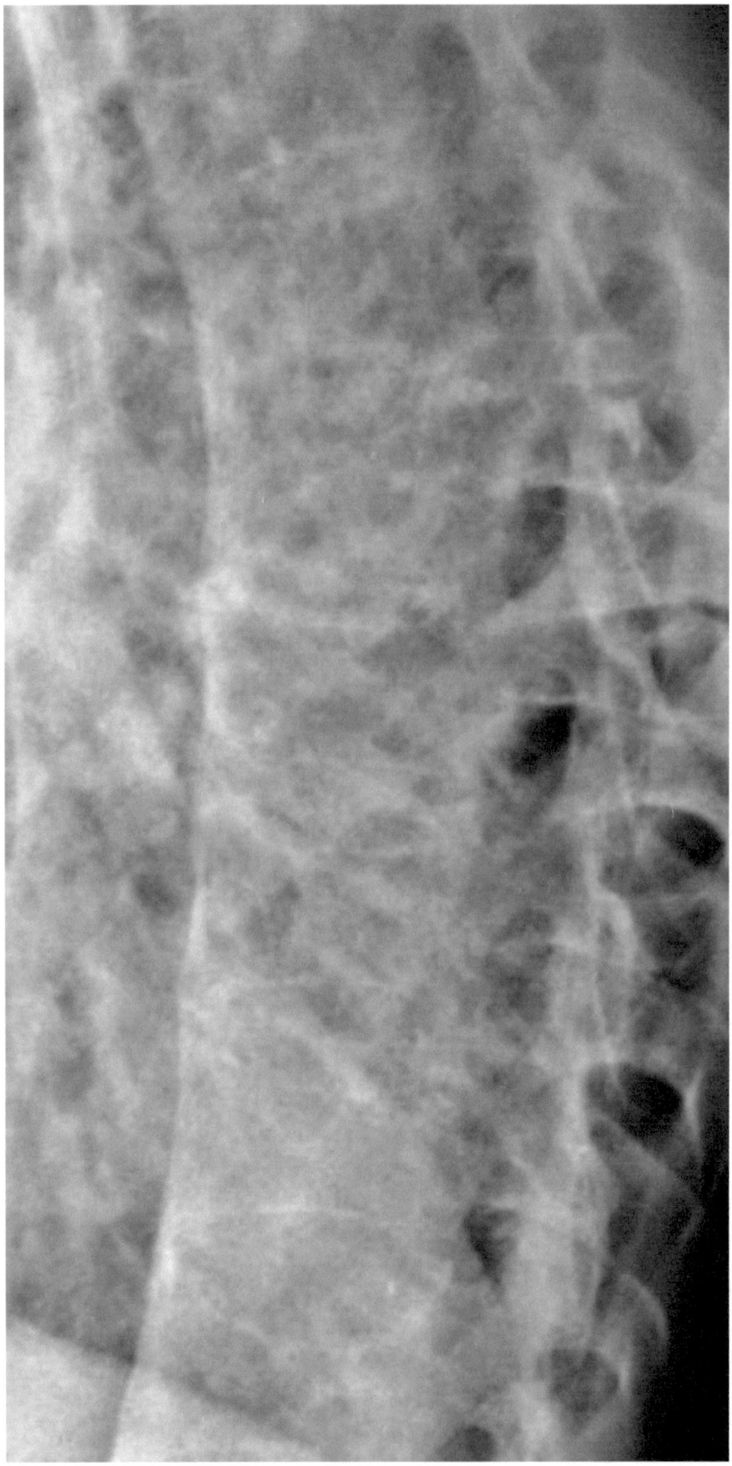

Fig 2. Bamboo stick.

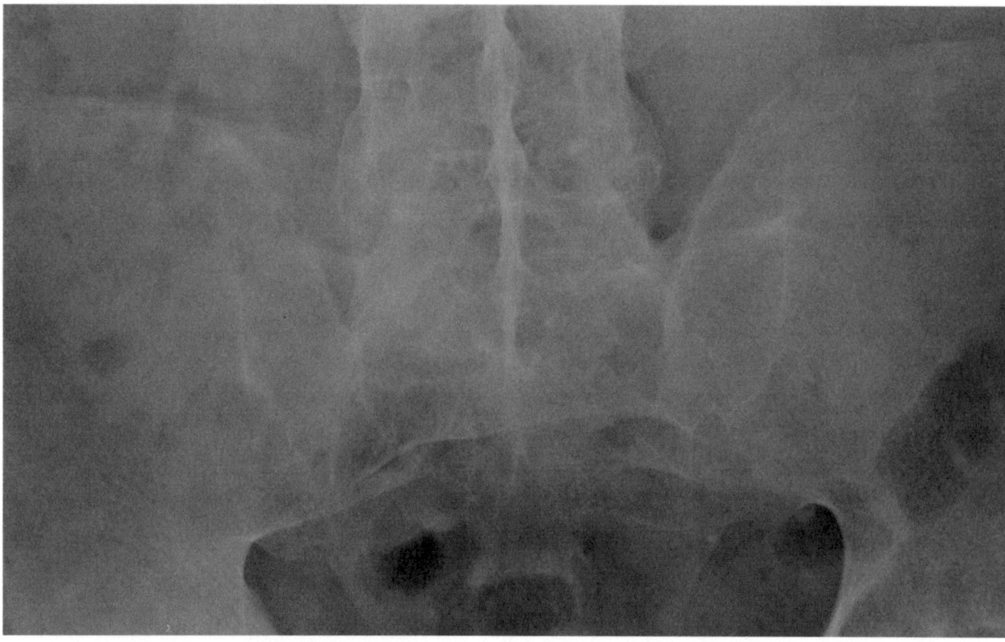

Fig. 3. Ankylosis caused by sacroiliits.

Up to 40% of all patients suffer from acute anterior uveitis at least once in their lifetime (Rosenbaum JT). Uveitis occurs usually unilateral, symptoms include pain, redness, reduced sight, photophobia, grittiness, myosis and increased lacrimation. It is self-limiting, but tends to reoccur. Untreated it may lead to complications like synechia and cataract. Patients have to be advised to see a doctor immediately after onset of the above mentioned symptoms.

Another extra-articular manifestation is aortitis and/or aortic regurgitation. Approximately 9% of ankylosing spondylitis patients are concerned. Aortitis can be seen in echocardiography showing thickening of the aortic wall and dilatation of the aortic root, thickening of the aortic valves causing aortic insufficiency (2-10% of the patients). 1-9% acquire a complete heart block, mainly located in the atrioventricular node (Bergfeldt L).

The lungs are usually only concerned indirectly because of involvement of the costovertebral and costotransverse joints and therefore reduction of chest expansion leading to reduced vital capacity. This can be detected by pulmonary function testing. But pulmonary participation like upper lobe fibrosis and pleural thickening has been described, these can be detected by high-resolution computed tomography (Maghraoui AE, Chaouir S, Abid A et al) (Souza AS, Muller NL, Marchiori E, Soares-Souza LV). These findings are usually clinically asymptomatic, yet fibrosis tends to progress over time.

4-9% of the patients develop a secondary renal amyloidosis as part of the autoimmune disease, yet primarily, renal involvement is rather uncommon in ankylosing spondylitis. Renal amyloidosis may occur in patients with long disease duration (Nabokov AV, Shabunin MA, Smirnov AV).

Due to chronic pain, patients with ankylosing spondylitis often depend upon painkillers. Especially non-steroidal anti-inflammatory drugs (NSAIDs) are prescribed, as these agents reduce pain, but also inflammation itself. Long-term intake of this medication is generally recommended, as trials have shown a significantly better effect on pain in comparison to placebo (Dougados M, Dijkmans B, Kan M, Maksymowych W, Van der Linden S, Brandt J) (Van der Heijde D, Baraf HS, Ramos-Remus C et al). Some studies even reported a decrease of spinal ossification, if the drug was taken on a regular basis (Boersma JW) (Wanders A, Van der Heijde D, Landewe R et al). On the other hand, NSAID induced nephropathy can occur in older patients with a longer disease duration and after several weeks or months of NSAID use, independent of the primal medical cause for painkillers. NSAIDs have to be discontinued in these cases. However, renal parameters should be checked on a regular basis in all patients with ankylosing spondylitis.

In up to half of the patients osteoporosis can be found, yet DEXA can be falsified by syndesmophytes, creating the impression of a higher bone density. Bone fracture caused by even minor traumatic events can lead to a sudden increase of pain. The same applies to fractures of the syndesmophytes themselves. Most frequently fractures of the cervical spine are observed, followed by the thoracolumbar region (Feldtkeller E, Vosse D, Geusens P, Van der Linden S). Osteoporosis may be induced by an imbalance between osteoblasts and osteoclasts in favour of the osteoclasts (Obermayer-Pietsch BM, Lange U, Tauber G et al). Decreased mobility may also play its part in the development of osteoporosis.

5. Disease impact

Fatigue and sleeping disorders are quite common in patients with ankylosing spondylitis (Jones SD, Koh WH, Steiner A, Garrett SL, Calin A) (Hultgren S, Broma JE, Gudbjornsson B, Hetta J, Lindqvist U), they can even lead to depression (Barlow JH, Macey SJ, Struthers GR) as well as reduced fitness and working capacity. Fatigue is a typical symptom of ankylosing spondylitis, therefore it has been included in the BASDAI, a patient´s questionnaire (Garrett S, Jenkinson T, Kennedy LG, Whitelock H, Gaisford P, Calin A). It seems to correlate with disease activity (Günaydin R, Göksel Karatepe A, Cesmeli N, Kaya T) and aggravates the difficulties patients already experience in daily life activities due to pain and reduced mobility. Sleep disturbance is caused by low back pain that typically begins at night and keeps the patient from having a restful sleep, but also by depression and anxiety. The combination of chronic disease, chronic pain and ensuing disability can lead to depression, for the patient is no longer able to perform activities of daily life the way he or she wishes to and may not be able to work full-time or even fears to lose his or her job because of reduced mobility and flexibility. Ankylosing spondylitis has a highly individual disease course and duration, some patients show only minor symptoms and restrictions, while others suffer very badly. Work disability is higher in patients with longer disease duration, inflammation of peripheral joints, lower level of education, high pain levels and physically straining jobs. Patients with long disease duration and difficult to treat back pain are more prone to develop depression than patients with no or only light pain and symptoms (Baysal O, Durmus B, Ersoy Y, Altay Z, Senel K, Nas K, Ugur M, Kaya A, Gür A, Erdal A, Ardicoglu O, Tekeoglu I Cevik R, Yildirim K, Kamnli A, Sarac AJ, Karatay S Ozgocmen S). The degree of disease activity also seems to correlate with anxiety and health status. Patients with higher disease activity scores were more anxious and more depressed (Martindale J, Smith J, Sutton CJ, Grennan D, Goodacre L, Goodacre JA).

Neurological symptoms are caused by complications of long-ongoing disease. Due to osteoporosis spinal fractures may occur, leading to suddenly increasing back pain in the afflicted region. If a fracture fragment is dislocated, it may injure the spinal cord and subsequently cause neurological symptoms. The cauda equina syndrome is evoked by dural ectasia, usually a late manifestation of the illness (Ahn NU, Ahn UM, Nallamshetty L, Springer BD, Buchowski JM), leading to sensory and / or motor loss of function and finally sphincter dysfunction. Patients may also develop pain in the rectum or the lower limbs. Atlantoaxial subluxation on the other hand may cause neurological symptoms in one or both arms. 2% of all patients with ankylosing spondylitis are concerned, but not all of them show signs of cord compression (Chou LW, Lo SF, Kao MJ, Jim YF, Cho DY). Subluxation may be caused by transverse or posterior longitudinal ligament damage or local atlantodental synovitis as well as somatic stress caused by increased kyphosis of the cervical spine.

6. Ankylosing spondylitis and other seronegative spondyloarthritides

Ankylosing spondylitis belongs to the group of seronegative spondyloarthritides together with psoriatic arthritis, reactive arthritis and unspecified spondyloarthritis. They all lack rheumatoid factor, thus being seronegative. Ankylosing spondylitis has also been seen in combination with psoriatic arthritis or enteropathic arthropathies like Crohn´s Disease and ulcerative colitis.

Peripheral asymmetrical arthritis is seen in approximately 50% of patients with psoriatic arthritis. As this disease can also include axial manifestations, a thorough skin examination has to be done in any patient with low back pain. 20 to 40% of patients with psoriatic arthritis suffer from sacroiliitis (Gladman DD, Shuckett R, Russell ML et al) (Torre Alonso JC, Rodriguez Perez A, Arribas Castrillo JM et al). There is also a tendency of cervical spine involvement and asymmetrical affliction (Jenkinson T, Armas J, Evison G et al). Psoriatic arthritis can cause monoarthritis, dactylitis, asymmetrical oligoarthritis and enthesitis, up to 25% of patients with psoriatic arthritis are HLA-B27 positive, but in patients with spinal inflammation up to 70% are HLA-B27 positive. On the other hand, there are patients who show no or only minimal skin affection at the onset of arthritis, making it even more difficult to find the right diagnosis. The transition between these two diseases is gradual and can differ greatly between two individuals. Some patients show definite signs and symptoms of ankylosing spondylitis with only marginal involvement of the skin and peripheral joints, others mainly present skin and joint affections with only little back pain. In these cases, it is quite easy to diagnose ankylosing spondylitis in combination with psoriasis or psoriatic arthritis with axial manifestations. But other individuals are not as easily diagnosed, especially if all symptoms are equally strong or weak or if there is no skin involvement at all. So sometimes it can be difficult even for the rheumatologist to differentiate between these two diseases. Yet this is of importance concerning the choice of treatment: while psoriatic arthritis can be treated with Disease Modifying Anti-Rheumatic Drugs (DMARDs) like Methotrexate or Leflunomide, these agents have no effect on peripheral arthritis caused by ankylosing spondylitis.

Spondyloarthritis can be found in both Crohn´s Disease and ulcerative colitis. The incidence lies at 1-12%. Up to 50% of the patients also develop peripheral arthritis. Both are autoimmune diseases, yet the pathogenesis is still largely unclear. Peripheral arthritis can appear before the onset of bowel symptoms, causing acute, but self-limiting attacks of monoarthritis or asymmetrical oligoarthritis as well as chronic arthritis. Hips and shoulders are less frequently affected as in ankylosing arthritis. A flare of the bowel disease can be accompanied by another flare of arthritis. Enthesitis of the Achilles tendon has been reported. Sacroiliitis can occur asymptomatic or with the typical signs of low back pain, stiffness and reduction of spinal mobility. Spondylitis is independent of gut flares. Up to 50% of patients with ankylosing spondylitis on the other hand are diagnosed with gut inflammation when examined by colonoscopy (De Kaiser F, Baeten D, Van De Bosch F et al).

Reactive arthritis is another disease belonging to the group of seronegative spondyloarthritides and usually leads to asymmetrical peripheral arthritis lasting for several months up to one or two years. Acute inflammation, swelling and pain of the joints, dactylitis and enthesitis are the main symptoms. Any joint can be affected, but most commonly knees, ankles and metatarsophalangeal joints. Later on, osteoarthritis may develop in formerly affected joints. Patients also suffer from fatigue, fever and malaise. Low back pain is rather common in these patients, caused by acute sacroiliitis, enthesitis and muscle tension. Spondylitis and sacroiliitis tend to be asymmetrical, but normally they do not lead to spinal fusion and ankylosis. There is a correlation between reactive arthritis, HLA-B27 and a previous infection (Khan MA) (Silman AJ, Hochberg MD), yet no germ can be found in any of the affected joints. Skin and mucous membrane lesions, sterile urogenital inflammation, sterile conjunctivitis, but also acute anterior uveitis and keratitis may occur (Saari KM). As ocular manifestations tend to reoccur, patients have to be advised to see an ophthalmologist immediately upon onset of ocular symptoms. X-ray will not be very helpful in acute sacroiliitis, but it can help to detect signs of previous sacroiliac inflammation. Back pain may persist even after disappearance of arthritis. In some patients ankylosing spondylitis subsequently evolves, but it is unclear whether reactive arthritis is the predecessor or if this is just a coincidence. Reactive arthritis tends to show a more aggressive and longer disease course when HLA-B27 positive, but at least 50% are HLA-B27 negative, so it should not be tested on a regular basis, as the result could be misleading.

7. Clinical measurements for ankylosing spondylitis

In order to evaluate pain, morning stiffness and functional ability two different questionnaires have been developed: the BASDAI (Bath Ankylosing Spondylitis Disease Activity Index) and the BASFI (Bath Ankylosing Spondylitis Functional Index). Both are questionnaires that have to be completed by the patient.

The BASDAI (Garrett S, Jenkinson T, Kennedy LG, Whitelock H, Gaisford P, Calin A) consists of 6 questions, they deal with fatigue, pain and morning stiffness during the last week. The questions have to be answered on a scale from 0 to 10. The patient has to tick the box with the appropriate number. 0 means no fatigue / pain / morning stiffness at all, 10 would be the worst possible case.

The BASFI (Calin A, Garrett S, Whitelock H et al) is meant to evaluate functional impairment. 10 questions are asked about the patient´s ability to dress, to bend forward, to reach up, to stand up, use the stairs, do physical labour, sports and a full day´s activities. Once again a scale from 0 to 10 is used. 0 means no problems at all, 10 means that the patient is not able to perform these activities.

As these two tests have to be filled out by the patient, they are very useful to evaluate how the patient is feeling overall and faring at work and at home. They can be redone at every visit to check, if there is an improvement or worsening of symptoms and mobility.

There are several easy to do measurements for the spine that can be evaluated at any visit and by every physician (Van der Heijde D, Bellamy N, Calin A, Dougados M, Khan MA, Van der Linden S). These examinations are important to check and control spinal function and flexibility, as ankylosing spondylitis is characterized by increasing ankylosis and loss of spinal flexibility and mobility. The rheumatologist can use these measurements to check on a possible progress of the illness or the success of an ongoing therapy. They can be easily done and redone at any given time. All that is necessary is a measuring tape and a pen.

The first test is called Schober (Schober P) (Viitanen JV, Heikkila S, Kokko ML, Kautiainen H). This gives evidence about the lumbal spine flexion. The patient has to stand straight, a sign is made over the spine at the height of the posterior superior iliac spines, a second sign 10 cm above the first (Figure 4). Then the patient has to bend forward with locked knees as far as possible, and the distance between the two marks is measured. A healthy and flexible lumbal spine shows an increase of this distance of at least 5 cm. An increase of 4 cm or less correlates with a restriction of movement of the lumbal spine.

A variation of the Schober test is the modified Schober test. When using the modified Schober test another mark is set 5 cm below the posterior superior iliac spines, then the distance between this point and the one 15 cm above is measured. There should be a difference of 20 cm at least (Mcrae IF, Wright V).

Lateral lumbar flexion can also be tested. The patient leans against the wall placing his or her hands to the side of his legs. The end of the middle finger is marked, then the patient is asked to bend laterally with straight knees towards the marked side as far as possible. The difference between start and endpoint of the middle finger is measured. A distance of more than 10 cm means normal lateral flexibility.

The next test is called Ott. Here the flexibility of the thoracic spine is measured. Once again, the patient has to stand upright. The seventh cervical spine is marked, then the second mark is applied 30 cm below the first one. Then the patient has to bend forward again as far as possible, and once again the distance between the two marks is measured. The distance should increase at least to 33 cm in order to show a normal movement of the thoracic spine.

Then the patient should stand against the wall, heels and shoulders touching the wall. The patient is asked to move his head backwards, until his occiput touches the wall (Heuft-Dorenbosch L, Vosse D, Landewe R, Spoorenberg A, Dougados M). Patients with decreased cervical movement are not able to do so, in this case the distance between the back of the head and the wall is measured. Any distance is pathological. Next the patient is asked to move his chin towards his breast, thus measuring the ventral flexibility of the cervical spine. The chin should touch the breast, any measurable distance is an indication for reduced agility of the cervical spine.

Next one can also measure the distance between fingertips and floor. In this case the patient has to bend his back forward with unbent knees as far as possible, until the fingertips touch the floor. This test is a general test of spinal flexion, but untrained people or patients with non-inflammatory diseases like spondylosis deformans or discopathy are quite often not able to reach the floor as well.

Another easy but very important test is the measurement of chest expansion. Chest circumference is measured at the height of the forth intercostal space in expiration, then in maximum inspiration. Normally there is a difference of 5 cm or more. Decreased chest expansion in patients with ankylosing spondylitis can lead to breath shortness, reduced exercise tolerance and reduced vital capacity of the lungs. Patients with a reduced chest expansion should be checked regularly by pulmonary function testing.

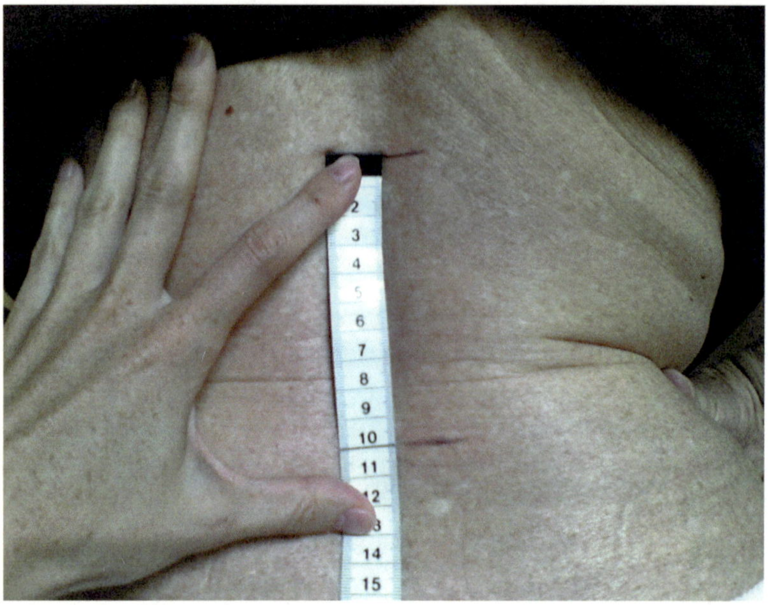

Fig. 4. Schober test.

8. Conclusion

Ankylosing spondylitis is a chronic inflammatory rheumatic disease. This disease - as all inflammatory rheumatic diseases - shows a great variability and individuality concerning symptoms, progress and outcome and is not limited to axial manifestation and affliction of the entheses, but may also involve peripheral joints, inner organs like the heart, lungs, kidneys and eyes and is associated with fatigue and depression.

So it can be quite difficult even for the rheumatologist to find the right diagnosis from the start. So every doctor should keep in mind to send each patient with low back pain during the night and in the morning , morning stiffness and reduced flexibility of the spine to a rheumatologist.

9. References

Ahn NU, Ahn UM, Nallamshetty L, Springer BD, Buchowski JM: Cauda equina syndrome in ankylosing spondylitis (the CES - AS syndrome): meta-analysis of outcomes after medical and surgical treatments. J Spinal Disord 2001; 14: 427-433

Barlow JH, Macey SJ, Struthers GR: Gender, depression and ankylosing spondylitis. Arthritis Care Res 1993; 6; 45-51

Baysal O, Durmus B, Ersoy Y, Altay Z, Senel K, Nas K, Ugur M, Kaya A, Gür A, Erdal A, Ardicoglu O, Tekeoglu I Cevik R, Yildirim K, Kamnli A, Sarac AJ, Karatay S Ozgocmen S: Relationship between psychological status and disease activity and quality of life in ankylosing spondylitis. Rheumatol Int 201 Jun; 31(6): 795-800

Bergfeldt L: HLA-B27- associated cardiac disease. Ann Intern Med 1997; 127: 621-629

Boersma JW: Retardation of ossification o the lumbar vertebral column in ankylosing spondylitis by means of phenybutazone. Scand J Rheumatol 1976: (5)1:60-64

Calin A, Garrett S, Whitelock H et al: A new approach to defining functional ability in ankylosing spondylitis: the development of the Bath Ankylosing Spondylitis Functional Index. J Rheumatol 1994; 21: 2281-2285

Chou LW, Lo SF, Kao MJ, Jim YF, Cho DY: Ankylosing spondylitis manifested by spontaneous anterior atlantoaxial subluxation. Am J Phys Med Rehabil 2002; 81: 952-955

De Kaiser F, Baeten D, Van De Bosch F et al : Gut inflammation and spondyloarthropathies. Curr Rheumatol Rep 2002; 4: 525-532

Dougados M, Dijkmans B, Kan M, Maksymowych W, Van der Linden S, Brandt J: Conventional treatments for ankylosing spondylitis. Ann Rheum Dis 2002; 61(suppl 3): iii40-50

Feldtkeller E, Vosse D, Geusens P, Van der Linden S: Prevalence and annual incidence of vertebral fractures in patients with ankylosing spondylitis. Rheumatol Int 2005; 26: 234-239

Francois RJ, Braun J, Khan MA : Entheses and enthesitis: a histopathologic rewiew and relevance to spondyloarthritis. Curr Opin Rheuamtol 2001; 13: 255-264

Garrett S, Jenkinson T, Kennedy LG, Whitelock H, Gaisford P, Calin A: A new approach to defining disease status in ankylosing spondylitis: the Bath Ankylosing Spondylitis Disease Activity Index. J Rheumatol 1994; 21: 2286-2291

Gladman DD, Shuckett R, Russell ML et al: Psoriatic arthritis (PSA) - an analysis of 220 patients. Q J Med 1987; 238: 127-141

Gladman DD: Clinical aspects of the spondyloarthropathies. Am J Med Sci 1998; 316: 234-238

Günaydin R, Göksel Karatepe A, Cesmeli N, Kaya T: Fatigue in patients with ankylosing spondylitis: relationships with disease-specific variables, depression and sleep disturbance. Clin Rheumatol 209 Sep; 28(9): 1045-51

Heuft-Dorenbosch L, Vosse D, Landewe R, Spoorenberg A, Dougados M: Measurement of spinal mobility in ankylosing spondylitis: comparison of occiput-to-wall and tragus-to-wall distance. J Rheumatol 2004; 31: 1779-1784

Hultgren S, Broma JE, Gudbjornsson B, Hetta J, Lindqvist U: Sleep disturbances in outpatients with ankylosing spondylitis: a questionnaire study with gender implications. Scand J Rheumatol 2000; 29: 365-369

Jenkinson T, Armas J, Evison G et al : The cervical spine in psoriatic arthritis: a clinical and radiological study. Br J Rheumatol 1994; 33: 255-259

Jones SD, Koh WH, Steiner A, Garrett SL, Calin A: Fatigue in ankylosing spondylitis : its prevalence and relationship to disease activity, sleep and other factors. J Rheumatol 1996; 23: 487-490

Khan MA, ed: Spondyloarthropathies. Rheum Dis Clin N Amer 1992, 18:1-276

Maghraoui AE, Chaouir S, Abid A et al: Lung findings on thoracic high-resolution computed tomography in patients with ankylosing spondylitis. Correlations with disease duration, clinical findings ad pulmonary function testing. Clin Rheumatol 2004; 23: 123-128

Martindale J, Smith J, Sutton CJ, Grennan D, Goodacre L, Goodacre JA: Disease and psychological status in ankylosing spondylitis. Rheumatology (Oxford) 2006 Oct; 45(10): 1288-93

McGonagle D, Gibbon W, Emery P: Classification of inflammatory arthritis by enthesitis. Lancet 1998; 352: 1137-1140

Mcrae IF, Wright V: Measurement of back movement. Ann Rheum Dis 1969; 28: 584-589

Moll J, Haslock I, Mac Rae IF, Wright V: Association between ankylosing spondylitis, psoriatic arthritis, Reiter´s syndrome, the intestinal arthropathies and Becet syndrome. Medicine 197; 53: 343-364

Nabokov AV, Shabunin MA, Smirnov AV: Renal involvement in ankylosing spondylitis (Bechterew´s disease). Nephrol Dial Transplant 1996: 11: 1172-1175

Obermayer-Pietsch BM, Lange U, Tauber G et al: Vitamin D receptor initiation codon polymorphism, bone density and inflammatory activity of patients with ankylosing spondylitis. Osteoporosis Int 2003; 14: 995-1000

Rosenbaum JT: Characterization of uveitis associated with spondyloarthritis. J Rheumatol 1989; 16: 792-796

Saari KM: The eye and reactive arthritis. In: Toivanen A, Toivanen P, eds: Reactive Arthritis. Boca Raton: CRC Press;1988, 113-124

Schober P: The lumbar vertebral column in backache. Munchener Medizinisch Wochenschrift 1937; 84: 336-338

Sieper J, Braun J, Rudwaleit M, Boonen A, Zink A: Ankylosing spondylitis: an overview. An Rheum Dis 2002; 61(suppl 3): iii8-18

Silman AJ, Hochberg MD: Epidemiology of Rheumatic Diseases. Oford: Oxford University Press; 1993

Souza AS, Muller NL, Marchiori E, Soares-Souza LV: Pulmonary abnormalities in ankylosing spondylitis: inspiratory and expiratory high-resolution CT findings in 17 patients. J Thorac Imaging 2004; 19: 259-263

Torre Alonso JC, Rodriguez Perez A, Arribas Castrillo JM et al: Psoriatic arthritis (PA): a clinical, immunological and radiological study of 180 patients. Br J Rheumatol 1991; 30: 245-250

Van der Heijde D, Baraf HS, Ramos-Remus C et al: Evaluation of the efficacy of etoricoxib in ankylosing spondylitis: results of a fifty-two-week, randomized, controlled study. Arthritis Rheum 2005; 52: 1205-1215

Van der Heijde D, Bellamy N, Calin A, Dougados M, Khan MA, Van der Linden S: Preliminary core sets for endpoints in ankylosing spondylitis. Assessments in Ankylosing Spondylitis Working Group. J Rheumatol 1997; 24: 2225-2229

Van der Linden SM, Valkenburg HA, De Jongh BM, Cats A: The risk of developing ankylosing spondylitis in HLA-B27 positive individuals. A comparison of relatives of spondylitis patients with the general population. Arthritis Rheum 1984: 27: 241-249

Viitanen JV, Heikkila S, Kokko ML, Kautiainen H: Clinical assessment of spinal mobility measurements in ankylosing spondylis: a compact set for follow-up and trials?. Clin Rheumatol 2000; 19: 131-137

Wanders A, Van der Heijde D, Landewe R et al: Nonsteroidal antiinflammatory drugs reduce radiographic progression in patients with ankylosing spondylitis: a randomized clinical trial. Arthritis Rheum 2005: 52(6): 1756-1765

Wolf J, Fasching P: Ankylosing spondylitis: Wien Med Wochenschr; 2010 May; 160(9-10): 211-4

Wright V: Seronegative polyarthritis. Amsterdam:North Holland Publishing Company: 1976

2

Ankylosing Apondylitis of Temporomandibular Joint (TMJ)

Raveendra Manemi[1], Rooprashmi Kenchangoudar[1] and Peter Revington[2]
[1]Dept. of Oral and Maxillofacial Surgery, Gloucestershire Royal Hospitals NHS Trust, Gloucester,
[2]Dept. of Oral and Maxillofacial Surgery North Bristol NHS Trust, Bristol
UK

1. Introduction

The ankylosing spondylitis (AS) (Bechterew's disease) is a chronic inflammatory rheumatoid disease with predilection in the axial structures. Often the first clinical indication of the condition is lumbo-sacral pain and discomfort with limited range of motion. The prevalence in Caucasian population is 1-2% with slight male predominance [1, 31, and 32]. Peak age of onset is between 20–30 years, with an average 5–6-year delay in diagnosis reported in the literature. A familial tendency has been strongly suggested by recent evidence. Immunologic activity is suggested by the presence of histocompatibility antigen HLA-B27 (in more than 90 percent of patients with this disease) and circulating immune complexes.

The disease course, although highly variable, will progress to severe disability in one third of patients. Progressive synovial changes eventually involve all of the axial joints including the temporomandibular joint [2]. Literature shows the temporomandibular joint (TMJ) is involved in 4% to 32% of cases [1, 31, and 32]. The severity of the disease may range from sore TMJ to complete ankylosis leading to restricted mouth opening. Ankylosis of the TMJ is exceptional; the involvement of TMJ has not been very well investigated. This chapter describes the incidence, clinical features, pathophysiology, signs, symptoms and current management of TMJ ankylosing spondylitis

2. Anatomy of TMJ

The Temporo-Mandibular joint (TMJ) is the joint of the jaw and is frequently referred to as TMJ [3]. There are two TMJs, one on either side, working in unison. The name is derived from the two bones which form the joint: the upper temporal bone which is part of the cranium (skull), and the lower jaw bone called the mandible. The unique feature of the TMJs is the articular disc. The disc is composed of fibrocartilagenous tissue (like the firm and flexible elastic cartilage of the ear) which is positioned between the two bones that form the joint. The TMJs are one of the only synovial joints in the human body with an articular disc, another being the sternoclavicular joint. The disc divides each joint into two. The lower joint compartment formed by the mandible and the articular disc is involved in rotational movement—this is the initial movement of the jaw when the mouth opens. The upper joint compartment formed by the articular disk and the temporal bone is involved in translational movement—this is the secondary gliding motion of the jaw as it is opened widely.

The part of the mandible which mates to the under-surface of the disc is the condyle and the part of the temporal bone which mates to the upper surface of the disk is the glenoid (or mandibular) fossa.

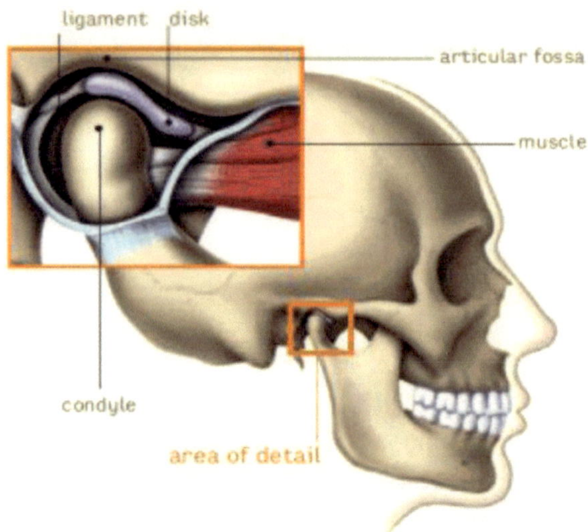

Fig. 1.

The TMJ is a hinge and gliding joint and is the most constantly used joint in the body. The round upper end of the lower jaw, or the movable portion of the joint, is called the condyle; the socket is called the articular fossa. Between the condyle and the fossa is a disk made of cartilage that acts as a cushion to absorb stress and allows the condyle to move easily when the mouth opens and closes.

3. Pathophysiology

Ankylosing spondylitis (AS) is a systemic rheumatic disease, meaning it affects the entire body. Approximately 90% of AS patients express the HLA-B27 genotype, meaning there is a strong genetic association. However, only 5% of individuals with the HLA-B27 genotype contract the disease. Tumor necrosis factor-alpha (TNF α) and Interleukin-1(IL-1) are also implicated in ankylosing spondylitis. Autoantibodies specific for AS have not been identified. Antineutrophil cytoplasmic antibodies (ANCA) are associated with AS, but do not correlate with disease severity.

TMJ involvement in patients with ankylosing spondylitis has been described previously in very few journals[16] Its reported frequency varies from 1% to 35%, depending on the diagnostic criteria, the population studied, and the tools used to assess TMJ involvement[17]. However, the majority of the reports included patients with long lasting ankylosing spondylitis from tertiary care centres, and while they focus on TMJ involvement, little information on the characteristics of the ankylosing spondylitis is given.

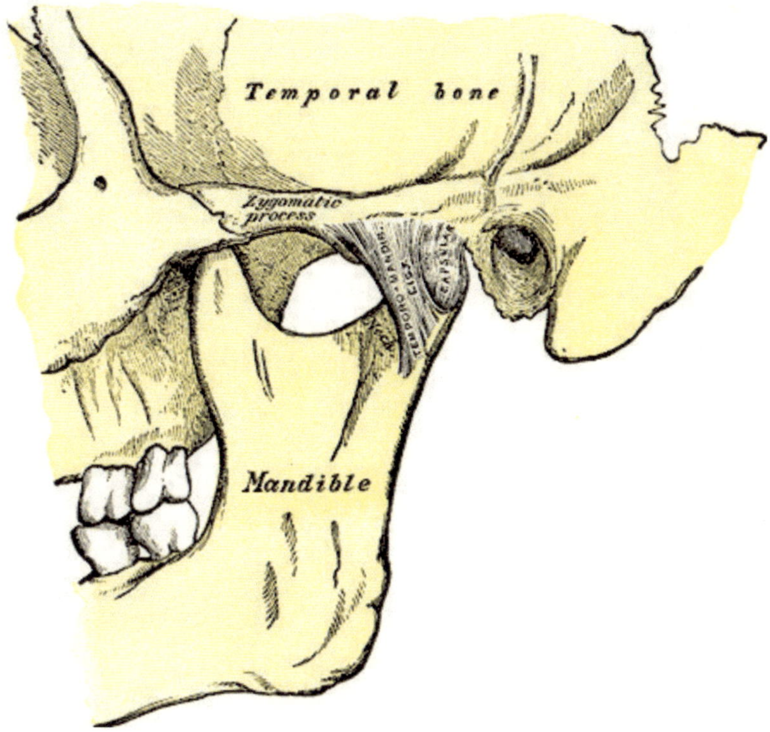

Fig. 2. Lateral view of TMJ (Courtesy: Gray's anatomy).

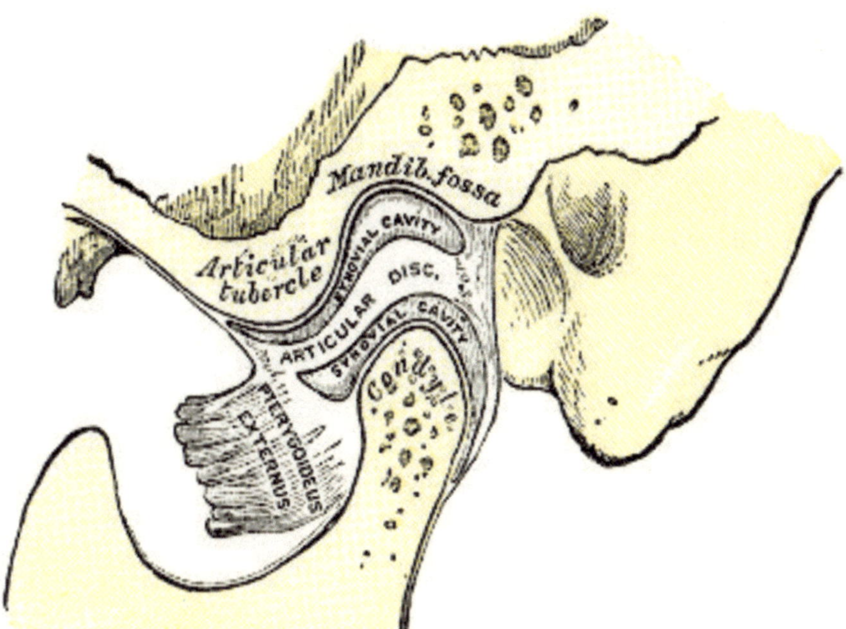

Fig. 3. Sagittal section of the articulation of the mandible. (Courtesy: Gray's anatomy).

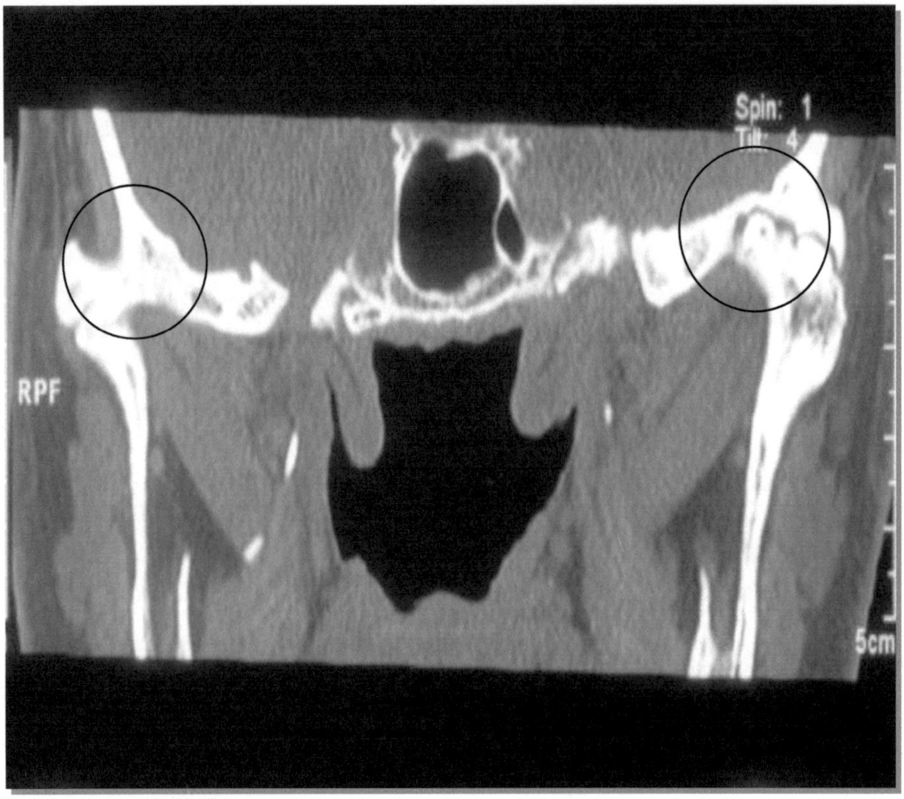

Fig. 4. CT scan shows complete ankylosis of bilateral TMJs in AS (marked areas showing reduced joint space and fusion of condylar head with glenoid fossa).

4. Signs and symptoms [4, 18]

- Chronic pain in the muscles of mastication described as a dull ache, typically unilateral may become bilateral in later stages.
- Pain may radiate to the ear and jaw and is worsened with chewing
- Headache and/or neck ache: In some cases, patients may complain of headache without localized pain in the temporomandibular joint.
- A bite that feels uncomfortable or different from usual
- Associated neck, shoulder, and back pain
- Increasing pain over the course of the day
- Limitation of jaw opening (normal range is at least 40 mm as measured from lower to upper anterior teeth) worsens as the disease progresses.
- Clicking or popping in the TMJ
- Tenderness to palpation of the TMJ

5. Diagnosis

This problem is diagnosed through a combination of clinical history, examination, imaging and the finding of HLA-B27 in the blood.

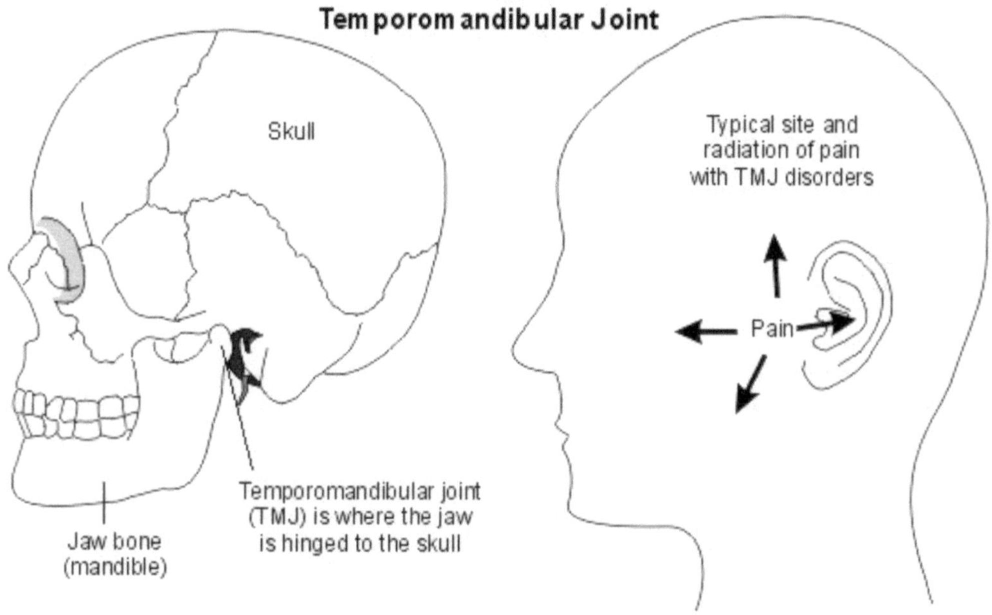

Fig. 5.

Radiographic findings in TMJ depend on the etiology, in cases of AS, rheumatoid arthritis and seronegative spondyloarthropathies, plain films show erosions, osteophytes, subchondral bony sclerosis, and condylar-glenoid fossa remodeling[1].It is diffcult to to differntiate AS of TMJ with other degenarative conditions affecting this joint as there is significant correlation between the radilogical findings of AS and other degenarative disorders[19]CT scans can explore both bony structures and muscular soft tissues. Of interest, there is utility with cone beam computed tomography (CBCT). The patient is scanned with the mouth open and closed. Specifically, CBCT can aid in the diagnosis of this condition along with history and physical examination.

Magnetic resonance imaging (MRI) is now clearly established as a sensitive and specific tool to detect sacroiliitis [20] but minimal literature found on MRI sensitivity of TMJs in AS hence MRI should be used as the study of choice if TMJ articular or meniscal pathology is suspected and an endoscopic or surgical procedure is contemplated.

Diagnostic arthroscopy is an invasive diagnostic approach and should be used mainly in patients suffering from internal TMJ derangements recalcitrant to conservative measures.TMJ can be approached via pre auricular incisions.

6. Management

The treatment modalities mainly aim for relief of the symptoms and may be to prevent the progression of the disease [21]. The management of AS includes non-pharmacological, pharmacological, invasive and surgical interventions that should be tailored to each patient's disease manifestations, current symptoms, clinical findings and prognostic indicators [22]. The non-surgical treatment of temporomandibular disorder secondary to AS continues to be the most effective way of managing over 80 per cent of patients who present with symptoms of temporomandibular pain and dysfunction. Non-steroidal anti-inflammatory drugs (NSAIDs) are recommended as first-line pharmacological treatment.

7. Non-pharmacological treatment

Non-pharmacological treatment of AS includes fabrication of intra-oral splint,physiothery and patient education.The most recent systematic review of physiotherapy for AS reviewed six randomised controlled trials (RCTs), showing that home exercise improved function in the short term compared with no intervention.

Fabrication and insertion of an Intra-oral Orthotic (also known as splint or bite-gaurd): The purpose of these Orthotics, which may be fitted to either the upper or lower jaws, and in some cases to both, is to re-position the condyle head in the joint space to a more normal position, thereby relieving the stresses, and pressures, being placed on the tissues of the joints, and their related supporting structures allowing them to heal.

Physiotherapy Therapy: These treatments might include Ultra-sound, TENS (transcutaneous electrical nerve stimulation) and home exercises.

Ultrasound therapy is part of a physical therapy treatment using sound waves at a remarkably exorbitant frequency to penetrate the skin deep to the soft tissue of painful area. It involves employing a hand held probe provided a rounded make every effort which is attached to an ultrasound machine. A gel would be rubbed onto the skin and the probe head will be moved over the affected area in small circular movements. The high-frequency (ultrasonic) waves are produced by vibration on the run of the probe. The waves travel with the skin bringing about vibration to the tissue in the affected area. The vibration causes a heating up of the tissue that has a beneficial effect on the TMJ. The ultrasound therapy is safe when administered by a professional or person who has had training as it can have its dangers of skin burns.

TENS in which a low voltage, low amperage current is applied to the preauricular region which is to relax the masticatory muscles, which are in a state of hyperactivity, fatigue or in spasm secondary to pain. It is like an electronic massage of the facial muscles.

In exercise rehabilitation program, patient has to roll back the tongue to touch the roof of the mouth and asked to open and close the jaw by holding the tongue in same position. In another technique patient is asked to slowly open and close the mouth by keeping the palm of the hand against chin with gentle pressure. These exercises mainly aid in improving the mouth opening and to strengthen the muscles of mastication and TMJ ligaments.

Patient education: has been shown to have short term benefit for function in AS in one controlled trial. There are no studies examining the effect of education on pain. Education and behavioural therapy have, however, been shown to be beneficial for other outcomes such as motivation and anxiety. Patient associations and self help groups have not been studied for their effect on pain or functional outcomes.

8. The pharmacological management

The pharmacological management of AS of TMJ is essentially same as general management of AS which include Nonsteroidal Anti-inflammatory Drugs (NSAIDs), Coxibs, and Corticosteroids. Literature also shows use of Disease-Modifying Antirheumatic Drugs (DMRDs) and anti-tumour necrosis factor (TNF) agents are recommended in the case of NSAID failure. There is insufficient evidence to support or not support the effectiveness of the reported drugs for the management of pain due TMD (Temporo-Mandibular Disorders). There is a need for high quality RCTs to derive evidence of the effectiveness of pharmacological interventions to treat pain associated with TMD [23] However it has been noticed that most patients respond well to medications given to reduce pain and inflammation, combined with mouth opening exercises to maintain adequate mouth opening and strengthen muscles of mastication to counteract possible ankylosis.

9. The surgical management

The surgical management is indicated in patients with marked trismus (decreased mouth opening) and in case of failure of other non surgical modalities. The surgical treatment may include injection of steroid, joint lavage and total joint replacement. TMJ intra-articular steroid injections use 0.5-1ml of Triamcinolone acetate or methyl prednilosone which is mixed with normal saline. These injections can be performed under local anaesthesia or general anaesthesia. Many patients reported quick relief of symptoms from steroid injections [24, 25] and joint lavage.

Total joint replacement is considered as a last resort if the other treatment modalities fail. The first TMJ total joint replacement was performed about twenty years ago [26]. The principles, which were learned in total hip and knee replacement, have been successfully applied to the TMJ. Prosthetic replacement of the TMJ is a procedure that has undergone a technological revolution over the last decade. In spite of the high frequency of TMJ involvement, ankylosis secondary to AS seems to seldom ensue, and relatively few patients develop such severe degenerative TMJ disease that they require total joint replacement. This is reflected in the paucity of literature on the topic, with approximately 11 cases reported worldwide involving the TMJs bilaterally [8, 26, and 27].

However, when the TMJ ankylosis occurs, it is an extremely disabling affliction that causes problems with mastication, digestion, speech, appearance, and access to routine dentistry. It also has an impact on the psychological development of the patient with concerns related to an inability to open the mouth. Therefore, in patients with ankylosing spondylitis, the total replacement of the TMJ with an alloplastic joint system has become the treatment of choice. These allow closer reproduction of the natural anatomy, avoids donor site morbidity, decreases the risk of reankylosis, and reduces operation time. Furthermore, they allow for immediate physiotherapy and rehabilitation with consequent increased benefit to the patient. [28].

TMJ concepts prosthesis (formerly Techmedica) has up to 17 years follow-up with 90% success rates [29]. These are computer-aided design/computer-aided manufacture (CAD/CAM) custom-made prostheses constructed on a stereolithographic model following a 3D CT scan. The glenoid fossa component is constructed from titanium mesh bonded to the articular surface of high-molecular-weight polyethylene. The condylar component head is cobalt-chrome alloy, and the remainder of the body is titanium and is secured to the ramus of the mandible by screws. Lorenz also makes a stock prosthesis with similar components to the TMJ concepts prosthesis. Whichever operative strategy is employed, it is important to note that these techniques all rely on aggressive postoperative physiotherapy to maintain optimal results [28].

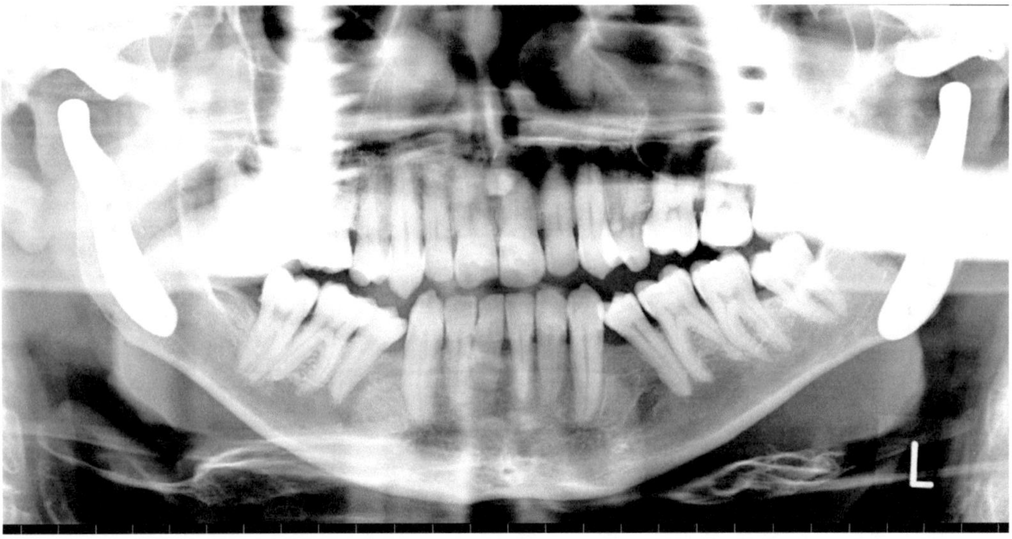

Fig. 6. Dental panoramic view showing bilateral TMJ replacement with TMJ prostheses in AS patient.

10. Discussion

Ankyolosing spondylitis has the tendency to involve fibro cartilaginous structures such as symphysis pubis, intervertibral discs, sternomanubrial and sternoclavicular joints. The involvement of TMJ has not been very well investigated and its incidence is disputed. Former studies have reported the involvement of the TMJ in AS between 4% and 32%. However, these studies were either only radiological [31] or used only insufficient clinical [32] or radiological [33] examination methods. Ehrlich (1930) reported on 753 cases, where

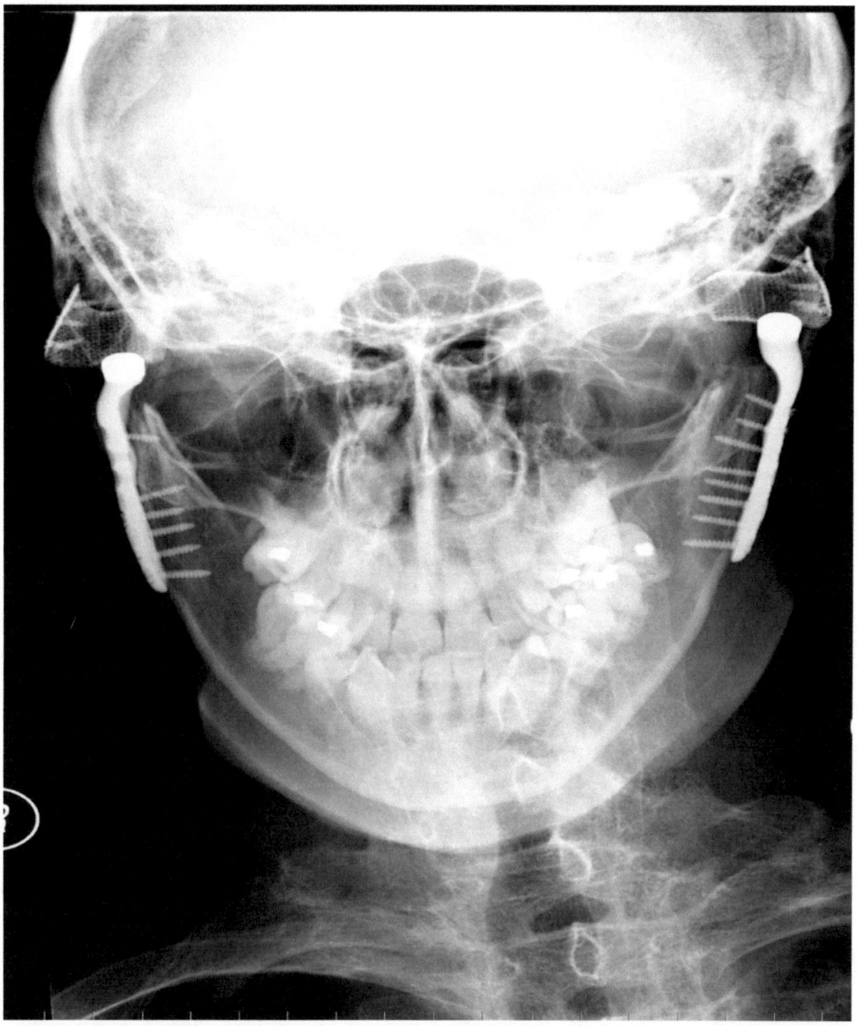

Fig. 7. Postero-Anterior (PA) mandible view showing total TMJ replacement using TMJ concepts prostheses.

he found 124 patients (16.5%). forestier et al (1951) found TMJ involvement in 6% of 200 patients. Nagel (1968) reviewed 1000 patients in which TMJ involvement was only 1%. [17]

Due disparity in clinical and radiological signs suggests that the TMJ rarely seems to be a severe problem for AS patients. It is felt that most TMJ symptoms may be secondary to muscle spasm, occlusal factors, and postural imbalance [34], and the literature is only sparsely populated with cases of true ankylosis of TMJ secondary to AS.

11. Conclusion

In conclusion we recommend routine clinical examinations of TMJ in patients with AS to detect rare complications like severe trismus and ankylosis. Both pharmacological and non pharmacological modalities are found to be effective in the treatment of AS of TMJ depending on the time and progression. One should have high index of suspicion of TMJ ankylosis in AS for an early detection. This could avoid the need of expensive and technique sensitive joint surgeries. Complementary explorations like joint lavage or arthroscopy should be undertaken in ankylosing spondylitis patients with clinical symptoms suggestive of TMJ lesions in order to establish the diagnosis and initiate treatment and avoid the development of ankylosis forms.

12. References

[1] M.C. Locher, M. Felder, H.F. Sailer Invovlement of TMJ in Ankylosing spondylitis (Bechterew's disease) *Journal of Cranio-Maxillofacial Surgery*, Volume 24, Issue 4, August 1996, Pages 205-213

[2] Ankylosing Spondylitis affecting TMJ-Case report; *International journal of Oral and maxillofacial Surgery.* Vol. 26, Supplement 1, 1997, Page 162

[3] Rodríguez-Vázquez JF, et al., JF; Mérida-Velasco, JR; Mérida-Velasco, JA; Jiménez-Collado, J (1998). "Anatomical considerations on the discomalleolar ligament". J *Anat.* 192 (Pt 4): 617–621.

[4] Robert.J, R.J.Loiselle TMJ Symptoms and Ankylosing Spondylitis. *JADA* 1972; 83.630-633.

[5] Miller GA, Page HL Jr, Griffith CR. Temporomandibular joint ankylosis: Review of the literature and report of 2 cases of bilateral involvement. *J Oral Surg* 1975; 33(10): 792-803.

[6] Guralnick WC, Kaban LB. Surgical treatment of mandibular hypomobility. *J. Oral Surg* 1976; 34(4): 343-8.

[7] Figueroa AA, Gans BJ, Pruzansky S. Long-term follow-up of mandibular costochondral graft. *Oral Surg Oral Med Oral Pathol* 1984; 58(3): 257-68.

[8] Moriconi ES, Popowich LD, Guernsey LH. Alloplastic reconstruction of the temporomandibular joint. *Dent Clin North Am* 1986; 30(2): 307-25.

[9] Kaban LB, Perrott DH, Fisher K. A protocol for management of temporomandibular joint ankylosis. *J Oral Maxillofacial Surg* 1990; 48(11): 1145-51; discussion 1152.

[10] Mauno Kononen, Bengt Wenneberg: Craniomandibular Disorders in Rheumatoid Arthritis, Psoriatic Arthritis and Ankylosing Spondylitis, *ACTA ODONTOL SCAND;* 1992,50:281-287.

[11] Chowk TK, Ng.WL. *Scand J Rheumatology.* 1997; 26(2): 133-4.

[12] Fonseca RJ. Oral and Maxillofacial Surgery: Temporomandibular Disorders. Philadelphia (PA): W.B. Saunders Company; 2000. p. 309-13.

[13] Ju Seop Song, Kwan Joon-Koh, ankylosing spondilitis associated with bilateral TMJ ankylosis. *Korean Journal of Oral and Maxillofacial Surgery* 2000,30. 217-222.

[14] Khan MA. 2002. *Ankylosing spondylitis:* The facts. Oxford University Press. ISBN 0192632825.

[15] Benazzou S, Maagoul R *Rev Stomatol Chir Maxillofac.* 2005 Nov; 106(5): 08-10.

[16] Qin L, Long X, Li X, Bilateral fibrous ankylosis of temporomandibular joint associated with ankylosing spondylitis: a case report. *Joint Bone Spine.* 2006 Feb 17;

[17] Manemi R V, Fasanmade A, Revington PJ; Bilateral ankylosis of the jaw treated with total alloplastic replacement using the TMJ concepts system in a patient with ankylosing spondylitis;*Br J Oral Maxillofac Surg.* 2009 Mar;47(2):159-61.

[18] Vivian Tsai; Rick Kulkarni; Temporomandibular Joint syndrome; *http://emedicine.medscape.com/article/809598-overview.* Feb 2010

[19] L. Miia J. Helenius , DDS, MB,a Dorrit Hallikainen, MD, DDS,b Ilkka Helenius, MD, PhD, Clinical and radiographic findings of the TMJ in patients with various rheumatic diseases. *Oral Surg Oral Med Oral Pathol Oral Radiol Endod* 2005; 99:455-63.

[20] Saeed A. Shaikh, MD, Ankylosing spondylitis: recent breakthroughs in diagnosis and treatment *J Can Chiropr Assoc.* 2007 December; 51(4): 249–260.

[21] Mansour.M, Cheema. G.S,Naqw A, Greenspan.A,Ankylosing spondylitis: a contemporary perspective on diagnosis and treatment. *Semin Arthritis Rheum.* 2007 Feb; 36(4):210-23. Epub 2006 Sep 29

[22] http://www.spine-health.com/conditions/arthritis/ankylosing-spondylitis-physical-therapy-and-exercise.

[23] Mujakperuo HR, Watson M, Morrison R, Macfarlane TV; Pharmacological interventions for pain in patients with temporomandibular disorders. *Cochrane Database Syst Rev.* 2010 Oct 6;(10):CD004715

[24] B Arabshahi, et al, *Arthritis Rheum. 2006;*

[25] S Ringold, et al. *J Rheumatol.* 2008; 35(6):1157-1164

[26] Speculand B, Hensher R, Powell D, Total prosthetic replacement of the TMJ: experience with two systems 1988-1997,*The British Journal of Oral & Maxillofacial Surgery 38,*360-369;2000

[27] Andrew M. Felstead, Peter J. Revington, Surgical management of TMJ Ankylosis in Ankylosing spondylitis, *Int J Rheumatol.* 2011;Published online 2011 March 24. doi: 10.1155/2011/854167

[28] Roychoudhury A, Parkash H, Trikha A. Functional restoration by gap arthroplasty in temporomandibular joint ankylosis a report of 50 cases. Oral Surgery, Oral Medicine, Oral Pathology, Oral Radiology, and Endodontics.1999;87(2):166–169

[29] Mercuri LG, Edibam NR, Giobbie-Hurder A. Fourteen-year follow-up of a patient-fitted total temporomandibular joint reconstruction system. Journal of Oral and Maxillofacial Surgery. 2007;65(6):1140–1148.

[30] Agarwal A. Preankylosing spondylitis. In: Moll JMH, editor. Ankylosing Spondylitis. Edinburgh, UK: Churchill Levingstone; 1980. pp. 69–75

[31] Maes HJ, Dihlmann W. Affection of the temporomandibular joints in spondylitis ankylopoeiticaBefall der Temporomandibulargelenke bei der Spondylitis ankylopoetica. Fortschritte auf dem Gebiete der Rontgenstrahlen und der Nuklearmedizin. 1968;109(4):513–516. [PubMed]

[32] Resnick D. Temporomandibular joint involvement in ankylosing spondylitis. Comparison with rheumatoid arthritis & psoriasis. Radiology. 1974; 112(3):587–591. [PubMed]

[33] Davidson C, Wojtulewski JA, Bacon PA, Winstock D. Temporo mandibular joint disease in ankylosing spondylitis.Annals of the Rheumatic Diseases. 1975;34(1):87–91. [PubMed]

[34] Crum RJ, Loiselle RJ. Temporomandibular joint symptoms and ankylosing spondylitis. The Journal of the American Dental Association. 1971;83(3):630–633. [PubMed]

3

Bone Mineral Density Changes in Patients with Spondyloarthropathies

Lina Vencevičienė[1], Rimantas Vencevičius[2] and Irena Butrimienė[3]

[1]*Vilnius University, Clinic of Internal Diseases, Family Medicine, Gerontology and Oncology*

[2]*Vilnius University, Clinic of Rheumatology, Traumatology, Orthopedics and Plastic and Reconstructive Surgery*

[3]*Vilnius University, Clinic of Rheumatology, Traumatology, Orthopedics and Plastic and Reconstructive Surgery; State Research Institute Centre for Innovative Medicine*

Lithuania

1. Introduction

The concept of inflammatory spondyloarthropathies (SpA) as an independent group of diseases was introduced approximately 15-20 years ago, when symptoms distinguishing these diseases from rheumathoid arthritis (RA) were defined precisely. SpA group includes 4 main diseases: ankylosing spondylitis (AS), psoriatic arthritis (PsA), reactive arthritis (ReA) and enteropathic arthropathies (EnA). Global prevalence of these diseases is .2-3.0 percent. Furthermore, SpA incidence in Lithuania is .64 percent (Adomaviciute et al., 2008). The incidence is higher in close relatives of patients with established human leucocyte antigen B27 (HLA B27). SpA is 2-3 times more common in males than in females (Khan, 2002; Sieper, 2002).

Although SpA and RA ethiology and pathogenesis differ, these immune arthritides are similar in their consequences, principles of diagnostic and treatment. Genetic predisposition to the disease and relation with infectious factors is characteristic to both SpA and RA diseases, however, the true causes remain unclear. It is known that tissue damage in these diseases is caused by reactions governed by immune processes. In addition, RA is the most investigated autoimmune, continuously progressing erosive-destructive poliarthritis. The incidence among adults ranges from .35 to 1.0 percent in various populations whilst in Lithuania it is about .55 percent (Adomavičiūtė et al., 2008). In both SpA and RA clinical outcomes depend primarily on various complications: cardiovascular abnormalities, infections, amyloidosis, osteoporosis.

Osteoporosis (OP) is a skeletal disease characterized by low bone mineral density (BMD) and poor bone quality that reduces bone strength and increases the risk of fractures. OP is a major public health concern, affecting approximately 200 million individuals worldwide, including a third of women aged 60 to 70 years. Fractures of the hip and spine are associated with increased morbidity and mortality (Johnell et al., 2005). Despite the high prevalence of OP and the availability of effective drugs to reduce the risk of fracture, it is underdiagnosed and undertreated (Feldstein et al., 2003). Patients with immune arthritides, who are at very high risk of fracture, are usually not evaluated for OP. It has been reported that in patients with SpA and RA decreased BMD is being diagnosed at a much younger age (Lane at al., 2002). These patients are affected not only by ordinary OP risk factors but also specific disease factors: activity and course of the disease, its duration, treatment with glucocorticoids (GC) and immunosuppressants, reduced mobility (Gratacos, 1999; Kroot, 2001; Baek, 2005).

Most of the publications analyzing BMD changes are related to RA. It was observed that RA is associated with local and systemic loss of bone mineral density (Sambrook, 1995; Gough, 1994) and also with increased risk of osteoporotic fracture (Cooper et al., 1995). The main factors associating RA and decrease of BMD are activity of the disease, physical disability and immobility, disease duration and use of gliucocorticoids (Dequeker, 1995; Kvien, 2000). According to other work in the field, pathologic fractures of spine vertebrae are more common in patients with SpA than RA (despite the formation of syndesmophytes and ossification of longitudinal ligaments that could probably "protect the spine" in SpA case) (Bessant, 2002; Brand, 2008). It is supposed that in both RA and SpA bone tissue is damaged due to reduced mobility, the activity of the disease and, most importantly, similar reactions caused by immune processes, which are characteristic to these diseases (Illei et al., 2000; Pettit, 2001).

Although in most cases SpA are investigated as a whole group of diseases with common clinical, radiological and genetic features, BMD was investigated mostly in patients with AS. According to other studies, the incident of OP in patients with AS is very different and ranges from 50 to 92% (Mitra, 2000; Capaci, 2003). Too little and controversial data concerning changes of BMD in other diseases belonging to SpA group were published (El Maghraoui, 2004; Speden, 2002).

Scientific novelty. This investigation for the first time evaluated and compared BMD at the lumbar spine and upper part of left and right femur in patients with SpA and RA and healthy people. Consistent patterns of BMD changes at the lumbar spine and upper parts of both femurs were assessed in patients with diseases belonging to SpA group (AS, ReA, EnA, PsA) and in SpA patients with various types of joint lesion. Relation between SpA specific factors - duration of the disease, physical disability and immobility, activity of the disease, medications in use and BMD changes at the lumbar spine and upper part of left and right femur was evaluated.

Absolute determination of consistent patterns of BMD changes at the lumbar spine and upper parts of both femurs in patients with various diseases belonging to SpA group (AS, ReA, EnA, PsA) and with various types of joint lesion together with, investigation of distinct clinical risk factors associated with BMD changes in SpA patients would allow to select patients for BMD test precisely, indicate the exact skeleton area for investigation, diagnose changes in bone mass earlier and timely apply effective preventive and/or treatment measures.

Aim of the research - to determine consistent patterns of BMD changes at the lumbar spine and upper part of left and right femur in patients with SpA (AS, ReA, PsA, EnA) and to assess the relation between changes of BMD and specific factors of the disease (duration of the disease, physical disability and immobility, activity of the disease, medications in use) using noninvasive method of BMD evaluation (dual-energy X-ray absorptiometry (DXA)).

Objectives of the research

- To investigate BMD changes at the lumbar spine and upper part of left and right femur in groups of patients with SpA, Ra and healthy subjects.
- To investigate BMD changes at the lumbar spine and upper part of left and right femur in patients with various diseases belonging to SpA group (AS, ReA, PsA, EnA) and in SpA patients with different type of joint lesions (only axial, only peripheral, both axial and peripheral).
- To analyse relation between the duration of SpA and BMD changes at the lumbar spine and upper part of left and right femur.
- To evaluate influence of physical disability and immobility on BMD changes in patients with SpA.
- To determine influence of medications in use: glucocorticoids and TNF-α blockers on BMD changes in patients with SpA.

Statements defended:

- BMD decrease at the lumbar spine and upper part of left and right femur is similar in patients with inflammatory joint diseases: SpA and RA.
- Impact of various diseases belonging to SpA group on bone mass changes is similar.
- SpA activity and physical disability and immobility are important prognostic factors for BMD decrease.

2. Study subjects and methods

2.1 Study population

Patients treated in the Department of Rheumatology of Vilnius University Hospital "Santariškių klinikos" in the period of December 2006 to June 2008 were invited to participate in this research. Patients arriving at Vilnius University Hospital "Santariškių klinikos" Family Health Center for the prophylactic examination were invited to take part in the control group of the research. A total of 136 patients with SpA, 104 patients with RA and 114 healthy people (control group) matching inclusion criteria, and not having any exclusion criteria stated below were involved in the investigation.

2.2 Inclusion criteria

- Age of subjects ranging from 20 to 75 years;
- People with RA diagnosis established according to rheumatoid arthritis diagnostic criteria of American College of Rheumatology (ARA'87) (diagnosis established by rheumatologist) (Arnett et al., 1988);
- Subjects with SpA diagnosis established according to diagnostic criteria approved by European Spondyloarthropathy Study Group (ESSG) (1991) (diagnosis established by rheumatologist);
- Subjects of control group - healthy individuals (Dougados et al., 1991);
- Subjects signed an *Informed Consent* form approved by Lithuanian bioethics committee. (The permission to perform this investigation was obtained from the Lithuanian bioethics committee (No.60; 2006-12-22)).

2.3 Exclusion criteria

- Subjects after hip joint replacement;
- Patients with other diseases (renal, liver, thyroid and parathyroid, and cancer) influencing calcium metabolism or interfering metabolism of bone tissue;
- Individuals treated with medications (anti-osteoporosis, thyroxin, insulin, anticoagulants, anticonvulsants, hormone replacement therapy, etc.) that may influence bone tissue metabolism, except medications used to treat underlying disease: disease modifiers, TNF-α blockers, GC and non-steroid anti-inflammatory drugs (data obtained from medical records and patient interviews);
- Pregnant women, vegetarians, alcohol addicts.

2.4 Research structure

Primary selection of patients was performed according to patients' medical history and data of clinical investigations (data from the hospital and out-patient records were used under the patients consent). Then, every patient completed one of the three questionnaires depending on the research subgroup he/she belonged to. The following questionnaire data were assessed: socio-demographic data - age, gender, education, profession, work environment; smoking, use of alcohol; bone fractures in subject and his close relatives; previous and current diseases; previously and currently used medications; calcium amount in the diet (mg/d); frequency of physical activities by month (at least 20 minutes physical exercises per day) and the age of the beginning and the end of menstrual cycle in femails.

In patients with SpA and RA: duration of the disease (in months) from the onset of the first symptoms and from the date the diagnosis was established; pain intensity assessment using 10 cm VAS scale; patient's general status assessment using 10 cm VAS scale.

In patients with SpA the following parameters were assessed: disease belonging to SpA group; type of joint lesion: axial, peripheric, both axial and peripheric; physical disability was assessed by completing Health Assessment Questionaire Modified for Spondyloarthropathies (HAQ-S) (Daltroy et al., 1990); immobility was assessed according to Bath Ankylosing Spondylitis Functional Index (BASFI) (Calin et al., 1994) and Bath Ankylosing Spondylitis Patient Global Score (BAS-G) (Jones et al., 1996); assessment of enthesis; movement of spine was assessed according to standardized SpA clinical measurements: lumbar side flexion, modified Schober's test, tragus to wall distance and intermalleolar distance (Jenkinson et al, 1994); activity of the disease according to patients self-assessment using Bath Ankylosing Spondylitis Disease Activity Index (BASDAI) (Garrett et al, 1994); activity of the disease evaluated by rheumatologist (Landewe et al, 2004). The linguistic and cultural adaptation of these questionnaires was made during the study. Internal consistency was high for functional and disease activity index (Cronbach alpha>/=0.80) and moderate for the Bath Ankylosing Spondylitis Patient Global Score (Cronbach alpha=0.58). High stability in regard to time was characteristic of all three questionnaires (intraclass correlation coefficient >0.95). A significant association between the separate questions of examined instruments, their joint results and other factors reflecting patient's health was established (Vencevičiene et al., 2009).

In patients with RA the following parameters were assessed: rheumatoid arthritis functional ARA classes; disease activity index DAS 28 and activity of the disease established by rheumatologist (Arnett et al., 1988).

Anthropometric measurements were performed on all patients: height, weight, BMI; laboratory tests: ESR, CRP, calcium blood level, HLA-B27 (in patients with SpA), RF (in patients with RA). Laboratory tests were performed in the Department of Laboratory Diagnostics of Vilnius University Hospital "Santariškių klinikos".

2.5 Evaluation of the bone mineral density

In all subjects BMD was measured by dual-energy X-ray absorptiometry (DXA) using osteodensitometer LEXXOS-DMS (software: V6, 20a, version of the year 2006). The anterior-posterior view of lumbar spine (L1-L4 vertebrae) and upper parts of both femurs were examined. BMD data were expressed as g/cm^2 and the number of standard deviations from the peak bone mass (T - score), and also the number of standard deviations of any individual result from the age and sex matched population mean (Z - score). Normal ranges were provided by manufacturers of the osteodensitometer. According to ISCD recommendations, BMD deviation was measured as Z-score, since most of the enrolled subjects were males less than 50 years old. Osteodensitometer quality test and measurement error test were performed every morning before work. Indications of the scan of spine vertebrae reference (phantom) fluctuated no more than 2 %, bias of the repeated measurement in spine vertebrae was not higher than 1.5 %, and in the upper part of femur-not higher then 2.1 %. All BMD measurements were performed by the principal investigator.

2.6 Data analysis

Statistical analysis was performed using SPSS 16 software. Mean (M) and standard deviation (SD) were used to describe quantitative characteristics of the research. Frequencies (n) and percents (%) were used for qualitative characteristics. Depending on applicable assumptions Student's t-test for independent samples was used to compare means of a particular qualitative characteristic of different samples. Analysis of variance ANOVA was used to compare quantitative variables of more than two samples (when variances were unequal Welch test statistics was used). When the hypothesis of the equality of means of two or more groups was rejected, pairwise comparison of this characteristic was additionally used. In that case Tukey HSD Post Hoc test was used. Differences of qualitative characteristics of experimental groups were assessed using Chi square test. Selected level of significance $\alpha = .05$.

To analyze relationship between SpA variables: the duration of disease, physical disability and immobility, activity of the disease and treatment with GC and TNF-α blockers and BMD changes linear regression models were developed. Stepwise selection of variables in the linear regression was used. Variables were included in the model when their p was $<.05$ and excluded when their p was $> .10$. When strong association between independent variables was observed (e.g., cumulative dose of GC and duration of use (calculated using Spearman correlation coefficient), only one of them was used for calculations. To assess probability that Z-score will be ≤ -2 in any site of examined skeleton logistic regression analysis was used.

3. Results

3.1 Characteristics of study groups

Three hundred fifty four subjects were enrolled in this research: 136 (38.4%) patients with SpA, 104 (29.4%) patients with RA and 114 (32.2%) healthy people (control group). The subjects of all groups were similar in BMI, physical activity and family history (all $p > .05$). No differences in disease activity determined by rheumatologist were observed between RA and SpA patients ($p > .516$). Subjects' differences in age (SpA patients: $M = 42.18 \pm 12.92$; RA patients: $M = 50.09 \pm 11.10$; $p < .001$), duration of the disease (SpA patients: $M = 112.09 \pm 94.54$; RA patients: $M = 148.49 \pm 109.60$; $p < .007$), and gender were determined. There were more males in SpA group compared with RA group ($p < .001$) and control group ($p < .001$); there were no differences in the number of males in RA group and control group ($p = .119$). No significant differences in the proportion of premenopausal and postmenopausal women in research groups were determined. (SpA vs. control group $p = .550$; SpA vs. RA $p = .112$; RA vs. control group $p = .600$).

3.2 BMD comparison in patients with SpA and RA and in control group subjects

The first objective of our research was to investigate BMD changes at lumbar spine and upper parts of the femurs in groups of patients with SpA, RA and healthy subjects.

BMD values at lumbar spine and upper part of the left and right femur (BMD expressed as g/cm^2 and Z-score) are presented in Table 1.

BMD	Research groups			p	Post hoc
	1	2	3		
	SpA (n = 136)	RA (n = 104)	Control (n = 114)		
BMDS	.873 (.128)	.866 (.125)	1.016 (.121)	< .001	3>1 (p <.001) 3>2 (p <.001)
BMDL	.849 (.121)	.832 (.131)	.998 (.113)	< .001	3>1 (p <.001) 3>2 (p <.001)
BMDR	.837 (.122)	.825 (.122)	.983 (.110)	< .001	3>1 (p <.001) 3>2 (p <.001)
ZS	-1.317 (.998)	-1.061 (1.096)	.045 (.941)	< .001	3>1 (p <.001) 3>2 (p <.001)
ZL	-1.133 (.949)	-1.014 (1.001)	.097 (.842)	< .001	3>1 (p <.001) 3>2 (p <.001)
ZR	-1.222 (.952)	-1.143 (1.161)	-.014 (.838)	< .001	3>1 (p <.001) 3>2 (p <.001)

Table 1. Comparison of BMD (g/cm^2) and Z-score (mean (SD)) between research groups SpA – patients with spondyloarthropathies; RA – patients with rheumatoid arthritis. Bone mineral density (BMD) expressed as g/cm^2 at spine (BMDS), left femur (BMDL) and right femur (BMDR); BMD expressed as Z-score in spine (ZS), left femur (ZL) and right femur (ZR).

In both SpA and RA patients a similar decrease of BMD (expressed as g/cm^2 and Z-score, unless otherwise stated) (Table 1) at lumbar spine and upper parts of the both femurs was determined. It was also established that in both SpA and RA patients mean BMD value in all examined skeletal sites was significantly lower than mean BMD value in control group subjects.

3.3 Homogenicity by BMD changes in patients with various diseases belonging to spondyloarthropathy group and with various types of joint lesions

The second objective of our research was to investigate BMD changes at lumbar spine and upper part of the left and right femur in patients with various diseases belonging to SpA group (AS, ReA, PsA, EnA) and in SpA patients with different type of joint lesions (only axial, only peripheral, both axial and peripheral).

Patients with SpA were allocated to the following subgroups: 54 (39.70%) patients with AS, 33 (24.3%) - with PsA, 29 (21.3%) - with EnA and 20 (14.7%) with ReA. The comparison of BMD value between these groups is presented in Table 2.

BMD	Disease belonging to SpA group				p
	AS (n = 54)	PsA (n = 33)	EnA (n = 29)	ReaA (n = 20)	
BMDS	.885 (.149)	.890 (.143)	.837 (.075)	.870 (.096)	.346
BMDL	.837 (.125)	.845 (.135)	.857 (.115)	.877 (.094)	.632
BMDR	.821 (.127)	.830 (.131)	.858 (.118)	.860 (.094)	.463
ZS	-1.301 (1.023)	-1.077 (1.258)	-1.631 (.484)	-1.298 (.868)	.179
ZL	-1.282 (.912)	-.991 (1.069)	-1.157 (.856)	-.928 (.965)	.392
ZR	-1.386 (.933)	-1.120 (1.032)	-1.158 (.891)	-1.040 (.954)	.418

Table 2. Comparison of BMD (g/cm^2) and Z-score (mean (SD)) between patients with various diseases of spondyloarthropathy group patients with ankylosing spondylitis (AS), psoriatic arthritis (PsA), reactive arthritis (ReA) and enteropathic arthropathy (EnA). Bone mineral density (BMD) expressed as g/cm^2 at spine (BMDS), left femur (BMDL) and right femur (BMDR); BMD expressed as Z-score in spine (ZS), left femur (ZL) and right femur (ZR).

Data presented in Table 2 do not demonstrate statistically significant BMD differences at lumbar spine and upper parts of the both femurs of patients with AS, PsA, EnA and ReA.

Patients with SpA were allocated to three subgroups depending on the type of joint lesion: patients with only axial lesion, only peripheral lesions and patients with both axial and peripheral lesion. Twenty five (18.4%) patients were allocated to the axial lesion group, 20 (14.7%) – to the peripheral lesion group, and both axial and peripheral lesion was diagnosed in 91 (66.9) patients. The comparison of BMD in SpA patients with various joint lesion types showed that there are no significant differences in BMD between subgroups at any examined sites of the skeleton (Table 3).

Summarizing data presented in Tables 2 and 3 it might be claimed that no significant differences in BMD mean values were found at any examined sites of the skeleton both comparing patients with various diseases belonging to SpA group and patients with different types of joint lesions. Therefore SpA group could be further analyzed as a homogeneous group without dividing it into subgroups by diseases.

BMD	Type of joint lesion			p
	Axial (n = 25)	Peripheric (n = 20)	Axial and peripheric (n = 91)	
BMDS	.859 (.158)	.846 (.080)	.883 (.128)	.416
BMDL	.836 (.147)	.882 (.100)	.845 (.117)	.391
BMDR	.818 (.149)	.875 (.103)	.833 (.117)	.269
ZS	-1.427 (1.289)	-1.541 (.668)	-1.237 (.952)	.384
ZL	-1.284 (1.122)	-.982 (.874)	-1.124 (.917)	.567
ZR	-1.408 (1.142)	-1.034 (.874)	-1.213 (.913)	.421

Table 3. Comparison of BMD (g/cm^2) and Z-score (mean (SD)) between patients with various types of joint lesions Bone mineral density (BMD) expressed as g/cm^2 at spine (BMDS), left femur (BMDL) and right femur (BMDR); BMD expressed as Z-score in spine (ZS), left femur (ZL) and right femur (ZR).

3.4 Variables associated with bone mineral density changes in patients with spondyloarthropathies

In order to determine variables related to BMD at lumbar spine and upper part of the left and right femur of patients with SpA, 90 models of multiple stepwise linear regression analysis were developed. One of the values of BMD (BMDS, BMDL, BMDR, ZS, ZL, ZR) served as dependent variable, and independent variables were controlled variables: age, gender (when BMD was expressed as g/cm^2), BMI, family history of fractures, various diseases belonging to SpA group, type of joint lesions and physical activity. Each time one of the specific SpA factors was involved into the model: duration of the disease calculated from the time of the manifestation of first symptoms and from the time the diagnosis was established; physical disability and immobility indicators: subjective (HAQ-S, BAS-G, BASFI) and objective (spine movement indicators: lumbar side flexion, modified Schober's test, tragus to wall distance and intermalleolar distance); disease activity indicators: BASDAI, ESR, CRP and disease activity determined by rheumatologist; medications in use: glucocorticoids and TNF-α blockers. Variables with highest determination coefficients of the equations of multiple stepwise linear regression obtained during the assessment of BMD at lumbar spine and upper part of the left and right femur were selected for the final multiple linear regression analysis:

- Age, gender (BMD expressed as g/cm^2), BMI;
- Duration of the disease calculated from the time of the manifestation of first symptoms;
- Indicators of patient's functional status: physical disability and immobility according to HAQ-S questionnaire, and reduction of spine movement assessed by the measurement of intermalleolar distance;
- Activity of the diseases determined by rheumatologist;
- Treatment: cumulative doses of glucocorticoids (g).

The summary of the final linear regression analysis model is presented in Table 4. Coding of the categorical variables is presented in Table 5.

Dependent variable	Independent variable	Regression coefficient (B) (standard error)	Beta	p
BMDS (R^2=.192; R^2 (adj.) = .168; p < .001)	DAR2	-.124 (.027)	-.459	< .001
	DAR1	-.066 (.026)	-.252	.012
	G2	.064 (.023)	.231	.006
	BMI	.005 (.002)	.189	.022
	constant	.773 (.063)		< .001
BMDL (R^2=.405; R^2 (adj.) = .382; p < .001)	DAR2	-.122 (.022)	-.480	< .001
	IM2	-.101 (.025)	-.290	< .001
	BMI	.006 (.002)	.244	.001
	DAR1	-.059 (.021)	-.240	.005
	Glucocorticoids	-.001 (.001)	-.141	.045
	Constant	.783 (.047)		< .001
BMDR (R^2=.443; R^2 (adj.) = .421; p < .001)	DAR2	-.115 (.022)	-.450	< .001
	IM2	-.121 (.024)	-.347	< .001
	BMI	.006 (.002)	.230	.001
	Glucocorticoids	-.002 (.001)	-.163	.017
	DAR1	-.046 (.020)	-.185	.025
	Constant	.775 (.046)		< .001
ZS (R^2=.294; R^2 (adj.) = .266; p < .001)	BMI	.061 (.015)	.313	< .001
	DAR2	-.919 (.196)	-.441	< .001
	DAR1	-.496 (.185)	-.247	.008
	Duration of the disease from first symptoms onset	.003 (.001)	.252	.003
	Glucocorticoids	-.019 (.007)	-.226	.006
	Constant	-2.608 (.418)		< .001
ZL (R^2=.388; R^2 (adj.) = .365; p < .001)	DAR2	-.922 (.177)	-.461	< .001
	BMI	.072 (.013)	.384	< .001
	DAR1	-.468 (.165)	-.243	.005
	Glucocorticoids	-.012 (.006)	-.146	.042
	IM2	-.400 (.199)	-.147	.046
	Constant	-2.399 (.373)		< .001
ZR (R^2=.384 R^2 (adj.) = .360; p < .001)	DAR2	-.853 (.178)	-.425	< .001
	BMI	.068 (.013)	.360	< .001
	IM2	-.550 (.200)	-.201	< .001
	Glucocorticoids	-.013 (.006)	-.160	.007
	DAR1	-.366 (.166)	-.189	.026
	Constant	-2.414 (.376)		< .001

Table 4. Multiple linear regression analysis of BMD (expressed as g/cm^2 and Z-score) at different sites of measurement (dependent variable), demographic and disease variables (independent variables). Bone mineral density (BMD) expressed as g/cm^2 at spine (BMDS), left femur (BMDL) and right femur (BMDR); BMD expressed as Z-score at spine (ZS), left femur (ZL) and right femur (ZR). IM – intermalleolar distance; DAR - activity of the disease determined by rheumatologist. The coefficient of determination R^2 and coefficient of determination corrected by the number of independent variables (R^2(adj.)), and p value close to the coefficient of determination is intended to test the hypothesis that regression is absent (hypothesis is discarded when $p < .05$); standard error determines standard deviation of the coefficient of regression; beta determines coefficient of regression of standardized data.

Variable	Coding	
Gender	**G1**	**G2**
Premonapausal females	0	0
Postmenopausal females	1	0
Males	0	1
Intermalleolar distance	**IM1**	**IM2**
0 – mild limitation of movement	0	0
1 – moderate limitation of movement	1	0
2 – severe limitation of movement	0	1
Activity of the disease determined by rheumatologist	**DAR 1**	**DAR 2**
2 – low activity	0	0
3 – moderate activity	1	0
4 – high activity	0	1

Table 5. Coding of the categorical variables in the regression analysis.

The analysis of Table 4 shows that main variable associated with BMD decrease at all examined sites of the skeleton is moderate and high disease activity which was determined by rheumatologist. Higher BMD values at all examined sites of the skeleton are determined by higher BMI of the patients with SpA (positive coefficient of regression). Spine BMD (expressed as Z-score) and both femurs BMD (expressed as g/cm^2 and Z-score) are significantly negatively affected by glucocorticoids. This means that higher cumulative glucocorticoid dose is associated with lower BMD at the spine and both femurs. Severe limitation of spine movement, assessed by the intermalleolar distance, is the significant negative variable for BMD changes at the upper part of the left and right femur (expressed as g/cm^2 and Z-score). The duration of the disease calculated from the onset of first symptoms was a significant variable associated with the changes in spine BMD (expressed as Z-score). It should be noted that lengthening of the duration of the disease is associated with higher Z-score at the spine (positive coefficient of regression was obtained). Male gender is another causative factor significantly positively affecting spine BMD changes (expressed as g/cm^2).

To summarise, it should be stated that the decrease of spine BMD is significantly associated with moderate and high activity of the disease determined by rheumatologist, and with the increase of cumulative dose of glucocorticoids; the decrease of upper part of both femurs BMD is associated with moderate and high activity of the disease determined by rheumatologist, the increase of cumulative dose of glucocorticoids and severe limitation of spine movement assessed by intermalleolar distance. Based on beta coefficients of significant variables it might be stated that the most precise prognostic variable for the decrease of BMD is increasing activity of the disease in patients with SpA determined by rheumatologist.

Analyzing BMD changes dependence from changes of established significant variables subjects of SpA group were allocated into subgroups according to these factors. Allocation was based on literature data and trends of changes of BMD and specific factors established by our research.

In order to clarify how BMD changes with the increase of the disease duration (assessed from the time of first symptoms) we allocated patients with SpA in three subgroups:

patients with the duration of the disease shorter than 100 months; patients with the duration of the disease from 100 to 200 months; and patients with the duration of the disease of more than 200 months. Results of the comparison BMD (expressed as g/cm^2 and Z-score) between subgroups presented in Table 6.

BMD	Duration of the disease from the time of first symptoms			p	Post hoc
	1	2	3		
	< 100 months (n = 75)	100-200 months (n = 35)	> 200 months (n = 26)		
BMDS	.878 (.105)	.852 (.158)	.890(.147)	.488	
BMDL	.886 (.100)	.804 (.123)	.803(.140)	< .001	1>2 (p = .002) 1>3 (p = .005)
BMDR	.875 (.096)	.795 (.138)	.782(.128)	< .001	1>2 (p = .002) 1>3 (p = .001)
ZS	-1.311 (.888)	-1.468 (1.163)	-1.131(1.016)	.422	
ZL	-.920 (.893)	-1.432 (.947)	-1.342(.986)	.013	1>2 (p = .021)
ZR	-1.004 (.878)	-1.489 (1.030)	-1.491(.922)	.011	1>2 (p = .031)

Table 6. Comparison of BMD (g/cm^2) and Z-score (mean (SD)) between patients with various disease duration (assessed from the time of first symptoms). Bone mineral density (BMD) expressed as g/cm^2 at spine (BMDS), left femur (BMDL) and right femur (BMDR); BMD expressed as Z-score in spine (ZS), left femur (ZL) and right femur (ZR).

Using analysis of variance (ANOVA) it was established that BMD (expressed as g/cm^2 and Z-score) at the both femurs significantly decreased when duration of the disease increased (assessed from the time of first symptoms). BMD at the spine not only decreases with the increase of the duration of disease, but even slightly increases, however, not significantly. We suppose that this is only „false-positive" effect occurred due to spine changes specific to SpA: syndesmophytes, calcification of longitudinal ligaments and calcification intervertebral discs and joint ankylosis in long-term SpA patients, and therefore no significant spine BMD (expressed as g/cm^2 and Z-score) differences between these subgroups were established measuring BMD by DXA anterior-posterior view. No significant BMD differences between subgroups of patients allocated according to the duration of the disease assessed from the time of diagnosis were established in any sites of the skeleton (all p > .05. data not shown). According to these data we may assume that the most significant loss of bone mass takes place in the beginning of disease when diagnosis is not established yet. When diagnosis is established, etiopathogenetic treatment starts strongly inhibiting local and systemic inflammation and associated osteoclast activity and demineralization of the bone tissue.

Another variable that allows for the suspected decrease of BMD (expressed as g/cm^2 and Z-score) at upper parts of both femurs is decrease in spine movement assessed by the intermalleolar distance. When SpA patients were allocated into subgroups according to standardized levels of limitation of movement, it was noticed that with the decline of spine movement (assessed by the intermalleolar distance) BMD decreased not only at both femurs (expressed as g/cm^2 and Z-score), but also at the spine (expressed as g/cm^2). The lowest femur BMD (expressed as g/cm^2 and Z-score) was determined in SpA patients with severe limitation of spine movement assessed by the intermalleolar distance (Table 7).

BMD	Level of limitation of spine movement			p	Post hoc
	0 (n = 73)	1 (n = 44)	2 (n = 19)		
BMDS	.899 (.112)	.857 (.124)	.813 (.171)	.019	2<0 (p = .024)
BMDL	.880 (.099)	.849 (.116)	.730 (.139)	< .001	2<0 (p < .001) 2<1 (p < .001)
BMDR	.871 (.100)	.840 (.103)	.698 (.145)	< .001	2<0 (p < .001) 2<1 (p < .001)
ZS	-1.184 (.929)	-1.448 (.877)	-1.522 (1.370)	.234	
ZL	-.980 (.879)	-1.145 (.873)	-1.692 (1.191)	.049	2<0 (p = .009)
ZR	-1.051 (.885)	-1.205 (.794)	-1.917 (1.238)	.002	2<0 (p < .001) 2<1 (p = .014)

Table 7. Comparison of BMD (g/cm^2) and Z-score (mean value (SD)) between SpA patients allocated according to the established limitation of spine movement assessed by the intermalleolar distance

Bone mineral density (BMD) expressed as g/cm^2 at spine (BMDS), left femur (BMDL) and right femur (BMDR); BMD expressed as Z-score in spine (ZS), left femur (ZL) and right femur (ZR); 0 - mild limitation of movement, 1 - moderate limitation of movement, 2 - severe limitation of movement.

Another significant and clinically important factor associated with BMD changes at the spine and both femurs is cumulative dose of GC. It is not known what cumulative dose of GC or duration of use of these medications become risk factors for the decrease of BMD. Therefore patients were conventionally allocated into 4 subgroups according to the following distribution of cumulative doses: untreated patients (n = 46); patients using cumulative dose of less than 1 g (n = 34) corresponding use of 5 mg/day during up to 6 months; patients using cumulative dose from 1 to 10 g (n = 36) corresponding use of 5 mg/day during up to 5 years; and patients using cumulative dose more than 10 g (n = 20) corresponding use of 5 mg/day longer than 5 years.

BMD	Cumulative glucocorticoid dose				p	Post hoc
	1	2	3	4		
	Untreated (n = 46)	< 1g (n = 34)	1-10 g (n = 36)	>10 g (n = 20)		
BMDS	.869 (.102)	.903 (.138)	.869 (.126)	.844 (.167)	.405	
BMDL	.881 (.110)	.873 (.122)	.830 (.106)	.769 (.133)	.002	4<1 (p = .002) 4<2 (p = .010)
BMDR	.868 (.112)	.856 (.113)	.827 (.101)	.747 (.150)	.001	4<1 (p = .001) 4<2 (p = .006)
ZS	-1.320 (.933)	-1.097 (.975)	-1.361 (.960)	-1.602 (1.160)	.333	
ZL	-.871 (.958)	-1.076 (.791)	-1.270 (.847)	-1.586 (1.180)	.028	4<1 (p = .024)
ZR	-.962 (.983)	-1.186 (.737)	-1.291 (.817)	-1.757 (1.226)	.017	4<1 (p = .009)

Table 8. Comparison of BMD (g/cm^2) and Z-score (mean value (SD)) between SpA patients allocated according to the cumulative glucocorticoid dose. Bone mineral density (BMD) expressed as g/cm^2 at spine (BMDS), left femur (BMDL) and right femur (BMDR); BMD expressed as Z-score in spine (ZS), left femur (ZL) and right femur (ZR).

Comparison of BMD (expressed as g/cm^2 and Z-score) between patients allocated according to cumulative glucocorticoid dose is presented in the Table 8. Analysis of the results using Turkey HSD test demonstrated that between first three groups (untreated patients, patients used < 1g and 1-10g cumulative dose of glucocorticoids) there are no statistically significant differences of BMD (expressed as g/cm^2 and Z-score) at the lumbar spine and upper part of the left and right femur. However, differences presented in the Table 8 are caused by the comparison of patients taking a cumulative dose of more than 10 g of glucocorticoids with untreated patients. Summarizing these results it may be said that higher than 10 g cumulative dose of glucocorticoids is associated with the decrease of BMD (expressed as g/cm^2 and Z-score) at the upper part of the left and right femur in patients with SpA.

The most important SpA factor associated with the loss of bone mass is the activity of SpA disease. In SpA group there were no patients with inactive disease determined by rheumatologist (score of activity = 1), and therefore patients were allocated into three subgroups according to the activity of disease: 2 - mild activity, 3 moderate activity, 4 - high activity. Comparison BMD between these subgroups presented in the Table 9.

BMD	Activity of the disease determined by rheumatologist			p	Post hoc
	2 (n = 35)	3 (n = 55)	4 (n = 46)		
BMDS	.937 (.112)	.878 (.116)	.819 (.133)	< .001	4<2 (p < .001) 4<3 (p =.015) 3<2 (p = .026)
BMDL	.927 (.093)	.865 (.110)	.771 (.107)	< .001	4<2 (p < .001) 4<3 (p < .001) 3<2 (p = .007)
BMDR	.909 (.087)	.860 (.109)	.754 (.113)	< .001	4<2 (p < .001) 4<3 (p < .001) 3<2 (p = .034)
ZS	-.809 (.899)	-1.301 (.837)	-1.722 (1.054)	< .001	4<2 (p < .001) 4<3 (p =.025) 3<2 (p = .016)
ZL	-.538 (.735)	-1.054 (.914)	-1.680 (.837)	< .001	4<2 (p < .001) 4<3 (p < .001) 3<2 (p = .005)
ZR	-.683 (.717)	-1.092 (.905)	-1.787 (.881)	< .001	4<2 (p < .001) 4<3 (p < .001) 3<2 (p = .028)

Table 9. Comparison BMD (g/cm^2) and Z-score (mean value (SD)) between SpA patients allocated according to the activity of the disease determined by rheumatologist Bone mineral density (BMD) expressed as g/cm^2 at spine (BMDS), left femur (BMDL) and right femur (BMDR); BMD expressed as Z-score in spine (ZS), left femur (ZL) and right femur (ZR); 2 - mild activity, 3 - moderate activity, 3 - high activity.

Analysis of the comparison data presented in Table 9 demonstrated that disease activity assessment performed by rheumatologist allows to suspect BMD changes in all sites of skeleton. In all analyzed sites (in lumbar spine and both femurs BMD expressed as g/cm^2 and Z-score) in patients with lower disease activity (2) BMD was higher in comparison with patients with moderate (3) activity of the disease, and in this group of patients BMD was higher than in patients with high (4) activity of the disease.

3.5 Factors predicting Z-score probability of ≤ - 2.0 at any site of skeleton

At the last step of the analysis of the results we performed forward stepwise (Wald) logistic regression analysis intended to find out which variables are the most predictive to event causing Z-score probability of ≤ - 2 at any site of skeleton. Assigning Z-score ≤ - 2.0 as one and Z-score > -2.0 as zero, logistic regression model will predict the probability of the event during which coded variable will obtain valuation of 1; in this case the probability will be designated as θ. Z-score of ≤-2.0 at least in one area of skeleton was determined in 43 patients with SpA (31.6 percent of all patients with SpA).

All variables analyzed in this research were entered into a forward stepwise logistic regression model: age, gender, BMI, family history of fractures, disease belonging to SpA group, type of joint lesion and physical activity; duration of the disease assessed from the time of the onset of first symptoms and from the time of the diagnosis; physical disability and immobility indicators: BAS-G, BASFI, HAQ-S, lumbar side flexion, modified Schober's test, tragus to wall distance and intermalleolar distance; indicators of the activity of the disease: ESR, CRP, BASDAI and disease activity determined by rheumatologist; cumulative dose of glucocorticoids and treatment with TNF-α blockers.

The following significant variables for event θ remained in the logistic regression model: moderate and high activity of the disease determined by rheumatologist, low BMI and positive family history of fractures. The results of the last step of logistic regression model are presented in Table 10.

Indices of the relevance of model	Regressor*	Coefficient of regression (B), (standard error)	Wald statistics	p	Exp (B)
χ^2 model compatibility criterion p < .001	DAR		17.852	<.001	
	DAR (2)	3.922 (1.091)	13.384	<.001	54.179
	DAR (1)	2.610 (1.077)	5.877	.015	13.602
Hosmer and *Lemeshow* χ^2 compatibility criterion p = .771	BMI	-.156 (.052)	9.025	.003	.856
	Positive family history of fractures	1.167 (.543)	4.618	.032	3.212
Coefficient of determination: *Negelkerke* R^2 = .407	constant	-.528 (1.607)	.108	.743	.590

Table 10. Logistic regression analysis of the event when Z-score probability at any site of skeleton will be ≤ - 2.0 at the analysis of SpA patient data. * DAR – activity of the disease determined by rheumatologist; coding of variables described in the Table 5.

The analysis demonstrated that correct probabilities for Z-score at any sites of the skeleton were established in 75.7 % of respondents.

4. Discussion

Skeletal remodeling in bone growth, maintenance, and repair is tightly regulated by a dynamic interaction between osteoclasts and osteoblasts. Recent advances in immunopathological mechanism of chronic inflammatory rheumatic disease highlighted the altered balance between bone loss and production by inflammation. T cells, natural killers, and cytokines that are involved in inflammatory process may also be responsible for the bone loss (Ritchlin et al., 2003). Many investigators have observed decreased BMD of the whole skeleton and increased femoral and vertebral fracture risk in patients suffering from both RA and SpA in comparison with healthy persons (Lodder, 2004; Huusko, 2001; Grisar, 2002). Up till now BMD changes were not being compared between SpA and RA patients.

An interesting observation from our study is that there was no statistically significant difference of BMD in any examined part of skeleton between the two groups of diseases, i.e. RA and SpA but the BMD difference between the control group and RA and SpA groups was statistically significant, the BMD being higher in all examined parts of skeleton of the control group. Analyzing BMD of SpA, RA and control groups the Z-score of the three groups were compared in order to exclude influence of age and gender, known OP risk factors, on BMD. The Z-score in all examined parts was similar for both RA and SpA groups while the Z-score difference in the same parts examined between the control group and both patient groups was statistically significant, the Z-score being higher in the control group. The findings support the hypothesis that inflammatory environment not only in joint synovial tissues but also in bone caused by autoimmune changes in RA and SpA patients induces a lot of molecular changes, RANKL and OPG equilibrium derangement and is one of the causes provoking not only local but also systemic osteoclastogenesis and related bone resorbtion (Suda, 1992; Franck, 2004; Golmia, 2002). The reduced BMD in case of both RA and SpA may also be explained by worsened mobility function (Szejnfeld, 1997; Faus-Riera, 1991), disturbances of calcium and vitamin D metabolism because of intestine injury and adverse effect of GC on bone tissue (Lange, 2005; Mielants, 1989).

Data on comparison of the BMD between healthy persons and patients diagnosed with SpA are scarce. As it was mentioned above the BMD of SpA patients was mostly investigated in AS. Several researchers have observed decreased BMD in AS patients compared with healthy persons (Will, 1989; Devogelaer, 1992; Sampaio-Barros, 2005). *K. Dheda* and colleagues, having examined 20 PsA patients, have not observed any statistically significant BMD reduction in PsA patients compared with healthy persons either in lumbar spine or in femur (Dheda et al., 2004). On the contrary *B. Frediani* and colleagues have found statistically significant BMD reduction both in vertebra and femur of PsA patients compared with corresponding skeleton parts of the control group (Frediani et al., 2001). Data on statistically significant BMD reduction in entire skeleton of EnA patients compared with the control group was published by several authors. (Frei, 2006; Reffitt, 2003). *J. Grisar* and colleagues investigated bone metabolism markers and BMD of AS, PsA and ReA patients. The investigators found statistically significant BMD decrease in the proximal femur of AS patients compared with PsA patients. There was no statistically significant difference of vertebral BMD of AS patients and both vertebral and proximal femoral BMD of PsA and ReA patients compared with the BMD of the control group. *J. Grisar* and colleagues conclude that in all forms of the above mentioned spondyloarthropathies accelerated resorbtion of bone tissue prevails regardless of the fact that decreased BMD was not observed in all examined disease patients compared with the control group (Grisar et al., 2002). We have not found any statistically significant BMD difference in AS, PsA, EnA and ReA patients in any part of the skeleton examined.

In our study we tried to define a correlation between BMD changes in lumbar spine and proximal femur and duration of the SpA.The SpA duration was calculated by the two following ways: from manifestation of the first symptoms and from the moment of clinical diagnosis statement. The results revealed that lenghthening disease duration calculated from manifestation of the symptoms is related to vertebral BMD growth and femoral BMD reduction. Agreeing with other authors (Donnelly, 1994; Reid, 1986; Mullaji, 1994), we think that vertebral BMD readings of patients with long disease duration measured by anterior-posterior view of DXA method are merely „deceptive". The lumbar spine often shows misleading high BMD values due to bridging syndesmophytes and ankylosis, which might mask osteoporosis in AS patients with an advanced disease (Donnelly, 1994; Karberg, 2005; Mullaji, 1994; Muntean, 2011).

Our previous investigations showed that SpA patients both with long and short disease duration have statistically significant lower proximal femoral and lumbar vertebral BMD compared with the control group (Venceviciene et al., 2008). Lengthening disease duration calculated from the moment of clinical diagnosis statement had no significant correlation to changes of vertebral and proximal femoral BMD. *R. Will* and colleagues have not found significant difference in the average lumbar vertebral BMD between patients suffering from AS longer than 10 years and the control group (Will et al., 1990). *E. S. Meirelles* and colleagues observed positive correlation between disease duration and changes of proximal femoral and lumbar vertebral BMD (Meirelles et al., 1999). Until now only one study that quantifies the magnitude of osteoporosis in population of early SpA patients is available (Van der Weijden et al., 2011). In this study all patients had a BMD measurement at a median of period 6.6 months after diagnosis. This study showed a high prevalence (47%) of low BMD in both femur and lumbar spine in SpA patients with early disease. In contrast with our study, no significant differences between the two groups with low and normal BMD were found in regard to time since diagnosis and disease duration (median of 6.3 years), counting from the very first symptoms of axial manifestations (Van der Weijden et al., 2011). Unfortunately the above mentioned study has some limitations: the BMD of patients was not compared with healthy persons. More to the point, a BMD and Z-score should be used instead of T-score to assess BMD changes in males under 50 years of age. The fact that low BMD is encountered in a young population with an early disease is very interesting. In most other studies, "early" often refers to patients who have not yet developed ankylosis or other radiological progression signs, or that these studies made use of disease durations as time since diagnosis and then referred to a disease duration of <10 years (Gratacos, 1999; Toussirot, 2001, Will, 1989). The issue of defining disease duration has been often debated in the AS literature. Today, the onset of the first symptoms is considered to be most important criteria (Davis et al., 2006). Taking into account the fact that AS is usually diagnosed 6-8 years after manifestation of the first symptoms we think that the most prominent decrease of the BMD takes place in the early pre-diagnosis period of the disease. Etiopathogenetic treatment begun after diagnosing the disease suppresses local and systematic inflammation and related activity of osteoclasts together with demineralization of the bone tissue.

In SpA, especially AS, other potential risk factors for bone loss occur, such as inflammation and mechanical factors -rigidity of the spine resulting in limited mobility and reduced physical activity due to pain and stiffness. Data about these risk factors, high disease activity variables such as ESR, CRP, BASDAI in relation with low BMD levels in different studies are not consistently reported (Karberg, 2005; Gratacos, 1999; Toussirot, 2001).

Acknowledging that high SpA activity is one of the most important risk factors for BMD reduction (Gratacos, 1999; Kim, 2006) and there being no currently standardized indicators of SpA activity we aimed to define which of the accessible disease activity indicators most frequently used in clinical practice might reflect BMD changes in SpA patients. We assessed disease activity on the basis of active disease diagnosis rated by the same rheumatologist, acute inflammatory phase indicators, ESR and CRP, and by subjective patient's evaluation of the disease activity using results of BASDAI questionnaire (Landewe et al., 2004). We found statistically significant association between decreased vertebral and both femoral BMD and moderate or hight SpA activity rated by the rheumatologist. There was no significant correlation between CRB, ESR, BASDAI and BMD changes in the examined skeleton parts.

On the contrary, *E. S. Meirelles* and colleagues have found no correlation between disease activity rated by the rheumatologist and BMD changes (Meirelles et al., 1999). *K. Capaci* and colleagues has proved that disease activity rated by physician on the basis of radiological signs of vertebral and hip destruction extent has no influence on the bone mass of AS patients (Capaci et al., 2003). Other authors have made similar conclusions to proving that acute inflammatory phase markers found once do not forecast either progression of radiological signs of SpA or reduction of BMD in different parts of skeleton. (Karberg, 2005; Toussirot, 2001; Muntean, 2011). Nevertheless, *J. Gratacos* and colleagues having carried out a two year perspective study and assessing AS disease activity by ESR, CRP and IL-6 blood concentration found that the subgroup of active disease patients had statistically significant reduction of BMD of femoral neck and lumbar spine but there were no significant BMD changes in the examined parts of the subgroup of non-active disease patients. (Gratacos, 1999). In another study disease activity parameters such as increased CRP and high BASFI and BASMI scores, correlated significantly with low bone mass in femoral neck as well as in lumbar spine (Van der Weijden et al., 2011). However, at the 12-month follow-up study hip bone loss was found to be associated with raised baseline C-reactive protein levels (Haugeberg et al., 2010).

Based on the previous research, as well as on the results of the present study, we conclude that active course of the disease and pronounced systemic inflammatory process without question has negative influence on BMD by different mechanisms which are insufficiently researched up to this time. We think that the contradiction that exists between our data and presented by other authors about the influence of disease activity on BMD changes may result from the difference in the groups of patients (the other authors mostly studied only AS patients) and methods used to assess disease activity. Furthermore, the role of pro-inflammatory cytokines might be important for the onset of osteoporosis because increased TNF-alpha levels have been found in patients with AS compared with subjects with non-inflammatory back pain, and correlations have been found between disease activity and markers associated with an increased bone metabolism (Lange et al., 2000). We, together with other authors think that cross-sectional laboratory acute inflammatory markers such as

CRP or ESR and results of BASDAI questionnaire which reflects the main SpA symptoms during the last week can not predict BMD changes (Karberg, 2005; Speden, 2002; Muntean, 2011). Only a physician rheumatologist's assessment of the entire case history including clinical, laboratory, radiological signs and taking regular care of the patient may accurately determine disease activity in the long course of disease activity. Disease activity according to our research data has a significant correlation with bone mass loss both in lumbar vertebral and femoral proximal regions.

We also tried to determine the influence of physical disability and disturbances of mobility function on BMD changes in lumbar vertebral and femoral proximal regions. Like other investigators we have found that patient's mobility function worsens with increasing duration of the illness (Falkenbach, 2002; Wei, 2007; Karatepe, 2005). It is known that SpA standardized indicators of spine mobility correlate with radiological changes such as impairment in sacroiliac joints and spine and the latter is an independent factor for the prediction of femoral BMD changes (Speden et al., 2002). We have established that the decrease of spine mobility determined by the modified Shober test shows possible reduction of femoral BMD. *H. J. Baek* and colleagues, having divided AS patients into two groups by spine flexibility index according to Schober test (correspondingly > 5cm and < 5cm), the group of patients with good mobility and the group of patients with bad mobility, have not found any BMD difference in lumbar spine between the groups while the proximal femoral BMD was statistically significantly lower in the bad mobility group in comparison with the good mobility group (Baek et al., 2005). We have obtained similar results by dividing SpA patients according to tragus-to-wall distance and lumbar lateral flexion measurement, then assessing the decrease in spine flexibility and comparing it's BMD. Statistically significant BMD difference was obtained only in the femur. Differently, the decrease in spine flexibility was determined by intermalleolar distance measurement, showed significant BMD reduction not only in femur but in spine too. We failed to find studies assessing correlation between spine flexibility indices such as lateral flexion, tragus-to-wall distance, intermalleolar distance (measuring spine flexibility in different parts of spine) and BMD changes.

It is worthy to note that many studies assessing mobility and physical disability of SpA patients are being carried out all over the world (Bostan, 2003; Zochling, 2006; Ward, 2002) but the research data about dependence of bone mass changes in different regions of skeleton on physical disability and disturbances of mobility are scarce and controversial. Several scientists insist that disturbances of mobility function have no influence on lowering BMD in AS patients (Mitra, 1999; Maillefert, 2001). *J. Gratacos* and colleagues failed to find the correlation between BMD reduction and the results of HAQ-S questionnaire evaluating physical disability of SpA patients. (Gratacos et al., 1999). Nevertheless *H. Franck* and colleagues found that patients having decreased BMD in different parts of the skeleton had significantly poorer mobility function indices (Schober index and results of BASFI questionnaire) in comparison with the group of patients having normal BMD (Franck et al., 2004). The results of our study however show that lessening of mobility function has no influence on spinal BMD. Changes in femoral BMD are best reflected by the physical disability of SpA patients assessed using HAQ-S questionnaire and disturbances of mobility function assessed by the BASFI questionnaire.

In agreement with other authors (Will, 1989; Mullaji, 1994) we have found that frequency of exercise of the patient had no significant influence on BMD changes in the parts of skeleton examined.

Summing up the results it is possible to state that reduction of BMD correlates with disturbances of mobility function that lessens during disease course as demonstrated by the results presented above. On the other hand, comparativelly good spine BMD results are probably „misleading". We as other researchers (Donnelly, 1994; Reid, 1986) support the statement that in the course of the disease, impairment of the spine begins in the form of calcification of longitudinal ligaments and intervertebral discs, formation of syndesmophytes and joint ankylosis. Apparently the decrease in spine mobility caused by changes in the spine may be associated with proximal femoral BMD changes.

The aim of our study was to clear up whether GC and TNF-α blockers can influence BMD changes for SpA patients. The effect of GC on bone mass of SpA patients is not sufficiently investigated. Some authors are of the opinion that GC cumulative doses is not a factor in the successful prognosis of BMD decrease [Bjarnason, 1997; Habtezion, 2002; Millard, 2001). Several clinical studies have shown that GC in doses of less than 7,5 mg/d does not incite more pronounced bone resorbtion (Bijlsma, 2000; Nishimura, 2000). *O. A. Malysheva* and colleagues have proved that the therapeutic GC dose of 7,5 mg/d has negative influence on BMD when being used longer than 48 weeks (Malysheva et al., 2008). Still A. Savickienė and colleagues have found that duration of GC use and their cumulative dose significantly correlated with lumbar spine BMD reduction in SpA patients (Savickienė et al., 2003). Negative GC influence on bone mass was also described by German researchers having determined that cumulative GC dose negatively correlates with BMD changes and serves as an independent factor for prognosis of BMD reduction in all parts of skeleton (Pollak, 1998; De Jong, 2002).

Considering the fact that GC treatment schemes (dose and duration of presciption) were changed several times we have conditionally divided SpA patients into 4 subgroups according to cumulative GC doses. We have compared BMD among the subgroups. We have not found statistically significant femoral and vertebral BMD difference among the first three subgroups (patients who have not used GC, used cumulative GC doses of <1g and 1-10g). Proximal femoral BMD of patients who used more than 10g of GC was statistically significantly less than BMD of patients who have not used GC. Similar results were obtained by the other group of researchers who proved that only cumulative GC doses exceeding 10 g has significant influence on BMD reduction in all parts of skeleton (Silvennoinen, 1995; Von Tirpitz, 1993).

A new group of drugs blocking cytokin TNF- α used for SpA treatment are called TNF- α blocking agents. This drug is effective in reducing disease symptoms, inflammatory processes and joint destruction (Braun, 2002; Brandt, 2000; Baeten, 2001; Breban, 2002; Gorman, 2002). It has been shown that TNF-blocking agents not only reduce signs and symptoms of disease activity in SpA, but also arrest hip and spine bone loss (Marzo-Ortega, 2003; Marzo-Ortega, 2005; Demis, 2002).

We compared BMD readings of patients treated with TNF-α blockers and patients who did not received TNF-α blockers and found no statistically significant BMD difference between the groups in all examined parts of the skeleton. While statistically significant influence of

TNF-α blockers on bone mass was not found it is still not possible to state that these drugs have no positive effect on suppression of bone tissue resorbtion. This cross-sectional study was not designed as an observation of TNF-α blockers effectiveness. On the other hand these drugs are only used to treat SpA of high activity after treatment with other disease modifying drugs and in cases with pronounced joint impairment. On the basis of the results of this study showing statistically significant negative influence of high disease activity on the BMD changes and „deceptive" BMD spine readings conditioned by long disease duration it is possible to assume that these factors could „hide" positive effect on bone caused by the TNF-α blockers. We hope that the further long term longitudinal studies with bigger observational cohort will prove the beneficial effect of TNF-α blockers for not merely reducing local and systemic inflammation but also their positive influence on the bone tissue of SpA patients.

Summing up all the results it is possible to state that only moderate or high SpA activity rated by the rheumatologist and GC cumulative dose are statistically significant specific factors which can predict reduction of BMD of lumbar spine in SpA patients.. It is important to note that the lengthening disease duration counted from the beginning of the first symptoms relates to augmentation of spinal BMD. Reduction of BMD of both proximal femurs was associated with moderate or high SpA activity rated by the rheumatologist, severe reduction of spine flexibility assessed by intermalleolar distance measurement and GC cumulative doses. The BMI is the only significant variable out of all other factors related to spinal and femoral BMD changes. It is necessary to point that increased BMI is related to higher vertebral and femoral BMD readings. The data of this study are in agreement with the data presented by the other authors that low BMI (< 19 kg/m^2) is related to possible nutritional deficiencies of vitamin D, calcium and protein and therefore, to BMD reduction (Ravn, 1999; Edelstein, 1993; Cetin, 2001). We have also determined the prognostic factors for SpA patients that need to be included into the group of reduced BMD (when the Z-score is ≤-2.0 in any part of the skeleton). Results of our study show that SpA patients whose disease activity rated by the rheumatologist is moderate or high and who have positive family history of OP fractures have a Z-score of ≤-2.0 found in any investigated part of the skeleton.

We have proved that SpA disease activity rated by the rheumatologist, spine flexibility assessed by intermalleolar distance measurement, cumulative GC doses, BMI, disease duration measured from the manifestation of symptoms and family history of OP fractures are important for evaluating the risk of BMD reduction for SpA patients. It is valuable for identifying those who should undergo testing for BMD and for what specific region of skeleton, and also for prescribing effective means for prevention and/or treatment.

5. Conclusions

- In patients with spondyloarthropathies BMD (expressed as g/cm^2 and Z-score) is the same as in patients with rheumatoid arthritis and is significantly lower in comparison with BMD of healthy subjects measured at the lumbar spine and upper part of left and right femur.
- Similar BMD changes at the lumbar spine and upper part of left and right femur are characteristic to SpA patients with various diseases belonging to SpA group.

- In SpA patients BMD changes do not depend on the predominant type of joint lesion.
- Duration of the disease reflects changes in BMD better when it is calculated not from the time of the establishment of clinical diagnosis, but from the time of onset of first clinical symptoms. Relations between the duration of the disease and BMD changes at the lumbar spine and upper part of left and right femur are different: BMD decreases at the upper parts of both femurs and increases at the spine with longer duration of the disease.
- High and moderate activity of the disease (established by rheumatologist) is associated with the elevated bone resorption at the lumbar spine and upper part of left and right femur. The relation between disease activity (which measured by ESR, CRP level and BASDAI questionnaire) and BMD decrease in any investigated area of skeletal system was not observed.
- BMD reduction at the lumbar spine and upper parts of both femurs is associated with the decrease of mobility of a SpA patient. Intermalleolar distance is the most precise indicant reflecting the relation between decrease of physical ability and mobility and BMD changes in all investigated areas of skeletal system: at the spine (BMD expressed as g/cm^2) and at the upper parts of both femurs (BMD expressed as g/cm^2 and Z-score); the lowest BMD at upper parts of both femurs is measured when reduction of spine movement is defined as severe.
- Significant negative association between cumulative dose of glucocorticoids and BMD changes at the lumbar spine and upper part of left and right femur were observed: BMD at the lumbar spine and upper parts of both femurs decrease with the increase of cumulative dose of glucocorticoids.

6. References

Adomaviciute, D; Pileckyte, M; Baranauskaite, A; Morvan, J; Dadoniene, J; Guillemin, F. Prevalence survey of rheumatoid arthritis and spondyloarthropathy in Lithuania. *Scand J Rheumatol*, Vol.37, No.2, (March 2008), pp. 113-119, ISSN 0300-9742

Arnett, FC; Edworthy, SM; Bloch, DA; McShane, DJ; Fries, FJ; Cooper, NS; Haeley, LA; Kaplan, SR; Liang, MH; Luthra, HS. The American Rheumatism Association 1987 revised criteria for the classification of rheumatoid arthritis. *Arthritis & Rheumatism*, Vol.31, No.3, (Mar 1988), pp. 315-324, ISSN 0004-3591

Baek, HJ; Kang, SW; Lee, YJ; Shin, KC; Lee, EB; Yoo, CD; Song, YW. Osteopenia in men with mild and severe ankylosing spondylitis. *Rheumatol Int*, Vol.26, No.1, (November 2005), pp. 30-34, ISSN 0172-8172

Baeten, D; Kruithof, E; Van den Bosch, F; Demetter, P; Van Damme, N; Cuvelier, C; De Vos, M; Mielants, H; Veys, EM; De Keyser, F. Immunomodulatory effects of anti-tumor necrosis factor alpha therapy on syvinium in spondyloarthropathy: histologic finding in eight patients from opel-label pilot study. *Arthritis Rheum*, Vol.44, No.1, (Jan 2001), pp. 186-195, ISSN 0004-3591

Bessant, R; Keat, A. How should clinicians manage osteoporosis in ankylosing spondylitis. *J Rheumatol*, Vol.29, No.7, (July 2002), pp. 1511-1519, ISSN 0315-162X

Bijlsma, JWJ; Jacobs, JWG. Hormonal preservation of bone in rheumatoid arthritis. *Rheum Dis Clin North Am*, Vol.26, No.4, (Nov 2000), pp. 897-910, ISSN 0889-857X

Bjarnason, I; Macpherson, A; Mackintosh, C; Buxton-Thomas, M; Forgacs, I; Moniz, C. Reduced bone mineral density in patients with inflammatory bowel disease. *Gut*, Vol.40, No.2, (Feb 1997), pp. 228-233, ISSN 0017-5749

Bostan, EE; Borman, P; Bodur, H; Barca, N. Functional disability and quality of life in patients with ankylosing spondylitis. *Rheumatol Int*, Vol.23, No.3, (May 2003), pp. 121-126, ISSN 0172-8172

Brand, C; Lowe, A; Hall, S. The utility of clinical decision tools for diagnosing osteoporosis in postmenopausal women with rheumatoid arthritis. *BMC Musculoskeletal Disorders*, Vol.9, (January 2008), pp. 13, ISSN 1471-2474

Brandt, J; Haibel, H; Cornely, D; Golder, W; Gonzalez, J; Reddig, J; Thriene, W; Sieper, J; Braun, J. Successful treatment of active ankylosing spondylitis with the anti-tumoral necrosis factor alpha monoclonal antibody infliximab. *Arthritis Rheum*, Vol.43, No.6, (Jun 2000), pp. 1346-1352, ISSN 0004-3591

Braun, J; Brandt, J; Listing, J; Zink, A; Alten, R; Golder, W; Gromnica-Ihle, E; Kellner, H; Krause, A; Schneider, M; Sörensen, H; Zeidler, H; Thriene, W; Sieper, J. Treatment of active ankylosing spondylitis with infliximab: a randomized controlled multicentre trial. *Lancet*, Vol.359, No.9319, (Apr 2002), pp. 1187-1193, ISSN 0140-6736

Breban, M; Vignon, E; Claudepierre, P; Devauchelle, V; Wendling, D; Lespessailles, E; Euller-Ziegler, L; Sibilia, J; Perdriger, A; Mezières, M; Alexandre, C; Dougados, M. Efficacy of inliximab in refractory ankylosing spondylitis: results of a six-month open-labeled study. *Rheumatolofy (Oxford)*, Vol.41, No.11, (Nov 2002), pp. 41: 1280-1285, ISSN 1462-0324

Calin, A; Garett, S; Whitelock, H; Kennedy, LG; O'Hea, J; Mallorie, P; Jenkinson, T. A new approach to defining functional ability in ankylosing spondylitis: the development of the Bath Ankylosing Spondylitis Functional Index. *J Rheumatol*, Vol.21, No.12, (Dec 1994), pp 2281-2285, ISSN 0315-162X

Capaci, K; Hepguler, S; Argin, M; Tas, I. Bone mineral density in mild and advanced ankylosing spondylitis. *Yonsei Med J*, Vol.44, No.3, (June 2003), pp. 379-384, ISSN 0513-5796

Cetin, A; Gokce-Kutsal, Y; Celiker, R. Predictors of bone mineral density in healthy males. *Rheumatol Int*, Vol.21, No.3, (Nov 2001), pp. 85-88, ISSN 0172-8172

Cooper, C; Coupland, C; Mitchell, M. Rheumatoid arthritis, corticosteroid therapy and hip fracture. *Ann Rheum Dis*, Vol.54, No.1, (January 1995), pp. 49-52, ISSN 0003-4967

Daltroy LH, Larson MG, Roberts WN, Liang MH. A modification of the Health Assesment Questionnaire for spondyloarthropathies. *J Rheumatol*, Vol.17, No.7, (Jul 1990), pp. 946-950, ISSN 0315-162X

Davis, JC; Dougados, M; Braun, J; Sieper, J; van der Heijde, D; van der Linden, S. Definition of disease duration in ankylosing spondylitis: reassessing the concept. *Ann Rheum Dis*, Vol.65, No.11, (Nov 2006),pp. 1518-1520, ISSN 0003-4967

de Jong, DJ; Mannaerts, L; van Rossum, LG; Corstens, FH; Naber, AH. Corticosteroid-induced osteoporosis: does it occur in patients with Crohn's disease? *Am J Gastroenterol*, Vol.97, No.8, (Aug 2002), pp. 2011-2015, ISSN 0002-9270

Demis, E; Roux, C; Breban, M; Dougados, M. Infliximab in spondyloarthropathy - influence on bone density. *Clin Exp Rheumatol*, Vol.20, No.6, (Nov-Dec 2002), pp. 185-186, ISSN 0392-856X

Dequeker, J; Westhovens, R. Low dose corticosteroid associated osteoporosis in rheumatoid arthritis and its praphylaxiz and treatment bones of contention. *J Rheumatol*. Vol.22, No.6, (Jun 1995), pp. 1013–1016, ISSN 0315-162X

Devogelaer, JP; Maldague, B; Malghem, J; Nagant de Deuxchaisnes, C. Appendicular and vertebral bone mass in ankylosing spondylitis. A comparison of plain radiographs with single- and dual- photon absorptiometry and with quantitative computed tomography. *Arthritis Rheum*, Vol.35, No.9, (Sep 1992), pp. 1062-1067, ISSN 0004-3591

Dheda, K; Cassim, B; Patel, N; Mody, Gm. A comparison of bone mineral density in Indians with psoriatic polyarthritis and healty Indian volunteers. *Clin Rheumatol*, Vol.23, No.1, (Feb 2004), pp. 89, ISSN 0770-3198

Donnelly, S; Doyle, DV; Denton, A; Rolfe, I; McCloskey, EV; Spector, TD. Bone mineral density and vertebral compression fracture rates in ankylosing spondylitis. *Ann Rheum Dis*, Vol.53, No.2, (Feb 1994), pp. 117-121, ISSN 0003-4967

Dougados, M; van der Linden, S; Juhlin, R; Huitfeldt, B; Amor, B; Calin, A. The European Spondyloarthropathy Study Group preliminary criteria for the classification of spondyloarthropathy. *Arthritis Rheum,* Vol.34, No.10, (Oct 1991), pp.1227: 1218, ISSN 0004-3591

Edelstein, SL; Barrett-Connor, E. Relation between body size and bone mineral density in elderly men and women. *Am J Epidemiol*, Vol.138, No.3, (Aug 1993), pp. 160-169, ISSN 0002-9262

El Maghraoui, A. Osteoporosis and ankylosing spondylitis. *Joint Bone Spine*, Vol.71, No.4, (July 2004), pp. 291-295, ISSN 1297-319X

Falkenbach, A; Franke, A; van Tubergen, A; van der Linden, S. Assessment of functional ability in younger and older patients with ankylosing spondylitis: performance of the Bath Ankylosing Spondylitis Functional Index. *Am J Phys Med Rehabil*, Vol.81, No.6, (Jun 2002), pp. 416-420, ISSN 0894-9115

Falkenbach, A; Franke, A; van der Linden, S. Factors associated with body function and disability in patients with ankylosing spondylitis: a cross-sectional study. *J Rheumatol*, Vol.30, No.10, (Oct 2003), pp. 2186-2192, ISSN 0315-162X

Faus-Riera, S; Martínez-Pardo, S; Blanch-Rubió, J; Benito-Ruiz, P; Duró-Pujol, JC; Corominas-Torres, JM. Muscle pathology in ankylosing spondylitis: clinical, enzymatic, electromyographic and histologic correlation. *J Rheumatol*, Vol.18, No.9, (Sep 1991), pp. 1268-1371, ISSN 0315-162X

Feldstein, A; Elmer, PJ; Orwoll, E; Herson, M; Hillier, T. Bone mineral density measurement and treatment for osteoporosis in older individuals with fractures: a gap in evidence-based practice guideline implementation. *Arch Intern Med*, Vol.163, No.18, (October 2003), pp. 2165-2167, ISSN 0003-9926

Franck, H; Meurer, T; Hofbauer, LC. Evaluation of bone mineral density, hormones biochemical markers of bone metabolism, and osteoprotegerin serum levels in patients with ankylosing spondylitis. *J Rheumatol*, Vol.31, No.11, (Nov 2004), pp. 2236-2241, ISSN 0315-162X

Frediani, B; Allegri, A; Falsetti, P; Storri, L; Bisogno, S; Baldi, F; Filipponi, P; Marcolongo, R. Bone mineral density in patients with psoriatic arthritis. *J Rheumatol*, Vol.28, No.1, (Jan 2001), pp. 138-143, ISSN 0315-162X

Frei, P; Fried, M; Hungerbuhler, V; Rammert, C; Rousson, V; Kullak-Ublick, GA. Analysis of risk factors for low bone mineral density in inflammatory bowel disease. *Digestion*, Vol.73, No.1, (Mar 2006), pp. 40-46, ISSN 0012-2823

Garrett, S; Jenkinson, T; Kennedy, LG; Whitelock, H; Gaisford, P; Calin, A. A new approach to defining disease activity in ankylosing spondylitis: The Bath Ankylosing Spondylitis Disease Activity Index. *J Rheumatol*, Vol.21, No.12, (Dec 1994), pp. 2286-2291, ISSN 0315-162X

Golmia, RP; Sousa, BD; Scheinberg, MA. Increased osteoprotegerin and decreased pyridinoline levels in patients with ankylosing spondylitis: comment on the article by Gratacos, et al. *Arthritis Rheum*, Vol.46, No.12, (Dec 2002), pp. 3390-3391, ISSN 0004-3591

Gorman, JD; Sack, KE; Davis, JD. Treatment of ankylosing spondylitis by inhibition of tumor necrosis factor alpha. *N Engl J Med*, Vol.346, No.18, (May 2002), pp. 1349-1356, ISSN 0028-4793

Gough, AK; Lilley, J; Eyre, S; Holder, RL; Emery, P. Generalized bone loss in patients with early rheumatoid arthritis. *Lancet*, Vol.344, No.8914, (July 1994), pp. 23–27, ISSN 0140-6736

Gratacos, J; Collado, A; Pons, F; Osaba, M; Sanmartí, R; Roqué, M; Larrosa, M; Múñoz-Gómez, J. Significant loss of bone mass in patients with early, active ankylosing spondylitis. *Arthritis Rheum*, Vol.42, No.11, (November 1999), pp. 2319-2324, ISSN 0004-3591

Grisar, J; Bernecker, PM; Aringer, M; Redlich, K; Sedlak, M; Wolozcszuk, W; Spitzauer, S; Grampp, S; Kainberger, F; Ebner, W; Smolen, JS; Pietschmann, P. Ankylosing spondylitis, psoriatic arthritis, and reactive arthritis show increased bone resorption, but differ with regard to bone formation. *J Rheumatol*, Vol.29, No.7, (Jul 2002), pp. 1430-1436, ISSN 0315-162X

Habtezion, A; Silverberg, MS; Parkes, R; Mikolainis, S; Steinhart, AH. Risk factors for low bone density in Crohn's disease. *Inflamm Bowel Dis*, Vol.8, No.2, (Mar 2002), pp. 87-92, ISSN 1078-0998

Haugeberg, G; Bennett, AN; McGonagle, D; Emery, P; Marzo-Ortega, H. Bone loss in very early inflammatory back pain in undifferentiated spondyloarthropathy: a 1-year observational study. *Ann Rheum Dis*, Vol.69, No.7, (Jul 2010), pp. 1364-1366, ISSN 0003-4967

Huusko, TM; Korpela, M, Karppi P; Avikainen, V; Kautiainen, H; Sulkava, R. Threefold increased risk of hip fractures with rheumatoid arthritis in Central Finland. *Ann Rheum Dis*, Vol.60, No.5, (May 2001), pp. 521-522, ISSN 0003-4967

Illei, GG; Lipsky, PE. Novel, non-antigen-specific therapeutic approaches to autoimmune/inflammatory diseases. *Curr Opin Immunol*, Vol.12, No.6, (December 2000), pp. 712-718, ISSN 0952-7915

Jenkinson, TR; Mallorie, PA; Whitelock, H; Kennedy, LG; Garrett, SL; Calin, A. Defining spinal mobility in ankylosing spondylitis (AS). The Bath Ankylosing Spondylitis AS Metrology Index. *J Rheumatol*, Vol.21, No.9, (Sep 1994), pp. 1694-1698, ISSN 0315-162X

Johnell, O; Kanis, J. Epidemiology of osteoporotic fractures. *Osteoporos Int*, Vol.16, No. 2, (March 2005), pp. 3-7, ISSN 0937-941X

Jones, SD; Steiner, A; Garrett, SL; Calin, A. The Bath Ankylosing Spondylitis Patient Global Score (BAS-G). *Br J Rheumatol*, Vol.35, No.1, (Jan 1996), pp. 66-71, ISSN 0263-7103

Karatepe, AG; Akkoc, Y; Akar, S; Kirazli, Y; Akkoc, N. The Turkish versions of the Bath ankylosing spondylitis and Dougados functional indices: reliability and validity. *Rheumatol Int*, Vol.25, No.8, (Oct 2005), pp. 612-618, ISSN 0172-8172

Karberg, K; Zochling, J; Sieper, J; Felsenberg, D; Braun, J. Bone loss is detected more frequently in patients with ankylosing spondylitis with syndesmophytes. *J Rheumato*, Vol.32, No.7, (Jul 2005), pp. 1290-1298, ISSN 0315-162X

Khan, MA. Ankylosing spondylitis: introductory comments on its diagnosis and treatment. *Ann Rheum Dis*, Vol.61, No.3, (December 2002), pp. 3-7, ISSN 00034967

Kim, HR; Kim, HY; Lee, SH. Elevated serum levels of solube receptor activator of nuclear factors-κB ligand (sRANKL) and reduced bone mineral density in patients in ankylosing spondylitis (AS). *Rheumatology (Oxford)*, Vol.45, No.10, (Oct 2006), pp. 1197-1200, ISSN 1462-0324

Kroot, EJ; Nieuwenhuizen, MG; de Waal Malefijt, MC; van Riel, PL; Pasker-de Jong, PC; Laan, RF. Change in bone mineral density in patients with rheumatoid arthritis during the first decade of the disease. *Arthritis Rheum, Vol.*44, No.6, *(Jun* 2001), pp. 1254-1260, ISSN 0004-3591

Kvien, TK; Haugeberg, G; Uhlig, T; Falch, JA; Halse, JI; Lems, WF; Dijkmans, BA; Woolf, AD. Data driven attempt to create a clinical algorithm for identification of women with rheumatoid arthritis at high risk of osteoporosis. *Annals of Rheumatic Diseases*, Vol.59, No.10, (October 2000), pp. 805-811, ISSN 0003-4967

Landewe, R; Rump, B; van der Heijde, D; van der Linden, S. Which patients with ankylosing spondylitis should be treated tumour necrosis factor inhibiting therapy? A survey among Ducth rheumatologists. *Ann Rheum Dis*, Vol.63, No.5, (May 2004), pp. 530-534, ISSN 0003-4967

Lane, NE; Rehman, Q. Osteoporosis in the rheumatic disease patient. *Lupus*, Vol.11, No.10, (November 2002), pp. 675-679, ISSN 0961-2033

Lange, U; Teichmann, J; Stracke, H. Correlation between plasma TNF-alpha, IGF-1, biochemical markers of bone metabolism, markers of inflammation/disease activity, and clinical manifestations in ankylosing spondylitis. *Eur J Med Res*, Vol.5, No.12, (Dec 2000), pp. 507-511, ISSN 0949-2321

Lange, U; Teichmann, J; Strunk, J; Müller-Ladner, U; Schmidt, KL. Association of 1.25 vitamin D_3 deficiency, disease activity and low bone mass in ankylosing spondylitis. *Osteoporosis Int*, Vol.16, No.12, (Dec 2005), pp. 1999-2004, ISSN 0937-941X

Lodder, MC; de Jong, Z; Kostense, PJ; Molenaar, ETH; Staal, K; Voskuyl, AE, Hazes, JM; Dijkmans, BA; Lems, WF. Bone mineral density in patients with rheumatoid arthritis: relation between disease severity and low bone mineral density. *Ann Rheum Dis*, Vol.63, No.12, (Dec 2004), pp. 1576-1580, ISSN 0003-4967

Maillefert, JF; Aho, LS; El Maghraoul, A; Dougados, M; Roux, C. Changes in bone density in patients with ankylosing spondylitis: a two-year follow-up study. *Osteoporosis Int*, Vol.12, No.7, (2001), pp. 605-609, ISSN 0937-941X

Malysheva, OA; Wahle, M; Wagner, U; Pierer, M; Arnold, S; Hantzschel, H; Baerwald, CG. Low-dose prednisolone in rheumatoid arthritis: adverse effects of various disease modifying antirheumatic drugs. *J Rheumatol*, Vol.35, No.6, (Jun 2008), pp. 979-985, ISSN 0315-162X

Marzo-Ortega, H; McGonagle, D; Haugeberg, G; Green, MJ; Stewart, SP; Emery, P. Bone mineral density improvement in spondyloarthropathy after treatment with etanercept. *Ann Rheum Dis*, Vol.62, No.10, (Oct 2003), pp. 1020-1021, ISSN 0003-4967

Marzo-Ortega, H; McGonagle, D; Jarrett, S; Haugeberg, G; Hensor, E; O'connor, P; Tan, AL; Conaghan, PG; Greenstein, A; Emery, P. Infliximab in combination with methotrexate in active ankylosing spondylitis: a clinical and imaging study. *Ann Rheum Dis*, Vol.64, No.11, (Nov 2005), pp. 1568-1575, ISSN 0003-4967

Meirelles, ES; Borelli, A; Camargo, OP. Influence of disease activity and chronicity on ankylosing spondylitis bone mass loss. *Clin Rheumatol*, Vol.18, No.5, (1999), pp. 364-368, ISSN 0770-3198

Mielants, H; Veys, EM; Cuvelier, C; De Vos, M. Subclinical involvement of the gut in undifferentiated spondyloarthropathies. *Clin Exp Rheumatol*, Vol.7, No.5, (Sep-Oct 1989), pp. 499-504, ISSN 0392-856X

Millard, TP; Antoniades, L; Evans, AV; Smith, HR; Spector, TD; Barker, JN. Bone mineral density of patients with chronic plaque psoriasis. *Exp Dermatol*, Vol.26, No.5, (Jul 2001), pp. 446-448, ISSN 0307-6938

Mitra, D; Elvins, DM; Collins, AJ. Biochemical markers of bone metabolism in mild ankylosing spondylitis and their relationship with bone mineral density and vertebral fractures. *J Rheumatol*, Vol.26, No.10, (Oct 1999), pp. 2201-2204, ISSN 0315-162X

Mitra, D; Elvins, DM; Speden, DJ; Collins, AJ. The prevalence of vertebral fractures in mild ankylosing spondylitis and their relationship to bone mineral density. *Rheumatology (Oxford)*, Vol. 39, No. 1, (January 2000), pp. 85–89, ISSN 1462-0324

Mullaji, AB; Upadhyay, SS; Ho, EK. Bone mineral density in ankylosing spondylitis. DEXA comparison of control subjects with mild and advanced cases. *J Bone Joint Surg Br*, Vol.76, No.4, (Jul 1994), pp. 660-665, ISSN 0301-620X

Muntean, L; Rojas-Vargas, M; Font, P; Simon, SP; Rednic, S; Schiotis, R; Stefan, S; Tamas, MM; Bolosiu, HD; Collantes-Estévez, E. Relative value of the lumbar spine and hip bone mineral density and bone turnover markers in men with ankylosing spondylitis. *Clin Rheumatol*, Vol.30, No.5, (May 2011), pp. 691-695, ISSN 0770-3198

Nishimura, J; Ikuyama, S. Glucocorticoid-induced osteoporosis: pathogenesis and management. *J Bone Miner Metab*, Vol.16, No.6, (2000), pp. 350-352, ISSN 0914-8779

Pettit, AR; Ji, H; von Strechow, D; Müller, R; Goldring, SR; Choi, Y; Benoist, C; Gravallese, EM. TRANCE/RANKL knowckout mice and protected from bone erosion in a serum transfer model of arthritis. *Am J Pathol*, Vol.159, No.5, (Nov 2001), pp. 1689-1699, ISSN 0002-9440

Pollak, RD; Karmeli, F; Eliakim, R; Ackerman, Z; Tabb, K; Rachmilewitz, D. Femoral neck osteopenia in patients with inflammatory bowel disease. *Am J Gastroenterol*, Vol.93, No.9, (Sep 1998), pp. 1483-1490, ISSN 0002-9270

Ravn, P; Cizza, G; Bjarnason, NH; Thompson, D; Daley, M; Wasnich, RD; McClung, M; Hosking, D; Yates, AJ; Christiansen, C. Low body mass index is an important risk factor for low bone mass and increased bone loss in early postmenopausal women.

Early Postmenopausal Intervention Cohort (EPIC) study group. *J Bone Miner Res*, Vol.14, No.9, (Sep 1999), pp. 1622-1627, ISSN 0884-0431

Reffitt, DM; Meenan, J; Sanderson, JD; Jugdaohsingh, R; Powell, JJ; Thompson, RP. Bone density improves with disease remission in patients with inflammatory bowel disease. *Eur J Gastroenterol Hepatol*, Vol.15, No.12, (Dec 2003), pp. 1267-1273, ISSN 0954-691X

Reid, DM; Nicoll, JJ; Kennedy, NS; Smith, MA; Tothill, P; Nuki, G. Bone mass in ankylosing spondylitis. *J Rheumatol*, Vol.13, No.5, (Oct 1986), pp. 932-935, ISSN 0315-162X

Ritchlin, CT; Haas-Smith, SA; Li P; Hicks, DG; Schwarz EM. Mechanisms of TNF-alpha- and RANKL-mediated osteoclastogenesis and bone resorption in psoriatic arthritis. *J Clin Invest*, Vol.111, No.6, (March 2003), pp. 821-831, ISSN 12639988

Sambrook, PN; Spector, TD; Seeman, E; Bellamy, N; Buchanan, RR; Duffy, DL; Martin, NG; Prince, R; Owen, E; Silman, AJ. Osteoporosis in rheumatoid arthritis. *Arthritis Rheum*, Vol.38, No.6, (June 1995), pp. 806–809, ISSN 0004-3591

Sampaio-Barros, PD; Filardi, S; Samara, AM; Marques-Neto, JF. Prognostic factors of low bone mineral density in ankylosing spondylitis. *Clin Rheumatol*, Vol.24, No.3, (Jun 2005), pp. 310-311, ISSN 0770-3198

Savickiene, A; Baranauskaite, A. Influence of glucocorticoids on bone mineral density in rheumatoid arthritis and seronegative spondyloarthropathies. *Medicina*, Vol.39, No.5, (2003), pp. 448-453, ISSN 1010-660X

Sieper, J; Braun, J; Rudwaleit, M; Boonen, A; Zink, A. Ankylosing spondylitis: an overview. *Ann Rheum Dis*, Vol.61, No.3, (Dec 2002), pp. 8-18, ISSN 0003-4967

Silvennoinen, JA; Karttunen, TJ; Niemela, SE; Manelius, JJ; Lehtola, JK. A controlled study of bone mineral density in patients with inflammatory bowel disease. *Gut*, Vol.37, No.1, (Jul 1995), pp. 71-76, ISSN 0017-5749

Speden, DJ; Calin, A; Ring, F; Bhalla, A. Bone mineral density, calnaceal ultrasound, and bone turnover markers in women with ankylosing spondylitis. *J Rheumatol*, Vol.29, No.3, (March 2002), pp. 516-521, ISSN 0315-162X

Suda, T; Takahashi, N; Martin, TJ. Modulation of osteoclast differentiation. *Endocr Rev*, Vol.13, No.1, (Feb 1992), pp. 66-80, ISSN 0163-769X

Szejnfeld, VL; Monier-Faugere, MC; Bognar, BJ; Ferraz, MB; Malluche HH. Systemic osteopenia and mineralization defect in patients with ankylosing spondylitis. *J Rheumatol*, Vol.24, No.4, (Apr 1997), pp. 683-688, ISSN 0315-162X

Toussirot, E; Michel, F; Wendling, D. Bone density, ultrasound measurements and body composition in early ankylosing spondylitis. *Rheumatology (Oxford)*, Vol.40, No.8, (Aug 2001), pp. 882-888, ISSN 1462-0324

van der Weijden, MA; van Denderen, JC; Lems, WF; Heymans, MW; Dijkmans, BA; van der Horst-Bruinsma, IE. Low bone mineral density is related to male gender and decreased functional capacity in early spondylarthropathies. *Clin Rheumatol*, Vol.30, No.4, (Apr 2011), pp. 497-503, ISSN 0770-3198

Venceviciene, L; Venalis, A; Sapoka, V; Butrimiene I. Bone mineral density in patients with spondyloarthropathies. *Medicinos teorija ir praktika*, Vol.14, No.3, (2008), pp. 275-282, ISSN 1392-1312

Venceviciene, L; Rugiene, R; Venalis, A; Butrimiene, I. Cross-cultural adaptation and validation of Lithuanian questionnaires for the spondyloarthropathies. *Medicina*, Vol.45, No.3, (May 2009), pp. 177-185, ISSN1010-660X von Tirpitz, C; Steder-Neukamm, U; Glas, K; Sander, S; Ring, C; Klaus, J; Reinshagen, M. Osteoporosis in inflammatory bowel disease - results of a survey among members of the German Crohn's and Ulcerative Colitis Association. *Z Gastroenterol*, Vol.41, No.12, (Dec 1993), pp. 1145-1150, ISSN 0044-2771

Ward, MM. Predictors of the progression of functional disability in patients with ankylosing spondylitis. *J Rheumatol*, Vol.29, No.7, (Jul 2002), pp. 1420-1425, ISSN 0315-162X

Wei, JC; Wong, RH; Huang, JH; Yu, CT; Chou, CT; Jan, MS; Tsay, GJ; Chou, MC; Lee, HS. Evaluation of internal consistency and re-test reliability of Bath ankylosing spondylitis indices in a large cohort of adult and juvenile spondylitis patients in Taiwan. *Clin Rheumatol*, Vol.26, No.10, (Oct 2007), pp. 1685-1691, ISSN 0770-3198

Will, R; Palmer, R; Bhalla, AK; Ring, F; Calin, A. Osteoporosis in early ankylosing spondylitis: A primary pathological event? *Lancet*, Vol.2, (Dec 1989), pp. 1483-1485, ISSN 0140-6736

Will, R; Palmer, R; Bhalla, A; Ring, F; Calin, A. Bone loss as well as bone formation is a feature of progressive ankylosing spondylitis. *Br J Rheumatol*, Vol.29, No.6, (Dec 1990), pp. 498-499, ISSN 0263-7103

Zochling, J; Braun, J; van der Heijde, D. Assessments in ankylosing spondylitis. *Best Pract Res Clin Rheumatol*, Vol.20, No.3, (Jun 2006), pp. 521-537, ISSN 1521-6942

4

Surgical Treatment After Spinal Trauma in Patients with Ankylosing Spondylitis

Stamatios A. Papadakis[1], Konstantinos Kateros[2], Spyridon Galanakos[1], George Machairas[1], Pavlos Katonis[3] and George Sapkas[4]
[1]D' Department of Orthopaedics, "KAT" General Hospital, Athens,
[2]A' Department of Orthopaedics, "G. Gennimatas" General Hospital, Athens,
[3]Department of Orthopaedics, University of Crete, Herakleion,
[4]A' Department of Orthopaedics, University of Athens, "Attikon" University Hospital, Haidari,
Greece

1. Introduction

Ankylosing Spondylitis (AS) is a chronic inflammatory disease which is characterized by pain and progressive stiffness and which spinal and sacroiliac joints are mainly affected. It affects mostly males, having a male-to-female ratio approximately 3-4:1 and the onset occur between the 15th and the 35th year of life (Bechterew, 1979; Calin, 1985; van der Linden et al., 2005).

Ankylosing Spondylitis transforms the flexible spinal column into a stiff rod; the stiffened spine cannot bear normal loads in comparison with a healthy spine. In addition, it has been established that bone mineral density loss occurs early in the AS disease course and is associated with inflammation correlated with increased bone resorption (van der Horst-Bruinsma, 2006). The kyphotic deformation of the spine that exists makes the ankylosing and osteoporotic spine susceptible to stress fractures under the impact of small forces and loads (van der Linden et al., 2005). The diffuse paraspinal ossification and inflammatory osteitis of advanced AS creates a fused, brittle spine that is susceptible to fracture (De Peretti et al, 2004; Einsiedel et al, 2006; Hanson and Mirza, 2000; van der Horst-Bruinsma, 2006; Taggard ans Traynelis, 2000;). Patients suffering from AS may undergo a fracture with minimal (Graham and Van Peteghem, 1989; Hanson and Mirza, 2000; Trent et al., 1988; Whang et al, 2009), or even no history of injury (Olerud et al., 1996; Westerveld et al., 2009; Yau and Chan, 1974).

The most frequent site, where a fracture is located is the cervical spine (75%) especially it's lower part, and the cervical-thoracic junction, following by the thoracolumbar junction (T10-L2). The drastic increase in stiffness at the cervicothoracic junction, combined with the lever arm of the fused cervical spine and weight of the head, makes fractures at the C6-C7 and C7-T1 levels most common. The lumbar and thoracic spines are more resistant to fracture because the anterior and posterior longitudinal ligaments are more thoroughly ossified than in the cervical spine. (Bohlman, 1979; Hanson and Mirza, 2000; Osgood et al., 1973; Surin,

1980; Taggard and Traynelis, 2000; Trent et al., 1988; Westerveld et al., 2009; Yau and Chan, 1974). Disruption of all the three columns of the spine predisposes to displacement and neurological injury (Gelman and Umber, 1978; Rasker et al., 1996).

When a fracture occurs in a patient with AS it should be considered as high-risk injury, especially when it is located in the cervical-thoracic junction of the spine (Fast et al., 1986; Sharma and Mathad, 1988). The most unstable types are shearing fractures. They may have severe neurological symptoms or may lead to haemothorax or rupture of the aorta, which are serious complications (Juric et al., 1990; Sharma and Mathad, 1988). Secondary neurological aggravation may be possible due to displacement of the fractured segments, which happens mainly in hyperextension injuries (Whang et al, 2009). Furthermore, where an interval occurs between trauma and the onset of neurologic signs or worsening of the neurologic picture the formation of an epidural hematoma should be suspected and excluded by means of an MRI scan (Thumbicat et al., 2007). Diagnosis can be difficult due to pre-existing spinal alterations (distortion of the normal spinal anatomy by ectopic bone formation, erosions, sclerosis, disk ossification, vertebral wedging). The standard radiographs are inadequate to fully evaluate shearing fractures due to osteoporosis, and the position of the shoulders (which are usually are located at a higher position). Thus, these fractures can be missed in the first examination and in the later stages, are characterized by vertebral corrosion, collapse and deformity. A misdiagnosed fracture can possibly lead to pseudarthrosis or Andersson lesion.

2. Diagnostic approach and clinical / radiological findings

The low grade of clinical suspicion makes the diagnosis difficult. The low imaging quality due to osteoporosis and the position of the shoulders (which usually are located in higher position) raise the difficulty level. Shearing fractures are possible to be missed in the first examination. All the available radiological tools should be used in order to validate the diagnosis, particularly when the injury concerns the occipital-cervical, the cervical-thoracic, the thoracolumbar or the lumbar-sacral junctions (Figures 1, 2, 3).

Plain radiographs (face, profile and oblique views) of the injured region may not reveal the fracture, giving only indirect information, such as widening of the disk space and discontinuity of the ossified paraspinal ligaments (Hanson and Mirza, 2000) which unfortunately are not able to set the diagnosis. In later stages these fractures are characterized by vertebral corrosion, collapse and deformity. A misdiagnosed fracture possibly leads to pseudarthrosis.

The neurological disorders may be established at the time of injury but it is not unusual to be established progressively with several days delay. It is not an exaggeration to say, that new back pain in patients with ankylosing spondylitis should be assumed to be caused by a fracture until proven otherwise (Einsiedel et al., 2006; Hanson and Mirza, 2000; Trent et al., 1988). Thus, thorough clinical and radiological assessment should be performed in these patients and should be repeated for the first few weeks, especially if the patient complains for indefinable pain or if neurological disorders are noted. The clinical doctor should always have in mind that the simple radiological evaluation of these injuries may not be able to reveal the fractures from the very first time. CT and MRI are valuable tools in order to reveal these fractures.

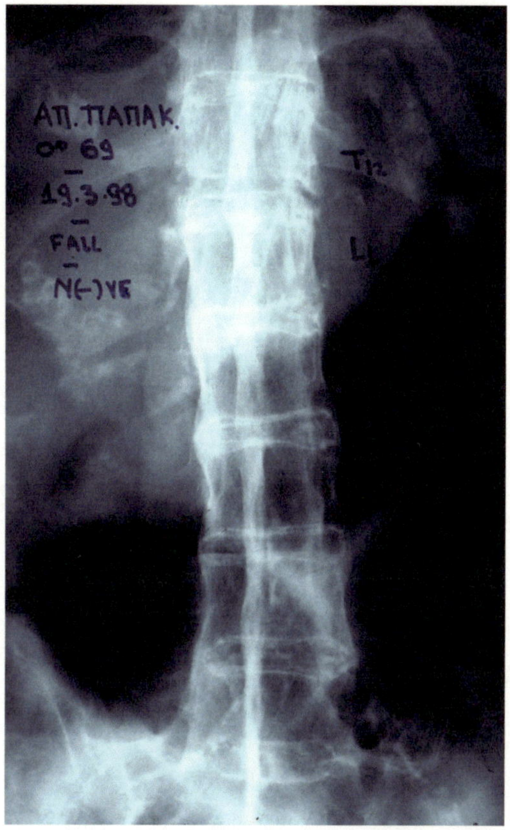

Fig. 1. Anteroposterior radiograph showing Chance type fracture due to a hyperextension injury at T12-L1 level.

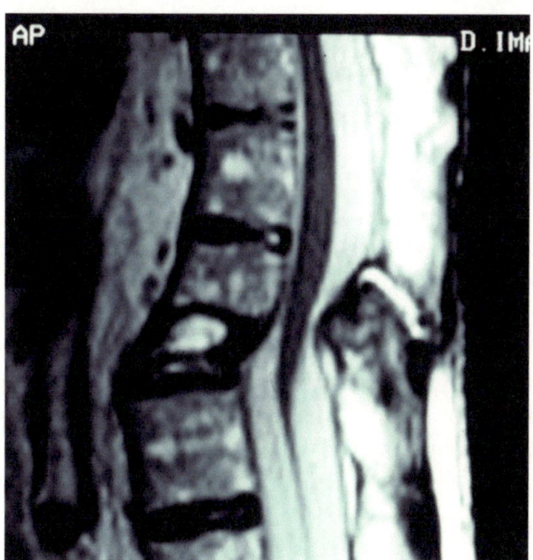

Fig. 2. Lateral MRI of the same case with a Chance type of fracture at T12-L1 level.

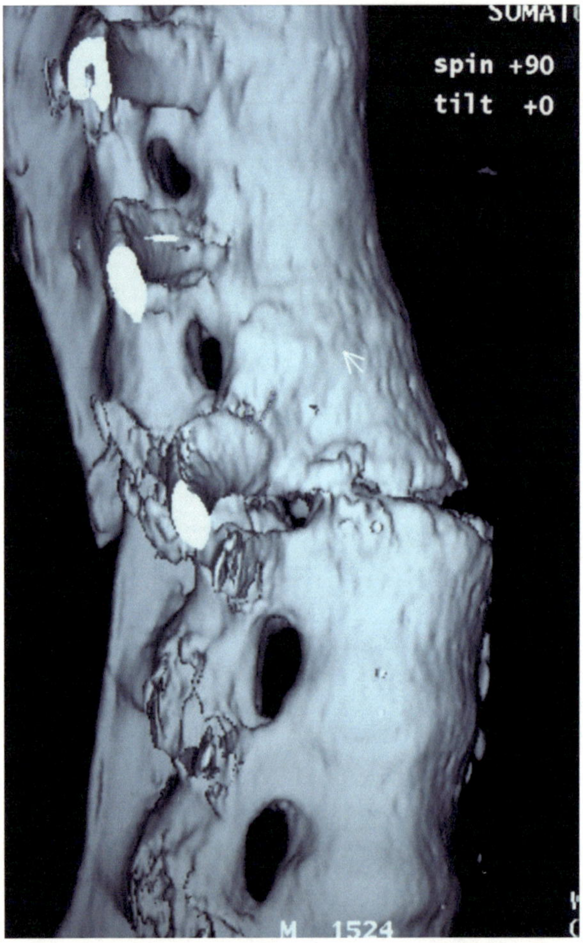

Fig. 3. Lateral 3D reconstruction image of the same case.

Preoperative evaluation of the cervical spine is essential when manipulating the neck during intubation and patient positioning. Physicians also must be aware that, because the atlanto-occipital joint is last to fuse, atlantoaxial instability may occur. Instability is usually demonstrated on lateral flexion-extension views of the neck, where the atlantodens and posterior atlantodens intervals are measured. An atlantodens interval >3.5 mm is indicative of instability. A difference of 7 mm indicates disruption of the alar ligaments, and a difference >9 to 10 mm or a posterior atlantodens interval >14 mm is associated with an increased risk of neurologic injury and usually requires surgical intervention (Kubiak et al, 2005). However, there are no guidelines for the management of atlantoaxial subluxation in patients with AS. Such management is similar to that performed in patients with rheumatoid arthritis (Ramos-Remus et al., 2006).

3. Surgical treatment

The majority of the cervical spine fractures occur at the level of the intervertebral disc and result in anatomic displacement and instability (Graham and Van Peteghem, 1987; Fox et al.,

1993; Kanter et al., 2008). Under these circumstances a potential neurological deficit is often and that necessitate early and aggressive surgical management with posterior and/or anterior fixation techniques to enable neural decompression, spinal stability, and optimal functionality (Broom and Raycroft, 1988; Deutsch and Haid, 2008).

A surgical intervention is necessary in cases of traumatic instability, significant deformity, and persistent degenerative radiculopathy with axial pain. In addition, selection of the patients that require surgical treatment is based on the degree of deformity, the level of pain and disability, and the medical status of the patient (Mundwiler et al., 2008).

3.1 Anesthesia options

It is well documented that a crucial step in airway management and prior to any surgical intervention, is a smooth and successful intubation (Hoh et al., 2008; Sciubba et al., 2008). The risks during obtaining airway access are significantly increased in patients with AS. The presence of large anterior cervical osteophytes may prohibit successful visualization of the larynx and may prevent endotracheal intubation due to significant mass obstruction. In addition, intubation may be impossible in cases in which the patient cannot extend his neck. Therefore, relatively minor flexion or extension forces during head positioning for intubation could lead to the creation of iatrogenic fractures or neurological injury by the intubation professional (Palmer, 1993). With modern anesthesia techniques, however, awake intubation allows for constant neurological monitoring during induction and insertion of an endotracheal tube. Fiberoptic visualization facilitates inserting a nasotracheal tube to secure airway access in patients with fixed cervical flexion (Hoh et al., 2008).

With endotracheal intubation, airway access is secured throughout the duration of the procedure. With a secured airway, the procedure can be performed in the prone position, facilitating placement of instrumentation, particularly at the upper thoracic levels, and reduces the risk of air embolism. General anesthesia also ensures patient comfort throughout the procedure. General anesthesia, however, impairs the ability to monitor neurological function, particularly immediately. While a wake-up test definitively demonstrates the patient's neurological function, expert anesthesia is required to perform a safe and timely evaluation. In a recent study, have been considered that as a special consideration for patients with AS, informed consent should include obtaining a consent for tracheotomy in the event that an obstructive cervical osteophyte or severe cervical flexion deformity prevent successful intubation (Cesur et al., 2005).

3.1.1 Patient positioning

Proper positioning of a patient with AS in the operating room or the ICU is imperative not only for the patient with an unstable fracture, but in all AS patients because of their increased risk of iatrogenic injury. During head positioning, the surgeon must take into account the sagittal alignment of the cervical spine, which may often be significantly kyphotic. When fractures already exist in these patients, inadequate assessment of the mass of the head and the extent of cervical kyphosis can have disastrous effects such as complete spinal cord damage and possible death (Hunter and Dubo, 1978; Sciubba et al., 2008).

In surgical procedures, preoperative halo placement and traction have shown success in improving stability during positioning (Chin and Ahn, 2007; Simmons et al., 2006;

Upadhyay et al., 1991). To allow a certain degree of freedom for patients with AS in the operating room or ICU, a number of adaptations to patient beds have been developed to accommodate prolonged immobilization. Such advances have particular relevance for the AS population because they allow the patient to maintain a more comfortable kyphotic condition with cervical traction.

3.1.2 Neurological monitoring

The ability to monitor the neurological status of any patient during positioning or surgical manipulation is extremely important in any spine surgery (Sciubba et al., 2008). In 1974 Scoliosis Research Society found that aggressive surgeries to correct deformities were associated with severe postoperative neurological deficits, and thus the society advised the universal use of intraoperative monitoring. In patients with AS, this statement is especially relevant. The surgeon must first decide whether the patient should receive general anesthesia at all. Because of the potentially hazardous nature of osteotomy procedures, a local anesthetic can be administered for frequent neurological assessments during deformity correction.

Urist (1958) was one of the first to report success with cervical osteotomy with the patient in the sitting position and with local anesthesia. Such operations carry a high risk of neurological complications due to the potential for iatrogenic cervical subluxation and spinal cord compromise, and thus continual feedback on neurological status provided by the awake patient is especially important (Belanger et al., 2005; Chin and Ahn, 2007). Nevertheless, performing these complex corrective spinal procedures on awake patients is a challenging task and is done on a rare basis.

Many complex spine surgeries however, require patients to be in the prone position for prolonged periods with extensive soft tissue exposure, making awake surgeries uncomfortable or completely infeasible for the patient. Hence, the wake-up test, which introduced by Vazuelle et al. in 1973, has been used to monitor the neurological status of patients undergoing prolonged spine deformity surgeries in the prone position.

Nowadays, placement of the patient in the prone position under general anesthesia is the preferred method for most spine surgeries, including those in patients with AS because it allows the surgeon easier access and manipulations of the spine, and the patient can tolerate a longer procedure (Bridwell et al., 2003, 2004; Hitchon et al., 2002, 2006; Langeloo et al., 2006).

Some surgeons feel that the cervical spine region is at a particularly high risk for neurovascular complications compared with the lumbar or thoracic area due to the higher level of the associated spine cord and accompanying vertebral arteries (Simmons et al., 2006). Therefore, if the decision has been made to proceed using general anesthesia, with or without the use of wake-up tests, many authors have stated that neurolophysiological monitoring is absolutely required (Chin and Ahn, 2007; Langeloo et al., 2006; Law, 1959). Common techniques include spinal cord evoked potentials introduced by Tamaki and Yamane, (1975), somatosensory cortical evoked potentials introduced by Nash and Brown, (1979), spinal somatosensory evoked potentials introduced by Shimoji et al. (1971), and muscle MEPs introduced by Merton and Morton, (1980). Unfortunately, such studies may not be sensitive enough to reliably predict neurological damage (Tamaki and Kubota, 2007).

Because there may exist discrepancies in sensitivity among the various monitoring techniques, it is now recommended that multiple and continuous neurological monitoring methods be used in addition to wake-up tests so that any false negatives provided by the electrophysiological recording are eliminated (Chin and Ahn, 2007; Tamaki and Yamane, 1975).

3.2 Management of a fracture

Conservative treatment either by prolonged bed rest in traction or in a cervical collar, or by early realignment and immobilization in a halo vest has been advocated because of supposed higher mortality after surgery (Graham and Van Peteghem, 1987). However, maintaining reduction is a major concern for conservative treatment: distraction, halo vest application, and transfer to a stretcher have led to secondary dislocation and neurological deterioration. Furthermore, immobilization in a halo has been associated with serious complications. Poor bone quality, vulnerable skin, and difficulty in achieving good alignment are additional arguments against the use of a halo (Schroder et al., 2003).

Surgical treatment is more commonly used, especially in patients with neurologic compromise, obscured visual fields, pseudarthrosis, or recurrent fracture. When traction or internal fixation is used to manage these injuries, the neck should be aligned to prefracture position, not necessarily to a normal position. Minor findings in patients with AS may be associated with substantial instability in the cervical spine, secondary to the altered biomechanics of the fused spine in addition to osteopenia and the concentration of forces at the cervico-occipital and cervico-thoracic junctions. The choice of the stabilization method is depending on the patient's personality, the type of the injury and the surgeon's experience. Currently, surgical stabilization with a rigid fixation is the choice of treatment that many surgeons perform (Figures 4, 5, 6).

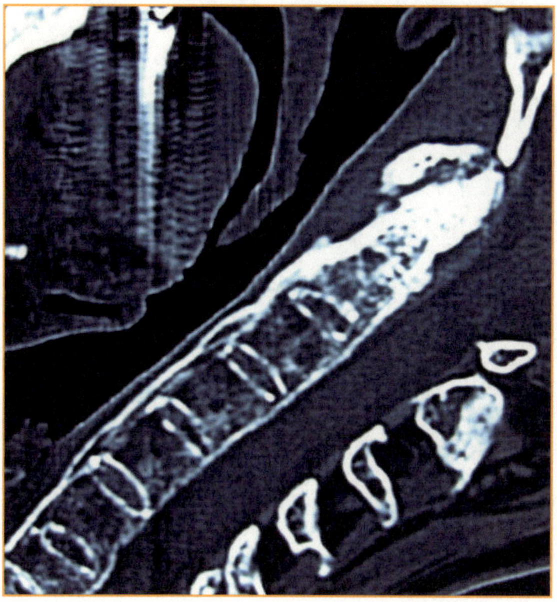

Fig. 4. CT image showing a fracture of the axis at the Cervical Spine.

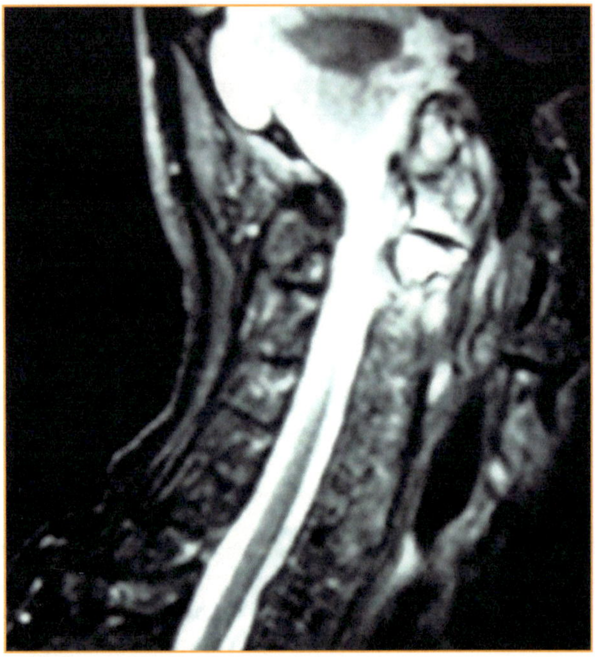

Fig. 5. MRI of the same patient with a fracture of the axis.

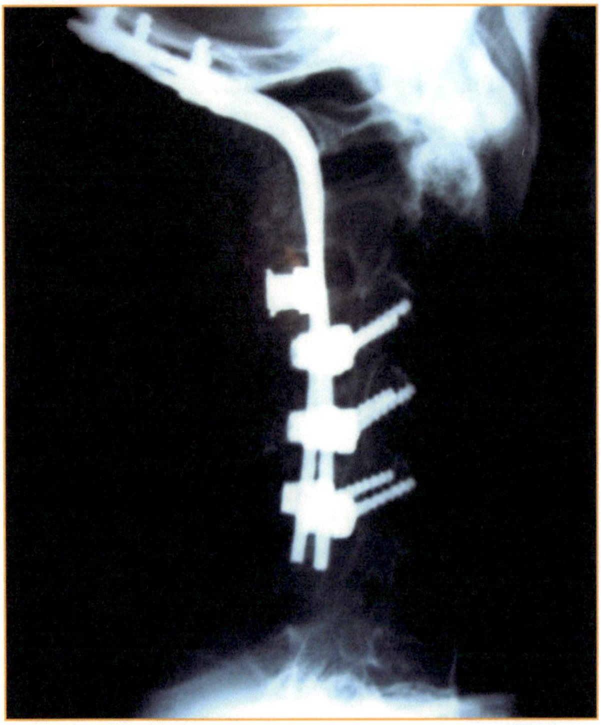

Fig. 6. The patient was treated with occipitocervical fusion by using a screw-rod stabilizing system.

In a review study by Westerveld et al., (2009) authors have recommended the follows:

1. Patients with an ankylosed spine have an increased fracture risk even after minor trauma,
2. Delayed diagnosis of fractures in patients with ankylosing spinal disorders often occur due to both doctor and patient related factors,
3. Fractures of the ankylosed spine tend to be unstable, because ossified ligaments and surrounding tissue also fracture,
4. An intrinsic unstable fracture configuration may lead to primary and secondary neurological deficit,
5. The clinical outcome of patients fracturing their ankylosed spine is worse compared to the general spine trauma population,
6. Surgical treatment may be favorable for patients with an ankylosed spine and spinal fracture, as this treatment option may be associated with lower complication and mortality rates and may lead to neurological improvement more frequently,
7. The presence of ankylosed spine segments should alert the treating physician for unstable spine fractures in every trauma patient,
8. In trauma registries ankylotic conditions of the spine should be registered separately, in order to acquire more knowledge on the patterns and prognosis of these injuries.

In a retrospective review of 12 patients with AS and 18 patients with diffuse idiopathic skeletal hyperostosis (DISH), authors mentioned that the treatment algorithm for managing spinal trauma is similar for both of these disorders, and the specific approach that is selected may be influenced by the type of injury, degree of spinal instability, and neurologic status of the individual (Wang et al., 2009). On the basis of these criteria, most of the injuries in those series were addressed with surgical intervention to more reliably stabilize the spine and prevent further neurologic decline. Although the operative rate observed for the AS group was higher than that of the DISH patients (83.3% vs. 66.7%, respectively), which may reflect the relatively greater neurologic impairment that was displayed by the subjects with AS, this difference was not found to be statistically significant. Even if it may not be feasible to formulate a definitive treatment protocol from the results of the above case series, it is clear that there are several important technical considerations that merit further discussion. As both of these diseases are associated with the development of kyphotic deformities, it is essential that the preinjury alignment of the spine be restored to achieve an adequate and hopefully stable reduction of the fracture. The authors recommended against any attempts to improve upon the preinjury sagittal alignment of these patients in the acute setting because aggressive manipulation may result in an unstable spinal construct that may subject the spinal cord or nerve roots to further harm; consequently, osteotomies and other corrective procedures should be delayed until the original injury has resolved so that they may be performed in a more controlled fashion. Although low-weight traction may be employed for selected cervical lesions to facilitate angular correction and postural positioning with wedge inserts may be useful for addressing any sagittal plane abnormalities associated with thoracolumbar injuries, the application of any type of distraction force is strictly contraindicated in these clinical scenarios because of the increased risk of precipitating a secondary neurologic insult at the level of an unstable spinal segment, particularly in the cervical spine.

It is generally assumed that the stabilization of cervical fractures is better performed with anterior and posterior support of the spine. Sapkas et al., (2009) presented their surgical experience of spinal fractures occurring in patients suffering from AS and to highlight the difficulties that exist as far as both diagnosis and surgical management. In this study, twenty patients suffering from ankylosing spondylitis were operated due to a spinal fracture. The fracture was located at the cervical spine in 7 cases, at the thoracic spine in 9, at the thoracolumbar junction in 3 and at the lumbar spine in one case (Table 1). Three of the cervical fractures were managed by both anterior and posterior approaches while all the rest were managed only by posterior approach, having no intra-operative complications, but one case with superficial wound infection and two cases (patients with cervical injuries) with loosening of posterior screws without loss of stability. Early mobilization was encouraged in all the patients. Cervical collars were used for 3-6 months, and thoracolumbar spinal orthoses were used for 6-12 months. Neurological defects were revealed in 10 patients. In four of them, neurological signs were progressively developed after a time period of 4 to 15 days. The initial radiological study was negative for a spinal fracture in twelve patients (60%). Authors noted that there was a statistically significant improvement of Frankel neurological classification between the preoperative and postoperative evaluation, only 35% of patients presented an improvement (10% from Frankel B to Frankel D, 10% from Frankel C to Frankel D, 10% from Frankel C to Frankel E and 5% from Frankel D to Frankel E) while 65% of patients were in stable condition (15% from Frankel A to Frankel A and 50% from Frankel E to Frankel E). The authors concluded that operative treatment for AS is useful and effective. It usually succeeds the improvement of the patients' neurological status. They also stated that taking into consideration the cardiovascular problems that these patients have, anterior and posterior stabilization aren't always possible, and in such cases, posterior approach can be performed and give excellent results, while total operation time, blood loss and other complications are decreased.

Olerud et al., (1996) believe that in the cervical spine, where implant loosening is a considerable problem, the failure of support is presented mainly in cases where only anterior or only posterior stabilization was applied because the stabilizing system may not be able to confront the forces which act on it. Thus, both anterior and posterior stabilization of the spine should be applied, especially for the cervical and the thoraco-lumbar spine. Nevertheless, in everyday practice posterior stabilization is usually performed. This is in order to reduce the possible causal factors of intra-operative and postoperative complications, taking into consideration that the most of these patients have cardiovascular and pulmonary disorders caused by restrictive ankylosis of the thoracic cage and prolonging the operating time by performing double stabilization and thoracotomy aggravates cardiovascular function. Moreover, the anterior approach to the cervical-thoracic junction is extremely difficult in these patients due to the great inclination and the kyphosis that exists at this region.

Long stabilizing systems that offer support to a greater area of the spine and the parallel use of braces postoperatively have been used in order to strengthen the stabilization. Serin et al., (2004) showed that four levels posterior fixation is superior to two levels posterior fixation and a four levels fixation plus offset hook is the most stable. Tezeren and Kuru (2005) demonstrated that final outcome regarding sagittal index and anterior body compression is better in the long segment instrumentation group than in the short segment instrumentation group.

#	Age (years)	Sex	Mechanism of injury	Level of fracture/Type	Neurological status preoperatively	Treatment/Levels of Fusion	Neurological status postoperatively
1	80	M	Fall	C2/Type II	Frankel C	Posterior instrumentation/ Occipito-C4	Frankel D
2	65	M	Fall	C2/Type I	Frankel E	Posterior instrumentation/ Occipito-C4	Frankel E
3	60	M	Fall	C6 - C7/A.3.1.1	Frankel E	Anterior + Posterior instrumentation/ C4-T2	Frankel E
4	38	M	Fall from height	C6 - C7/A.2.3.1	Frankel C	Anterior + Posterior instrumentation/ C4-T2	Frankel E
5	67	M	Fall	C6-C7/B.3.2.2	Frankel C	Posterior instrumentation/ C4-T2	Frankel E
6	69	F	Fall	C6 - C7/C.2.2.1	Frankel A	Anterior + Posterior instrumentation/ C4-T2	Frankel A
7	55	M	Fall	C6 - C7/A.3.1.1	Frankel E	Posterior instrumentation/ C4-T2	Frankel E
8	39	M	Fall	T5 - T6/ A.3.3.1	Frankel D	Posterior instrumentation/ T3-T8	Frankel E
9	23	F	Fall	T8/A.3.2.3	Frankel E	Posterior instrumentation/ T6-T10	Frankel E
10	53	M	Fall	T8 - T9/B.2.2.2	Frankel C	Posterior instrumentation/ T6-T11	Frankel D
11	65	F	Fall	T8 - T9/B.1.1.1	Frankel E	Posterior instrumentation/ T6-T11	Frankel E
12	57	M	Fall	T9/A.3.2.3	Frankel E	Posterior instrumentation/ T7-T11	Frankel E
13	64	M	Fall	T10 - T11/C.2.2.1	Frankel A	Posterior instrumentation/ T8-L1	Frankel A
14	79	M	Fall	T10 - T11/A.3.2.1	Frankel B	Posterior instrumentation/ T8-L1	Frankel D
15	40	M	Fall	T10 - T11/C.2.1.3	Frankel A	Posterior instrumentation/ T8-L1	Frankel A
16	52	M	Car Accident	T11 - T12/B.1.1.1	Frankel E	Posterior instrumentation/ T9-L2	Frankel E

17	69	F	Fall	T12 - L1/A.3.2.3	Frankel E	Posterior instrumentation/ T10-L2	Frankel E
18	38	M	Fall	T12 - L1/A.3.2.3	Frankel E	Posterior instrumentation/ T10-L2	Frankel E
19	40	M	Fall	T12 - L1/B.1.1.1	Frankel E	Posterior instrumentation/ T10-L2	Frankel E
20	55	M	Fall	L1 - L2/ B.1.1.1	Frankel B	Posterior instrumentation/ T12-L4	Frankel D

Table 1. Patients' data. (Adapted from Sapkas et al, BMC Musculoskeletal Disorders 2009 2, 10(1), 96)

3.2.1 Perioperative complications

1. Intraoperative blood loss: Operations involving patients with AS have been associated with increased perioperative blood loss (Nash and Brown, 1979; Palm et al., 2002). It may partly be caused by high intra-abdominal pressures due to difficulties in patient positioning (de Kleuver, 2006).
2. Trauma to dura mater: Due to chronic inflammation of the disease adhesions between dura meter, ligamentum flavum and bone may exist, making easier possible lacerations and tears of the dura.
3. Poor bone quality and internal fixation: The spine in AS is osteoporotic, due to the chronic inflammation and the bone atrophy. The consumption of corticosteroid drugs in the long run takes a serious part in this process making implant loosening a considerable problem.

4. Conclusions

Even minor injuries may cause fractures in an ankylosing spine. Patients with AS who sustain injuries of the spine are at greater risk of developing neurological impairment. These neurological disorders may be established at the time of injury but it is not unusual for them to become progressively, with several days delay. It is not an exaggeration to say that new back pain in patients with AS should be assumed to be caused by a fracture until proven otherwise. Thus, thorough clinical and radiological assessment should be performed in these patients and should be repeated for the first few weeks, especially if the patient complains of indefinable pain or if neurological disorders are noted. Accident and Emergency physicians should always bear in mind that simple radiological evaluation of these injuries may not be able to reveal fractures at first. CT and MRI are valuable tools in order to reveal these fractures.

The operative treatment of these injuries is useful and effective for these patients. It usually succeeds the improvement of the patients' neurological status, apart from cases where paraplegia is already established. However, the operative treatment is very demanding, especially when the cervical spine is concerned. Both anterior and posterior stabilization offer better support. Taking into consideration the cardiovascular and pulmonary problems that these patients have, anterior and posterior stabilization aren't always possible. There is a need for wider multicenter studies to get a correct picture of the incidence and the problems encountered in management of vertebral column trauma in AS.

5. References

Bechterew, VM. (1979). The classic stiffening of the spine in flexion, a special form of disease. *Clinical Orthopaedics and Related Research*, Vol.143, (September 1979), pp. 4-7

Belanger, TA.; Milam, RA IV.; Roh. JS.; & Bohlman, HH. (2005). Cervicothoracic extension osteotomy for chin-on-chest deformity in ankylosing spondylitis. *Journal of Bone and Joint Surgery Am*, Vol.87, No.8, (August 2005), pp. 1732–1738

Bohlman. HH. (1979). Acute fractures and dislocation of the cervical spine. An analysis of three hundred hospitalized patients and review of the literature *Journal of Bone and Joint Surgery Am*, Vol.61, No.8, (December 1979), pp. 1119-1142

Bridwell, KH.; Lewis, SJ.; Edwards, C.; Lenke, LG.; Iffrig, TM.; Berra, A.; Baldus, C.; & Blanke, K. (2003). Complications and outcomes of pedicle subtraction osteotomies for fixed sagittal imbalance. *Spine (Phila Pa 1976)*, Vol.28, No.18, (September 2003), pp. 2093–2101

Bridwell, KH.; Lewis SJ.; Rinella A.; Lenke LG.; Baldus C.; & Blanke K. (2004). Pedicle subtraction osteotomy for the treatment of fixed sagittal imbalance. Surgical technique. *Journal of Bone and Joint Surgery Am*, Vol.26, (March 2004) (1 Suppl), pp. 44–50

Broom MJ.; & Raycroft, JF. (1988). Complications of fractures of the cervical spine in ankylosing spondylitis. *Spine (Phila, Pa 1976)*, Vol.13, No.7, (July 1988), pp. 763–766

Calin A. (1985). Ankylosing spondylitis. *Clinics in Rheumatic Diseases*, Vol.11, No.1 (April 1985), Review, pp. 41-60

Cesur M.; Alici HA.; & Erdem, AF. (2005). An unusual cause of difficult intubation in a patient with a large cervical anterior osteophyte: a case report. *Acta Anaesthesiologica Scandinavica*, Vol.49, No.2, (February 2005), pp. 264–266

Chin, KR.; & Ahn, J. (2007). Controlled cervical extension osteotomy for ankylosing spondylitis utilizing the Jackson operating table: technical note. *Spine (Phila Pa 1976)*, Vol.32, No.17, (August 2007), pp. 1926–1929

De Peretti, F.; Sane, JC.; Dran, G.; Razafindratsiva C.; & Argenson C. (2004). Ankylosed spine fractures with spondylitis or diffuse idiopathic skeletal hyperostosis: diagnosis and complications. *Revue de Chirurgie Orthopédique et Réparatrice de l'Appareil Moteur*, Vol.90, No.5, (September 2004), pp. 456-465.

Deutsch, H.; & Haid Jr, RW. (2008). Cervical ankylosing spondylitis, in Mummaneni PV.; Lenke LG.; & Haid Jr, RW (eds): Spinal Deformity: A Guide to Surgical Planning and Management. St. Louis: Quality Medical Publishing, 2008, pp 307–330, ISBN: 978-1-57626-189-7

Einsiedel, T.; Schmelz, A.; Arand, M.; Wilke, HJ.; Gebhard, F.; Hartwig, E.; Kramer, M.; Neugebauer, R.; Kinzl, L.; & Schultheiss, M. (2006). Injuries of the cervical spine in patients with ankylosing spondylitis: experience at two trauma centers. *Journal of Neurosurgery Spine*, Vol.5, No.1, (July 2006), pp. 33-45.

Fast, A.; Parikh, S.; & Marin, EL. (1986). Spine fractures in ankylosing spondylitis. *Archives of Physical Medicine and Rehabilitation*, 67:595-597. Sep;67(9):595-597.

Fox, MW.; Onofrio, BM.; & Kilgore, JE. (1993). Neurological complications of ankylosing spondylitis. *Journal of Neurosurgery,* Vol.78, No.6, (June 1993), pp. 871–878

Gelman, MI.; & Umber, JS. (1978). Fractures of the thoracolumbar spine in ankylosing spondylitis. *American Journal of Roentgenology,* Vol.130, No.3, (March 1978), pp. 485-491.

Graham, B.; & Van Peteghem, PK. (1989). Fractures of the spine in ankylosing spondylitis. Diagnosis, treatment, and complications. *Spine (Phila Pa 1976),* Vol.14, No.8, (August 1989), pp. 803–807

Hanson, J.; & Mirza, S. (2000). Predisposition for spinal fracture in Ankylosing spondylitis. *American Journal of Roentgenology,* Vol.174, No.1, (January 2000), pp. 150.

Hitchon, PW.; From, AM.; Brenton, MD.; Glaser, JA.; & Torner, JC. (2002). Fractures of the thoracolumbar spine complicating ankylosing spondylitis. *Journal of Neurosurgery,* Vol.97, (2 Suppl), (September 2002), pp.218–222

Hitchon, PW.; Torner, J.; Eichholz, KM.; & Beeler, SN. (2006) Comparison of anterolateral and posterior approaches in the management of thoracolumbar burst fractures. *Journal of Neurosurgery Spine,* Vol.5, No.2, (August 2006), pp. 117–125

Hoh, DJ.; Khoueir, P.; & Wang, MY. (2008). Management of cervical deformity in ankylosing spondylitis. *Neurosurgical Focus,* Vol.24, No.1:E9.

van der Horst-Bruinsma, IE: Clinical aspects of ankylosing spondylitis. In *Ankylosing Spondylitis. Diagnosis and Management.* Edited by van Royen BJ.; & Dijkmans BAC. New York, London: Taylor and Francis; 2006, pp. 45-70

Hunter, T.; & Dubo, H. (1978). Spinal fractures complicating ankylosing spondylitis. *Annals of Internal Medicine,* Vol.88, No.4, (April 1978), pp. 546–549

Juric, S.; Coumas, JM.; Giansiracuse, DF.; & Irwin, RS. (1990). Hemothorax—an unusual presentation of spinal fracture in ankylosing spondylitis. *Journal of Rheumatology,* Vol.17, No.2, (February 1990), pp. 263-266

Kanter, AS.; Wang, MY.; & Mummaneni, PV. (2008). A treatment algorithm for the management of cervical spine fractures and deformity in patients with ankylosing spondylitis. *Neurosurgical Focus,* Vol.24, No.1, E11

Kubiak, EN.; Moskovich, R.; Errico, TJ.; & Di Cesare, PE. (2005) Orthopaedic management of ankylosing spondylitis. *Journal of the American Academy of Orthopaedics Surgeons,* Vol.13, No.4, (July-August 2005), pp. 267-78

Langeloo, DD.; Journee, HL.; Pavlov, PW.; & de Kleuver, M. (2006) Cervical osteotomy in ankylosing spondylitis: evaluation of new developments. *European Spine Journal,* Vol.15, No.4, (April 2006, Epub 2005 June), pp. 493–500

Law, WA: Osteotomy of the cervical spine. (1959). *Journal of Bone and Joint Surgery Br,* Vol.41, (August 1959), pp. 640–641

van der Linden, S.; van der Heijde, D.; & Braun, J. (2008). *Ankylosing Spondylitis.* In *Harris: Kelley's Textbook of Rheumatology.* 8th edition. Philadelphia: WB Saunders Co, pp. 1169-1189, ISBN: 978-1-4160-3285-4

Merton, PA.; & Morton, HB. (1980). Stimulation of the cerebral cortex in the intact human subject. *Nature* Vol.285, No.5762, (May 1980), p. 227

Mundwiler, ML.; Siddique, K.; Dym, JM.; Perri, B.; Johnson, P.; & Weisman, MH. (2008). Complications of the spine in ankylosing spondylitis with a focus on deformity correction. *Neurosurgical Focus,* Vol.24, No.1, E6, Review

Nash, CL Jr.; & Brown, RH. (1979). The intraoperative monitoring of spinal cord function: its growth and current status. *The Orthopedic Clinics of North America,* Vol.10, No.4, (October 1979), pp. 919–926

Olerud, C.; Frost, A.; & Bring, J. (1996). Spinal fractures with ankylosing spondylitis. *European Spine Journal,* Vol.5, No.1, pp. 51-55.

Osgood, C.; Martin, L.; & Ackerman, E. (1973). Fracture dislocation of the cervical spine with ankylosing spondylitis. *Journal of Neurosurgery,* Vol.39, No.6, (December 1973). pp. 764-769.

Palm, O.; Moum, B.; Ongre, A.; & Gran, JT. (2002). Prevalence of ankylosing spondylitis and other spondyloarthropathies among patients with inflammatory bowel disease: a population study (the IBSEN study). *Journal of Rheumatology,* Vol.29, No.3, (March 2001), pp. 511–515

Palmer, AR: Tracheal intubation and cervical injury. (1993). *Canadian Journal of Anaesthesia* Vol.40, May, (5 Pt 1), pp. 470–471

Rasker, JJ.; Prevo, RL.; & Lanting, PJH. (1996) Spondylodiscitis in ankylosing spondylitis, infection or trauma? A description of six cases. *Scandinavian Journal of Rheumatology,* Vol.25, No.1, pp. 52–57.

Sapkas, G.; Kateros, K.; Papadakis, SA.; Galanakos, S.; Brilakis, E.; Machairas, G.; Katonis, P. (2009). Surgical outcome after spinal fractures in patients with ankylosing spondylitis. *BMC Musculoskeletal Disorders,* Vol.2, No.10, (August 2009), p. 96

Schroder, J.; Liljenqvist, U.; Greiner, C.; & Wassmann, H. (2003). Complications of halo treatment for cervical spine injuries in patients with ankylosing spondylitis—report of three cases. *Archives of Orthopaedic and Trauma Surgery* Vol.123, No.(2-3), (April 2003, Epub 2003 Mar 25), pp. 112–114

Sciubba, DM.; Nelson, C.; Hsieh, P.; Gokaslan, ZL.; Ondra, S.; & Bydon, A. (2008). Perioperative challenges in the surgical management of ankylosing spondylitis. *Neurosurgical Focus,* Vol.24, No.1:E10.

Serin, E.; Karakurt, L.; Yilmaz, E.; Belhan, O.; & Varol, T. (2004). Effects of two-levels, four-levels, and four-levels plus offset-hook posterior fixation techniques on protecting the surgical correction of unstable thoracolumbar vertebral fractures: a clinical study. *European Journal of Orthopaedic Surgery and Traumatology,* Vol.14, No.1, pp. 1-6.

Sharma, RR.; & Mathad, NV. (1988). Traumatic spinal fracture in ankylosing spondylitis (a case report). *Postgraduate Medicine,* Vol.34, No.3, (July 1988), pp. 193-195.

Shimoji, K.; Higashi, H.; & Kano, T. (1971). Epidural recording of spinal electrogram in man. *Electroencephalography and Clinical Neurophysiology,* Vol.30, No.3, (March 1971), pp. 236–239

Simmons, ED.; DiStefano, RJ.; Zheng, Y.; & Simmons, EH. (2006) Thirty-six years experience of cervical extension osteotomy in ankylosing spondylitis: techniques and outcomes. *Spine (Phila, Pa 1976),* Vol.31, No.26, (December 2006), pp. 3006–3012

Surin, V. (1980). Fractures of the cervical spine in patients with ankylosing spondylitis. *Acta Orthopaedica Scandinavica,* Vol.51, No.1, (February 1980), pp. 79-84.

Taggard, D.; & Traynelis, V. (2000). Management of cervical spinal fractures in ankylosing spondylitis with posterior fixation. *Spine* (Phila, Pa 1976), Vol.25, No.16, (August 2000), pp. 2035–2039.

Tamaki, T.; & Kubota, S. (2007). History of the development of intraoperative spinal cord monitoring. *European Spine Journal*, Vol.16, Suppl 2, (November 2007, Epub 2007 Aug) pp. S140-6. 1.

Tamaki, T.; & Yamane, T. (1975). Proceedings: Clinical utilization of the evoked spinal cord action potential in spine and spinal cord surgery. *Electroencephalography and Clinical Neurophysiology*, Vol.39, No.5, (November 1975), pp. 539

Tezeren, G.; & Kuru, I. (2005). Posterior fixation of thoracolumbar burst fracture: short-segment pedicle fixation versus long-segment instrumentation. *Journal of Spinal Disorders and Techniques*, Vol.18, No.6, (December 2005), pp. 485-488.

Thumbikat, P.; Hariharan, RP.; Ravichandran, G.; McClelland, MR.; & Mathew, KM. (2007). Spinal cord injury in patients with ankylosing spondylitis. A 10-Year Review. *Spine* (Phila, Pa 1976), Vol.32, No.26, (December 2007), pp. 2989–2995.

Trent, S.; Armstrong, GW.; & O'Neil, J. (1988). Thoracolumbar fractures in ankylosing spondylitis. High-risk injuries. *Clinical Orthopaedics and Related Research*, Vol.227, (February 1988), pp. 61-66.

Upadhyay, SS.; Ho, EK.; & Hsu, LC. (1991). Positioning for plain spinal radiography producing paraplegia in a patient with ankylosing spondylitis. *British Journal of Radiology*, Vol.64, No.762 (June 1991), pp. 549–551

Urist, MR. (1958). Osteotomy of the cervical spine; report of a case of ankylosing rheumatoid spondylitis. *Journal of Bone and Joint Surgery Am*, Vol.40, No.4 (July 1958), pp. 833–843

Vauzelle, C.; Stagnara, P.; & Jouvinroux, P. (1973). Functional monitoring of spinal cord activity during spinal surgery. *Clinical Orthopaedics and Related Research*, Vol.93, (June 1973), pp. 173–178

Westerveld, LA.; Verlaan, JJ.; & Oner, FC. (2009). Spinal fractures in patients with ankylosing spinal disorders: a systematic review of the literature on treatment, neurological status and complications. *European Spine Journal*, Vol.18, No.2, (February 2009, Epub 2008 Sep 13), pp. 145-156

Whang, PG.; Goldberg, G.; Lawrence, JP.; Hong, J.; Harrop, JS.; Anderson, DG.; Albert, TJ.; & Vaccaro, AR. (2009). The management of spinal injuries in patients with ankylosing spondylitis or diffuse idiopathic skeletal hyperostosis: a comparison of treatment methods and clinical outcomes. *Journal of Spinal Disorders and Techniques*, Vol.22, No.2, (April 2009), pp. 77-85

Yau, A.; & Chan, R. (1974). Stress fracture of the fused lumbo-dorsal spine in ankylosing spondylitis. *Journal of Bone and Joint Surgery* Br, Vol.56, No.4, (November 1974), pp. 681-687

Part 2

HLA and Non-MHC Genes, Immune Response, and Gene Expression Studies

5

HLA-B27 and Ankylosing Spondylitis

Wen-Chan Tsai
Kaohsiung Municipal Ta-Tung Hospital,
Kaohsiung Medical University
Taiwan

1. Introduction

Ankylosing spondylitis (AS) is a chronic inflammatory disease with potential disabling outcomes. Clinically, patients presented with inflammatory lower back pain, enthesis and alternated buttock pain (van der Linden & van der Heijde, 1998). Bernard Corner (1666-1698) was the first physician who published the clinical features of AS in his medical thesis (Baker & Weisman, 2006). In the late 19th century, 3 independent physicians: Marie, Strupell, and Bechterew were able to describe the specific radiographic change in those patients by the help of the invention of radiology (Bywaters, 1983). But, still clinically, the boundary between AS and rheumatoid arthritis was unclear. Thanks to the discovery of rheumatoid factor which was strongly associated with rheumatoid arthritis, the distinction between these two arthritides became crystal clear. In those patients with inflammatory lower back pain and seronegative for rheumatoid factor, the diagnosis of ankylosing spondylitis became more popular in the early 1960 (Zeider et al., 2011). In 1963, American Rheumatism Association proposed a new nomenclature and classification for the rheumatic diseases. In this new edition, AS was specified as a complete different disease entity from rheumatoid arthritis (Blumberg et al., 1964). In addition to those different clinical characteristics, such as bone proliferation in enthesis site and sacroiliitis, in AS patients from those of patients with rheumatoid arthritis, AS is also known for its high association with HLA-B27. It has been known for more than 30 years since this association was discovered at 1973 (Schlosstein, 1973; Brewerton et al., 1973), although afterward, researchers found several HLA antigens were associated with other diseases (Invernizzi, 2011; McElroy, 2011; Piga, 2011), the strongest of any HLA antigens associated with human disease is HLA-B27 molecule. Hence, the roles of HLA-B27 in the pathogenesis and clinical manifestation of ankylosing spondylitis were among most frequent discussed topics in the past three decades.

2. Structure, subtypes and epidemiology of HLA-B27

HLA-B27 is one of the HLA class I molecules which are highly polymorphic and plays major role in protective immunity against intracellular parasites including virus and bacteria (Bjorkman et al., 1987). Traditionally, HLA class I molecule is considered to present peptide antigens to cytotoxic (CD8+) T cells. X-ray crystallographic studies revealed that extracellular structure of heavy chain of class I molecule contained three components: α-1, α-2 and α-3 domains. α-1 and α-2 together with a β pleated intervening sequence to form a peptide binding groove. α-3 domain is the membrane-proximal portion of the heavy chain which interact with CD8 of cytotoxic T cells. Besides binding peptides, class I molecule must associate non-covalently with beta2-microglobulin to form the tri-molecule complex on the cell surface. In lack of any one of these molecules, the molecular stability of this tri-molecule complex will be weak and easy to be degraded (Natarajan et al., 1999; Madden et al., 1991). Through their different amino acid compositions at binding groove, different HLA class I antigens has their own specific selectivity of binding peptides (Madden et al., 1992). In addition, to the selectivity of binding peptides, differences in the amino acid composition also influence the strength of association between heavy chain and beta2-microglobulin. (David, 1997).

HLA-B27 is a unique HLA class I molecule, not only because of its high association with AS but also has characteristically different amino acid composition from other class I molecules. In brief, there are two important characteristic structures which are different from others: the presence of B pocket and the free thiol group of Cys67 (Madden, 1995; Powis et al, 2009). In the presence of B pocket in the binding groove, B27 anchoring peptides had a very specific P2 residue: arginine. Free thiol Cys67 residue made B27 molecule easy to form homodimer in the extracellular domain which has great impact on its physiological role (Allen et al, 1999). There is an astonishing distribution of HLA-B27 gene among world population, with highest prevalence in northern territory of the earth, Eskimos and Native American in the circumpolar area and north Canada were known for their high carrier rate and some of the world's highest prevalence rates of spondyloarthropathies are described in these groups (Peschken & Esdaile, 1999; Boyer et al., 1997). It was shown that the distribution of HLA-B27 had a tendency of a decreasing north-south gradient of prevalence and was speculated that the peculiar geographic distribution of HLA-B27 might reflect a genetic selection for better survival from microbial infection (Piazza et al., 1980) (Figure 1).

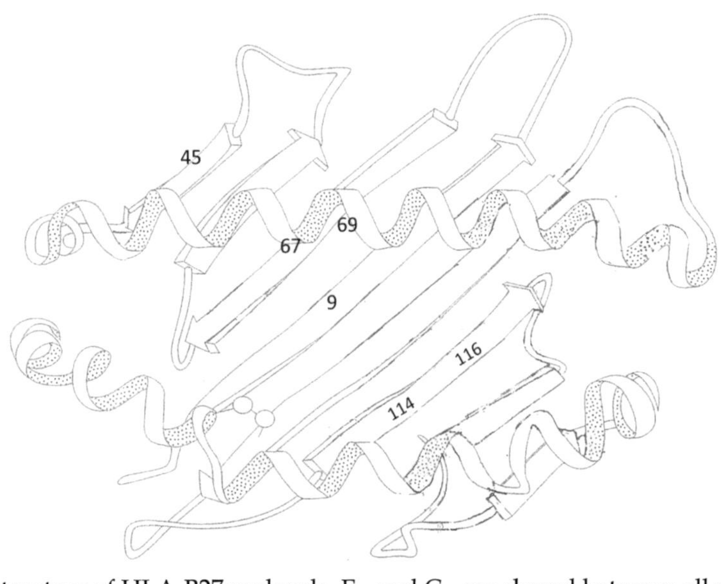

Fig. 1. The structure of HLA-B27 molecule. E_{45} and C_{67} are shared between all predisposing alleles. The presence of unpaired C_{67} made B27 molecule easy to form homodimers. In addition, the presence of H_9 in the floor of β pleated sheet is critical for the stability of the heavy chain/β2-microglobulin complex.

Till July 2011, 82 HLA-B27 subtypes were described based on nucleotide differences (International IMunoGene Tics information system [IMGT], 2011). Most nucleotide changes locate at exons 2 and 3 which encode the α-1 and α-2 domains. HLA-B*27:05 is the most prevalent subtype and present in almost every population in the world. It was thought that HLA-B*27:05 was the ancestor subtype, all other subtypes could have evolved from HLA-B*27:05 by point mutation (B*27:03), reciprocal recombination (B*27:07, B*27:09) and gene conversion (B*27:01, B*27:02, B*27:04, B*27:06). Following the ethnic migration and genetic evolution, HLA-B27 evolved into three ancestral pathways. Each pathway developed into a specific pattern. The first pattern was characterized by amino acid substitutions in the α-1 domain. HLA-B*27:02 was the most frequent allele, followed by HLA-B*27:03. This pattern is found largely in Africa, Middle Eastern and European groups. The second pattern contains a constant substitution at α-1 domain and variable substitutions at α-2 domain. HLA-B27:04 was the most prevalent subtype. This pattern is largely found in Eastern Asian such as Chinese, Thai and Korean. The third pattern contains a similar α-1 domain as HLA-B*27:05 and variable substitution at α-2 domain. In which, HLA-B*27:07 is the most prevalent subtype. This pattern is largely found in Middle East, but also in Turkey and Greece (Reveille & Maganti, 2009) (Figure 2).

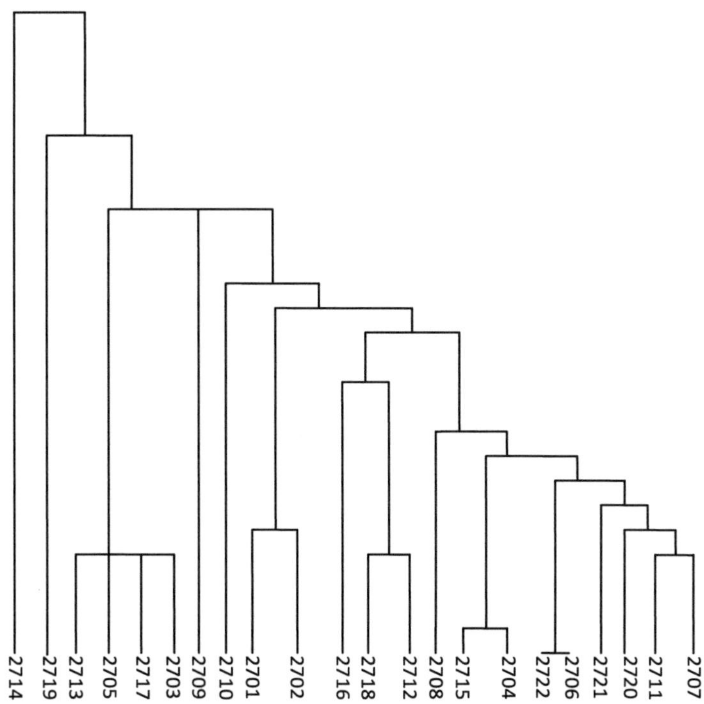

Fig. 2. Phylogenetic trees for the most common HLA-B27 subtypes (Adapted and modified from Blanco-Gelaz et al., 2001).

It is interesting to note that not all subtypes are associated with AS. In addition to B*27:05, most alleles such as B*27:01, B*27:02, B*27:03, B*27:04, B*27:10, B*27:13, B*27:14, B*27:15 are documented to be associated with ankylosing spondylitis (Taurog, 2007). In Chinese population, B*27:04 seemed to play major role in the pathogenesis of AS. Meta-analysis results showed a positive association between B*27:04 and susceptibility to AS in Han population (Zang et al., 2011). Also in the Taiwanese population, susceptibility to AS was determined by the presence of HLA-B*27:04 (Hou et al., 2007). In contrast, two subtypes, B*27:06 and B*27:09 have been reported not to be associated with AS and even considered to play a protective role. B*27:06 is a common subtype in countries such as Indonesia, Singapore and Thailand. In Singapore Chinese, B*27:06 had a significant negative association with AS (Ren et al., 1997). The same result also was reported from Taiwanese patients (Chen et al., 2002). Similarly, B*27:09, a rare subtype primarily found in Sardinia island and southern Italy, was found to have negative association with AS (Fiorillo et al., 2003). In addition to B*27:06 and B*27:09, other HLA-B27 alleles such as B*27:08 in Venezuela and B*27:07 in Cyprus were claimed not to be associated with AS (Armas et al., 1999). But these results are not universal, in other populations the same alleles have been found in AS patients (Cipriani et al., 2003; Varnavidou-Nicolaidou et al., 2004; Paladini et al., 2005). (Table 1)

B27 subtype	Ethnic distribution	Association with AS
B*27:05	Most ethnic groups	+
B*27:02	Caucasians, Central American, American Indians	+
B*27:03	Africans	+
B*27:04	Asians	+
B*27:06	Asians	–
B*27:07	Caucasians, Cyprus, middle east	+
B*27:08	Caucasians, Central Americans	+
B*27:09	Sardinian, Italy	–

Table 1. The ethnic distribution and ankylosing spondylitis association of most frequent subtypes of HLA-B27.

3. Hypotheses of the role of HLA-B27 in the pathogenesis of ankylosing spondylitis

Since the discovery of the high association of HLA-B27 with AS, models have been proposed to explain the role of B27 in the pathogenesis of AS. Several aspects of research were made including epidemiology studies, analysis of molecular structure, transgenic animal models and analysis of environmental factors. Using these tools, during the past three decades, several hypotheses had been raised successfully to explain some aspects of this association, but still, like the story of blind men and elephant, each hypothesis touch tangentially different appendages of the animal. The correct description fit all aspects of the elephant remained unsolved.

In most population, B27 carry-rate was more than 80%in patients with ankylosing spondylitis. However, B27 carry-rate in patients with ankylosing spondylitis was less than 50% in some areas. For example, among African Americans, 50% of patients with ankylosing spondylitis possess HLA-B27 (Akkoc & Khan, 2006). Focus had been put on the effect and level of gene expression of B27 on disease presentation. It was reported that disease developed earlier in patients who were HLA-B27+ than those HLA-B27- (Wu et al., 2009). B-27+ patients had higher incidence of anterior uveitis and hip joint involvement (Khan et al., 1977; Feldtkeller et al., 2003). The level of HLA-B27 mRNA had been claimed to be correlated with clinical disease activity in Chinese patients (Liu, 2006). It is interesting to find that in animal study, the copy number of HLA-B27 genes seemed to be a critical factor in determining the expression of a arthritis phenotype (Mammer et al, 1990). However, the effect of B27 homozygosity on the risk of disease development was controversial (van der Linden et al., 1984; Kim et al., 2009; Jaakkola et al., 2006). On the other hand, only a small percentage of B27-carriers developed AS. Twin studies suggest that susceptibility to AS is more than 90% inherited. HLA-B27 accounts for more than 50 % of this inheritance (Brown et al., 2000; Brown et al., 1997). Other genes must be involved in the disease development. A genome-wide study identified several other candidate genes such as ERAP1, IL-23R, IL1R2, ANTXR2, TNFSF15, TNFR1 and TRADD (Australo-Anglo-American Spondyloarthritis consortium [TSAC]; Reveille et al., 2010; Wellcome Trust Case Control Consortium [TASC]; Burton et al., 2010). Many of these candidate genes are hot topics for research recently (Campbell et al., 2011; Chen et al., 2011; Layh-Schmitt & Colbert, 2008; Brown, 2010).

According to the above finding, theories of the disease pathogenesis were proposed. Hypotheses including molecular mimicry, arthritogenic peptide, free heavy chain and unfolded protein response were considered main streams of hypotheses.

3.1 Theory of molecular mimicry and arthritogenic peptides

A striking finding of the similarity of 6 consecutive amino acids of HLA-B27 to 6 consecutive amino acids of nitrogenase from *Klebsiella pneumonia* made researchers to propose that after the microbial infection, our immune system mis-recognized self-antigens as a target and launched an autoimmune response (Schwimmbeck & Oldstone, 1998). A Finnish group also identified that two bacterial proteins shared homology with HLA-B27, namely YadA (Yersinia adhesin) and OmpH, outer surface proteins of Yersinia and Salmonella, respectively (Lahesmaa et al., 1991). Further support of this hypothesis is the finding that HLA class II antigen associated with rheumatoid arthritis shared the same amino acid sequences with some viral antigens (Albani & Carson, 1996). Data from serologic studies also indicated that patients with AS had high incidence of antibodies against microbial pathogens (Ewing et al., 1990). This study indicate that AS patient sera contain antibodies which were reactive to K. pneumoniae nitrogenase peptides and HLA B27.1 peptides, and that there are at least two epitopes in the alpha 1 domain at the groove region, that are autoantigenic. However, not all reports are consistent, later reports did not support the finding of antibodies against self-antigens in patients with AS (de Vries et al., 1992).

As mentioned before, the unique amino acid composition, especially in the peptide -binding groove, made B27 molecule distinct. The presence of B pocket fits only arginine inside. This finding together with the knowledge of highly polymorphism of B27 alleles which were differentially associated with AS pave a new way to search for the presence of arthritogenic peptides with the ability to provoke arthritis. All these alleles differed from each other by only one or few amino acid changes, but interestingly, the association with AS were quite different. Most HLA-B27 alleles are found at a very low frequency, their association with AS are largely unknown. B*27:05 is an ancestral type and associated with AS in almost every population in the world. B*27:04 is very prevalent in Asian country and also is thought to make individual susceptible to AS. On the contrary, B*27:03, B*27:06 and B*27:09 were considered to play a protective role. Rare incidence of these allele-carriers developed AS. B*27:03 was initially thought not to be associated with AS and only was prevalent in Black African population where B*27:05 is also not associated with AS (Hill et al., 1991). Certainly, other genes might be involved in the pathogenesis. Recently, AS patients possessing B*27:03 were found (Reveille et al., 2000). B*27:09 were found in healthy inhabitants of Sardinian island but not in patients, who only carry B*27:05. Although a case of AS possess B*27:09 together with B*14:03, another AS-associated allele in black Africans reported (Cauli et al., 2007). The amino acid sequence of B*27:09 differed from that of B*27:05 only in residue 116 (His vs Asp) .(de Castro, 2009) . Self-peptide pVIPR binds to B*27:05 in dual conformation but only one conventional form can be bound to B*27:09 (Hulsmeyer M et al., 2004). This different binding link might provoke different T cell response. B*27:06 is found mainly in Southeastern Asia among healthy control, while other B27 alleles were associated with AS. B*27:03 differs from B*27:05 by the Y59H change located in the A pocket. B*27:04 and B*27:06 are closely related differ only by two amino acid changes, namely H114D and D116Y. Different amino acid sequences in the binding groove will change the polar-nonpolar interaction of heavy chain with peptides, hence causes different peptides anchoring to the groove. It was postulated that some disease-causing alleles of HLA-B27 selectively bound arthritogenic peptides derived from several intracellular parasites which were claimed to be triggering agents in reactive arthritis. Even more, some investigators found that peptides derived from self antigen, including peptide from HLA-B27 itself and cartilage were found to trigger CD8+ T cell response (Kuhne et al., 2009; Atagunduz et al., 2005). Three self peptides derived from cartilage/bone proteins showed homology to sequence of protein from arthritogenic bacteria. One of them, peptide PRGLLAWISR derived from chondoitin sulfate N-acetygalatosaminyltransferase 1 shared 8 amino acids with FhuB protein from *Yersinia Enterocolitica* and 7 amino acids with intracellular attenuator protein A from *Salmonella Typhimurium* (Dror LB et al., 2010). The presence of self peptide in the HLA binding groove with homologous sequence from arthritogenic bacteria forms the cornerstone of molecular mimicry. It is interesting to note that in addition to HLA-B27, HLA-B39 had similar B pocket was found to be associated with ankylosing spondylitis in those who were HLA-B27 negative. It was considered to harbor same peptide repertoire with HLA-B27 (Yamaguchi et al, 1995). Another observation is that HLA-B*14:03 is a major MHC molecule associated with AS in Africa, it differs from HLA-B*27:05 at 18 positions and shares only 3-5% peptide repertoires (Lopez-Larrea et al., 2002). Two important papers showed that CD8+ cytotoxic T cells are not essential for the arthritis to develop. In these observations, May et al use monoclonal antibody to deplete CD8+ T cells from peripheral circulation, however, arthritis and colitis still develop in the HLA-B27 transgenic rat (May et al.,2003). In addition, the same conclusion was obtained by the chemical deletion of CD8a gene expression which eliminated CD8+ T cells from peripheral blood (Taurog et al, 2009). The other observation revealed that CD4+ T cells, when transferred to athymic nude rat which had high level of HLA-B27/hβ2m expression in the bone marrow, developed arthritis (Taurog et al., 1999).

3.2 Free heavy chain theory

Another models focus on the molecular stability of tri-molecular complex indicating that due to unique amino acid composition at interface between HLA-B27 and beta2-

microglobulin, the tri-molecular complex is not stable enough. Only HLA-B27 was found to be able to express as free form. Amino acid residue 9 in the floor of β pleated sheet is critical for the stability of the heavy chain/β2-microglobulin complex. All the HLA-B27 subtypes contain histidine at this site, interestingly, two other classs I molecules, HLA-B73 and HLA-B40, which had been reported in a few cases of spondyloarthropathies, were found to have histidine at amino acid residue 9 (David, 1997). Histidine at this position was claimed to weaken the non-covalent interaction between heavy chain and β2-microglobulin. The unstable structure made HLA-B27 dissociate from beta2-microglobulin and presented as free form on the cell surface. It was proposed that free HLA-B27 bound different peptides from those stable forms. Higher percentage of free heavy chain-carrying monocytes was found in the peripheral blood and synovial fluid in patients with AS compared to normal population. The level of free heavy is correlated with sedimentation rate (Tsai et al., 2002). In addition, as mentioned before, in the presence of unpaired Cys67 free heavy chains have been shown to form homodimer. Expression of heavy chain homodimer on the surface of cell lines and AS patients' peripheral blood mononuclear cells was observed. (Kollnberger et al., 2002)

This HC homodimer was found to bind to NK inhibitory receptors KIR3DL1 and KIR3DL2 and LILRA1, LILRB2 alleles on the surface of NK, T and B cells. Patients with ankylosing spondylitis have higher level of Th17 cells expressing KIR3DL2 and responsive to B27 HC homodimer (Bowness et al., 2011). This hypothesis postulates that through this interaction, NK cells, B cells and T cells were activated to induce the inflammatory reaction.

3.3 Unfolded protein response theory

In the last decade, another new theory was proposed calling "unfolded protein response". In this theory, researcher proposed that due to its unique structure, i.e.; the presence of B pocket and free form, HLA-B27 molecule is not properly folded in the endoplasmic reticulum. The accumulation of unfolded proteins in the endoplasmic reticulum induced stress reaction in the organelle and hence triggered inflammatory response. Most evidences came from animal study. Khare et al found high incidence of joint inflammation and ankylosis when HLA-B27 was transgenic into β2-microglobulin deficient mice (Khare et al., 1995). Later, investigator found a deficiency in class I molecule expression either due lack of peptides (TAP^{-}/TAP^{-}) or β2-microglobulin was able to induce spontaneous inflammatory joint disease (Kinsbury et al, 2000). In animal study, transgenic rats were found to have increased IL-23 secretion when unfolded protein response was triggered by B27 molecule in the presence of pattern recognition receptor agonist (Colbert et al., 2010). This finding reminds us that IL-23R was found to be a susceptibility gene from genome-wide scan. Another observation from genome-wide scan shows that one of the peptide-trimming peptidase: ERAP1 is associated with AS. Defect in the function of ERAP1 might delay the folding process of HLA class I molecules (Evans et al., 2011). Patients with AS were found to have high level of chaperon proteins which were related to the folding process of class I molecules in their macrophage derived from peripheral joint (Dong et al., 2002).

4. Conclusion

In conclusion, the high association of HLA-B27 with ankylosing spondylitis paved the path to the resolution of pathogenesis of this disease. Identification of this important finding might open ways to design new treatment modalities and prevent the occurrence of the disease. Evidence from both epidemiology and transgenic animal studies further widen our vision. Although none of the above theories can explain all the phenomena we observed before, newer data from genome-wide scan can further supplement the missing link.

5. References

Akkoc N, Khan MA. 2006. Epidemiology of ankylosing spondylitis and related spondyloarthropathies. In Ankylosing Spondylitis and the Spondyloarthropathies: A Companion to Rheumatology. Weisman MH, Reveille JDvan der Heijde D. pp 117-131, Mosby-Elservier London.

Albani S, Carson DA. A multistep molecular mimicry hypothesis for the pathogenesis of rheumatoid arthritis. Immunology today 1996;17(10):466-70

Allen RL, O'Callagran CA, McMichael AJ, et al. Cutting edege. HLA-B27 can form a novel beta2-microglobulin-free heavy chain homodimer structure. J Immunol 1999;162:5045-8.

Arms JB, Gonzalez S, Martinez-Borra J et al.. Susceptibility of ankylosing spondylitis is independent of the BW4 and BW6 epitopes of the HLA-B27 alleles. Tissue antigens.1999;53(3):237-43.

Atagunduz P, Appel H, Kuon W, Wu P, Thiel A, Kloetzel PM, Sieper J.

Australo-Anglo-American Spndyloarthritis consortium (TASC); Reveille, L. D. et al, Genomewide association study of ankylosing spondylitis identifies non-MHC susceptibility loci. Nat. Genet. 42,123-127(2010).

Baker SA, Weisman MH. Introduction to unifying concepts of spondyloarthropathy, including historical aspects of the disease. In:Weisman M, van der Heijde D, Reveille J, editors. Ankylosing spondylitis and the spondyloarthropathies. Philadelphia, PA: Mosby Elsevier;2006. Pp1-6.

Bjorkman PJ, Saper MA, Samraoui B, et al. Structure of the human class I histocompatibility antigen HLA-A2. Nature 1987;329:506-12

Blanco-Gelaz MA, Lopez-Vazquez A, Garcia-Fernandez S, et al. Genetic variability, molecular evolution, and geographic diversity of HLA-B27. Human Immunol 2001;62:1042-50.

Blumberg B, Bunium JJ, Calkins E, et al. ARA nomenclature and classification of arthritis and rheumatism. Arthritis Rheum 1964;7:93-7.

Bowness P, Ridley A, Shaw J, et al. Th17 cells expressing KIR3DL2+ and responsive to HLA-B27 homodimers are increased in ankylosing spondylitis. J Immunol 2011;186:2672-80.

Boyer GS, Templin DW, Bowler A, Lawrence RC, Heyse SP, Everett DF, Cornoni-Huntley JC, Goring WP. Class I HLA antigens in spondyloarthropathy: observations in Alaskan Eskimo patients and controls. J Rheumatol. 1997 Mar;24(3):500-6.

Brewerton DA, Hart FD, Nicholls A, Caffrey M, James DCO, Sturrock RD. Ankylosing spondylitis and HLA-B27. Lancet 1973:1;904-7.

Brown MA, et al. Susceptibility to ankylosing spondylitis in twins: the role of genes, HLA, and the environment. Arthritis Rheum. 1997;40:1823-28.

Brown MA. Genetics of ankylosing spondylitis. Curr Opin Rheum 2010;22:126-32.

Brown, M.A., Lavel, S. H., Brophy, S. & Calin, A. Recurrence risk modeling of the genetic susceptibility to ankylosing spondylitis. Ann. Rheum. Dis.59, 883-886(2000).

Bywaters EGL. Histological perspectives in the etiology of ankylosing spondylitis. Brit J Rheumatol 1983;22 (suppl 2):1-4.

Campbell EC, Fettke F, Bhat S, Morley KD, Powis SJ. Expression of MHC class I dimers and ERAP1 in an ankylosing spondylitis patient cohort. Immunology. 2011 Jul;133(3):379-85.

Cauli A, Vacca A, Mameli A et al. A Sardinian patient with ankylosing spondylitis and HLA-B*2709 co-occurring with HLA-B1403. Arthritis Rheum 2007:56;2807-9.

Chen IH, Yang KL, Lee A, Huang HH, Lin PY, Lee TD. Low frequency of HLA- B*2706 in Taiwanese patients with ankylosing spondylitis. Eur J Immunogenet. 2002 Oct;29(5):435-8.

Chen R, Yao L, Meng T, Xu W. The association between seven ERAP1 polymorphisms and ankylosing spondylitis susceptibility: a meta-analysis involving 8,530 cases and 12,449 controls. Rheumatol Int. 2011 Jan 13. [Epub ahead of print]

Cipriani A, Rivera S, Hassanhi M, Marquez G, Hernadez R, Villalobos C, et al. HLA-B27 subtypes determination in patients with ankylosing spondylitis from Zulia, Venezuela. Human Immunol 2003;64:745-9.

Colbert RA, Delay ML, Klenk EI et al. From HLA-B27 to spondyloarthritis: a journey through the ER. Immunol Rev 2010;233:181-202

David CS. The mystery of HLA-B27 and disease. Immunogenetics 1997;46:73-7

de Castro JA. HLA-B27-bound peptide repertoires: their nature, origin and pathogenetic relevance. Adv Exp Med Biol. 2009;649:196-209

de Vries DD, Dekker-Saeys AJ, Gyodi E, Bohm U, Ivanyi P. Absence of autoantibodies to peptides shared by HLA-B27.5 and Klebsiella pneumoniae nitrogenase in serum samples from HLA-B27 positive patients with ankylosing spondylitis and Reiter's syndrome. Ann Rheum Dis 1992;51:783-9.

Dong, W. et al. Upregulation of 78-kDa glucose-regulated protein in macrophages in peripheral joints of active ankylosing spondylitis. Scand. J. Rheunatol. 2002;29: 2159-2164.

Dror LB, Barnea E, Beer I et al. The HLA-B2705 peptidome. Arthritis Rheum 2010;62:420-9.

Evans DM, Spencer CC, Pointon JJ et al.. Interaction between ERAP1 and HLA-B27 in ankylosing spondylitis implicates peptide handling in the mechanism of HLA-B27 in disease susceptibility. Nature genet .2011;43(8):761-7.

Ewing C, Ebringer R, Tribbick G, Geysen HM. Antibody activity in ankylosing spondylitis sera to two sites on HLA B27.1 at the MHC groove region (within sequence 65-85), and to a Klebsiella pneumoniae nitrogenase reductase peptide (within sequence 181-199). J Exp Med. 1990 May 1;171(5):1635-47.

Feldtkeller E, Khan MA, van der Linden et al.. Age at disease onset and diagnosis delay in HLA-B27 negative vs positive patients with ankylosing spondylitis. Rheumatol Int 2003;23:61-66.

Fiorillo MT, Cauli A, Carcassi C, Bitti PP, Vacca A, Passiu G, Bettosini F, Mathieu A, Sorrentino R. Two distinctive HLA haplotypes harbor the B27 alleles negatively or positively associated with ankylosing spondylitis in Sardinia: implications for disease pathogenesis. Arthritis Rheum 2003;48:1385-9.

Hammer RF, Maika SD, Richardson JA, et al. Spontaneous inflammatory disease in transgenic rat expressing HLA-B27 and human β2m: an animal model of HLA-B27-associated human disorder. Cell 1990,63:1099-1112.

Hill AV, Allsopp CE, Kwiatkowski D, Anstey NM, Greenwood BM, McMichael AJ. HLA class I typing by PCR: HLA-B27 and an African B27 subtype. Lancet. 1991 Mar 16;337(8742):640-2.

HLA-B27-restricted CD8+ T cell response to cartilage-derived self peptides in ankylosing spondylitis. Arthritis Rheum. 2005 Mar;52(3):892-901

Hou TY, Chen HC, Chen CH, Chang DM, Liu FC, Lai JH. Usefulness of human leucocyte antigen-B27 subtypes in predicting ankylosing spondylitis: Taiwan experience. Intern Med J. 2007 Nov;37(11):749-52.

Hulsmeyer M, Fiorillo MT, Bettosini F et al. Dual, HLA-B27 subtype-dependent conformation of a self-peptide. J Exp Med 2004;199:271-81.

IMGT/HLA database allele search tool [Internet. Accessed July 21. 2011] Available from:http://www.ei.ac.uk/cgi-bin/imgt/hla/allele.cgi.

Invernizzi P. Human leukocyte antigen in primary biliary cirrhosis: An old story now reviving. Hepatology. 2011 May 11. [Epub ahead of print]

Jaakkola E, Herzberg I, Laiho K, Barnardo MC, Pointon JJ, Kauppi M, Kaarela K, Tuomilehto-Wolf E, Tuomilehto J, Wordsworth BP, Brown MA. Finnish HLA studies confirm the increased risk conferred by HLA-B27 homozygosity in ankylosing spondylitis. Ann Rheum Dis. 2006 Jun;65(6):775-80.

Khan MA, Kushner I, Braun WE. Comparison of clinical features in HLA-B27 positive and negative patients with ankylosing spondylitis. Arthritis Rheum 1977;20:909-912.

Khare SD, Luthra HS, David CS. Spontaneous inflammatory arthritis in HLA-B27 transgenic mice lacking β2-microglobulin: a model of human spondyloarthropathies. J Exp Med 1995;182:1153-8

Kim TJ, Na KS, Lee HJ. Lee B, Kim TH. HLA-B27 homozygosity has no influence on clinical manifestations and functional disability in ankylosing spondylitis. Clin Exp Rheumatol 2009:27:574-9.

Kinsbury DJ, Mear JP, Witte DP. Development of spontaneous arthritis in β2-microglobulin-deficient mice without expression off HLA-B27: association with deficieny of endogenous major histocompatibility complex I expression. Arthritis Rheum 2000;43:2290-6.

Kollnberger S, Bird L, Sun MY, Retiere C, Braud VM, McMichael A, et al. Cell-surface expression and immune receptor recognition of HLA-B27 homodimers. Arthritis Rheum 2002;46:2972-82.

Kuhne M, Erben U, Schulze-Tanzil G, Köhler D, Wu P, Richter FJ, John T, Radbruch A, Sieper J, Appel H. HLA-B27-restricted antigen presentation by human chondrocytes to CD8+ T cells: potential contribution to local immunopathologic processes in ankylosing spondylitis. Arthritis Rheum. 2009 Jun;60(6):1635-46

Lahesmaa R, Skurnik M, Vaara M, Leirisalo-Repo M, Nissilä M, Granfors K, Toivanen P. Molecular mimickry between HLA B27 and Yersinia, Salmonella, Shigella and Klebsiella within the same region of HLA alpha 1-helix. Clin Exp Immunol. 1991 Dec;86(3):399-404.

Layh-Schmitt, G. & Colbert, R. A. The interleukin-23/interlukin-17 axis in spondyloarthritis. Curr. Opon. Rheunatol. 20,392-397(2008).

Liu SQ, Yu HC, Gong YZ, Lai NS. Quantitative measurement of HLA-B27 mRNA in patients with ankylosing spondylitis-correlation with clinical activity. J Rheumatol 2006;33:1128-32.

Lopez-Larrea C, Mijivawa M, Gonzalez S et al. Association of ankylosing spondylitis with HLA-B1403 in a western African population. Arthritis Rheum 2002;46:2968-71.

Madden DR, Gorge JC, Strominger JL, et al. The structure of HLA-B27 reveals nonamer self-peptides bound in a extended conformation. Nature 1991;352:321-5.

Madden DR, Gorge JC, Strominger JL, et al. The three-dimentional structure of HLA-B27 at 2.1 Å resolution suggest a general mechanism for the tight peptide binding to MHC Cell 1992;70:1035-44.

Madden DR. The three-dimensional structure of peptide-MHC complexes. Ann Rev Immunol 1995;13:587-622.

May E, et al. CD8αβ T cells are not essential to the pathogenesis of arthritis or colitis in HLA-B27 transgenic rats. J Immunol 2003;170:1099-1105.

McElroy JP, Oksenberg JR. Multiple sclerosis genetics 2010. Neurol Clin. 2011 May;29(2):219-31

Natarajan K, Li H, Mariuzza RA, et al. MHC class I molecule structure and function. Rev Immunogenet 1999:1:32-46.

Paladini F, Taccari E, Fiorillo MT, Cauli A, Passiu G, Mathieu A, et al. Distribution of HLA-B27 subtypes in Sardinia and Continental Italy and their association with spondyloarthropathies. Arthritis Rheum 2005;52:3319-21.

Peschken CA, Esdaile JM. Rheumatic diseases in North America's indigenous peoples. Semin Arthritis Rheum. 1999 Jun;28(6):368-91.

Piazza A, Menozzi P, Cavalli-Sfprza LL. The HLA-A,B gene frequencies in the world: migration or selection? Hum Immunol 1980;1:297-304.

Piga M, Mathieu A. Genetic susceptibility to Behcet's disease: role of genes belonging to the MHC region. Rheumatology (Oxford). 2011 Feb;50(2):299-310.

Powis SJ, Santos SG, Antoniou AN. Biochemical features of HLA-B27 and antigen processing. Adv Exp Med Biol. 2009;649:210-6

Ren EC, Koh WH, Sim D, Boey ML, Wee GB, Chan SH. Possible protective role of HLA-B*2706 for ankylosing spondylitis. Tissue Antigens. 1997 Jan;49(1):67-9.

Reveille JD, Inman R, Khan M, et al. Family studies in ankylosing spondylitis: microsatellite analysis of 55 concordant sib pairs. J Rheumatol 2000;27:5.

Reveille JD, Maganti RM. Subtypes of HLA-B27: history and implications in the pathogenesis of ankylosing spondylitis. Adv Exp Med Biol 2009;649:159-76.

Schlosstein L, Terasaki PI, Bluestone R, Pearson CM.High association of an HL-A antigen, W27, with ankyloing spondylitis. N Engl J Med 1973:288:704-6.

Schwimmbeck PL, Oldstone MB. Molecular mimicry between human leukocyte antigen B27 and Klebsiella. Consequences for spondyloarthropathies. Am J Med. 1988 Dec 23;85(6A):51-3.

Taurog JD et al. Inflammatory disease in HLA-B27 transgenic rats. Immunol Rev 1999;169:209-223.

Taurog JD. The mystery of HLA-B27: if it isn't one thing, It's another. Arthritis Rheum 2007:56:2478-81.

Taurog JD et al. Spondyloarthritis in HLA-B27/human beta2-microglobulin-transgenic rats is not prevented by lack of CD*. Arthritis Rheum 2009;60:1977-84.

Tsai WC, Chen CJ, Yen JH et al.. Free HLA class I heavy chain-carrying monocytes - a potential role in the pathogenesis of spondyloarthropathies. J Rheumatol 2002;29:966-72.

Van der Linden SM, Valkenburg HA, de Jongh BM, Catshe risk of developing ankylosing spondylitis in HLA-B27 positive individuals: a comparison of relatives of spondylitis patients with the general population. Arthritis Rheum 1984;27:241-9.

Van der Linden S, van der Heijde D. Ankylosing spondylitis, clinical features. Rheum Dis Clin North Am 1998;24:663-76.

Varnavidou-Nicolaidou A, Karpasitou K, Georgiou D, Stylianou G, Kkkoftou A, Michalis C, et al. HLA-B27 in the Greek Cypriot population: distribution of subtypes in patients with ankylosing spondylitis and other HLA-B27-related diseases. The possible protective role of B*2707. Human Immunol 2004;65:1451-4.

Wellcome Trust Case Control Consortium; (TASC); Burton, P. R. et al. Association scan of 14,500 nonsynonymous SNPs in four diseases identifies autoimmunity variants. Nat. Genet, 39, 1329-1337(2007).

Wu Z, Lin Z, Wei Q, Gu J. Clinical features of ankylosing spondylitis may correlate with HLA-B27 polymorphism. Rheumatol Int 2009;29:389-92.

Yamaguchi A, Tsuchiya N, Mitsui H, Shiota M, Ogawa A, Tokunaga K, Yoshinoya S, Juji T, Ito K. Association of HLA-B39 with HLA-B27-negative ankylosing spondylitis and pauciarticular juvenile rheumatoid arthritis in Japanese patients. Evidence for a role of the peptide-anchoring B pocket. Arthritis Rheum 1995;38:1672-7.

Zeider H, Calin A, Amor B. A historical perspective of the spondyloarthritis. Curr Opin Rheumatol 2011;23:327-33.

Zhang L, Liu JL, Zhang YJ, Wang H. Association between HLA-B*27 polymorphisms and ankylosing spondylitis in Han populations: a meta-analysis. Clin Exp Rheumatol. 2011 Mar-Apr;29(2):285-92.

6

Humoral Immune Response to *Salmonella* Antigens and Polymorphisms in Receptors for the Fc of IgG in Patients with Ankylosing Spondylitis

Ma. de Jesús Durán-Avelar[1], Norberto Vibanco-Pérez[1], Angélica N. Rodríguez-Ocampo[1], Juan Manuel Agraz-Cibrian[1], Salvador Peña-Virgen[2] and José Francisco Zambrano-Zaragoza[1]

[1]*Unidad Académica de Ciencias Químico Biológicas y Farmacéuticas-Universidad Autónoma de Nayarit,*

[2]*Unidad de Reumatología-Instituto Mexicano del Seguro Social HGZ No. 1 Tepic, Nayarit, Mexico*

1. Introduction

Ankylosing Spondylitis (AS) is the prototype of an interrelated group of rheumatic diseases now named spondyloarthritides (SpA), otherwise known as spondyloarthropathies. Clinical features of this disease include inflammatory back pain, asymmetrical peripheral oligoarthritis, enthesitis, and specific organ involvement, such as anterior uveitis, psoriasis and chronic inflammatory bowel disease (Braun & Sieper, 2007).

AS is a chronic inflammatory disease primarily affecting the spine. Its major clinical features include sacroiliitis, loss of spinal mobility and spinal inflammation. The chronic inflammation leads to fibrosis and ossification, where bridging spurs of bone known as syndesmophytes form, especially at the edges of the inter-vertebral discs, thus producing the ankylosing (Ebringer & Wilson, 2000).

AS is a disease that affects more men than women, with a ratio of 2:1 (Feldtkeller *et al.*, 2003). The prevalence of the disease is between 0.1 and 1.4 %in general population. Studies conducted in different countries have shown that the incidence of AS is between 0.5 and 14 per 100,000 people per year (Braun & Sieper, 2007).

The diagnosis of AS is based more on clinical features than laboratory tests. Table 1 shows the criteria for diagnosing AS, according to the modified New York criteria (van der Linden et al., 1984). Further, in 1990, Amor and colleagues proposed the first set of classification criteria for the entire group of spondyloarthritis, allowing a patient to be classified as having spondyloarthritis whatever the presenting symptoms (Amor *et al.*, 1990). A different set of criteria for the entire group of spondyloarthritis was developed by the European Spondyloarhropathy Study Group (Dougados *et al.*, 1991), with inflammatory back pain and peripheral arthritis as major entry criteria. Recognition of the drawbacks of criteria focused on a specific subtype, the Assessment of Spondyloarthritis International Society did a large cross-sectional study to propose new criteria on the basis of the two main clinical features identified in daily practice—eg, axial symptoms and peripheral involvement (Dougados & Baeten, 2011).

Clinical criteria	
-	Lower back pain and stiffness for longer than 3 months, which improve with exercise but are not relieved by rest
-	Restriction of the movement of the lumbar spine in both the sagital and frontal planes
-	Restriction of chest expansion relative to normal values correlated with age and sex
Radiological criterion	
-	Sacroiliitis grade ≥2 bilaterally, or grade 3-4 unilaterally
Definite ankylosing spondylitis is present if the radiological criterion is associated with at least one clinical criterion	

Table 1. Modified New York criteria, 1984, for ankylosing spondylitis (Braun & Sieper, 2007).

Sacroiliitis on imaging* plus one or more features of spondyloarthritis†
Or
HLA-B27 plus two or more other features of spondyloarthritis†
*Active (acute) inflammation on MRI highly suggestive of sacroiliitis associated with spondyloarthritis or definite radiographic sacroiliitis according to modified New York criteria.
†Inflammatory back pain, arthritis, enthesitis (heel), uveitis, dactylitis, psoriasis, Crohn's disease or ulcerative colitis, good response to non-steroidal anti-inflammatory drugs, family history for spondyloarthritis, HLA-B27, or elevated C-reactive protein (a spondyloarthritis feature in the context of chronic back pain).

Table 2. Assessment of Spondyloarthritis International Society (ASAS) classification criteria for axial spondyloarthritis in patients with back pain for 3 months or more and age at onset younger than 45 years (Dougados & Baeten, 2011).

Although AS is of unknown aetiology, it is considered an autoimmune disease in which environmental and genetic factors are involved. There is a strong association with HLA-B27, as approximately 95% of AS patients are positive for this antigen. However, this association does not explain the cause of the disease. It has been reported that the risk of developing AS is about 5% for HLA-B27-positive subjects, but substantially higher for HLA-B27-positive relatives. However, most HLA-B27-positive individuals remain healthy. The HLA-B27 subtypes most clearly associated with AS are HLA-B*2705 B*2702, B*2704 and B*2707. The HLA-B*2706 and B*2709 subtypes do not appear to be associated with AS (Reveille & Arnett, 2005).

In addition, evidence of the importance of HLA-B27-bacteria interaction comes from work in animals, where HLA-B27-transgenic rats developed SpA-like features, but many transgene copies are needed to transfer the disease. Environmental factors also play a role, since HLA-B27-transgenic rats bred in a germ-free environment do not develop the disease, though gut flora contribute to the development of colitis (Braun & Sieper, 2007).

On the other hand, about 10-20% of HLA-B27-positive patients with reactive arthritis develop AS after 10-20 years. A possible central role of bacteria in the pathogenesis of SpA is further supported by the relation between Crohn's disease, HLA-B27 positivity, and ankylosing spondylitis, as 54% of HLA-B27-positive patients with Crohn's disease develop AS, but only 2.6% of HLA-B27-negative patients develop this disease. Leakage of the gut mucosa, as a result of the inflammation caused by colitis such as that found in Crohn's disease, leads to an interaction of the immune system with gut bacteria. In about 50% of patients with AS, chronic macroscopic or microscopic mucosal lesions resembling Crohn's disease have been detected in the gut mucosa (Braun & Sieper, 2007).

In this study, we provide support for the hypothesis of the interaction between an environmental factor (a bacterial antigen) and a genetic factor (a receptor for the Fc fragment of IgG).

2. Environmental factors involved in the pathogenesis of ankylosing spondylitis

It has been postulated that infectious agents play a crucial role as triggering factors for some autoimmune diseases, such as rheumatoid arthritis and ankylosing spondylitis. However, the mechanisms by which these microbial antigens become involved in the aetiopathogenesis of the disease remain unknown, though abundant data suggest this possibility.

Humoral immune responses against bacteria such as *Klebsiella pneumoniae, Salmonella typhimurium, Shigella flexneri, Yersinia enterocolitica* and *Campylobacter jejuni* have been analyzed in patients with SpA, and it has been suggested that some microbial agents have a role in the disease.

Klebsiella pneumoniae has been considered the main microbial agent implicated as a triggering factor for the aetiopathogenesis of AS (Rashid & Ebringer, 2007). It has been reported that IgA antibodies to *Klebsiella pneumoniae* are significantly elevated in AS patients compared to healthy subjects (Blankenberg-Sprenkels *et al.*, 1998; Tani *et al.*, 1997). Moreover, an association between the heat shock protein (HSP) of 60 kDa from *Klebsiella pneumoniae* and AS has been evidenced because of the significantly higher levels of IgG antibodies in proportion to this protein observed in AS patients compared to control groups (Cancino-Diaz *et al.*, 1998; Parra-Campos *et al.*, 1996), while the cellular immune response, measured as lymphoproliferation (LP) against this protein, has also been reported (Dominguez-Lopez *et al.*, 2000).

Other HSPs have been associated with HLA-B27-positive subjects, because of the higher levels of IgG antibodies observed, compared to HLA-B27-negative subjects, in particular HSP60 from *Klebsiella pneumoniae* and *Salmonella typhi* (Dominguez-Lopez *et al.*, 2002).

The antibody response against the lipopolisaccharide (LPS) of *Klebsiella pneumoniae, Escherichia coli, Salmonella typhimurium* and *Salmonella enteritidis* has been evaluated by

ELISA, indicating that only the LPS from *Klebsiella pneumonaiae* and *Escherichia coli* are associated with AS, on account of the higher levels of IgG and IgA antibodies observed (Ahmadi *et al.*, 1998).

The association of *Salmonela spp.* with AS is supported by the presence of DNA from *Salmonella sp.* in the synovial fluid of patients with SpA (Pacheco-Tena *et al.*, 2001). On the other hand, the behaviour of *Salmonella typhimurium* is modified by the presence of HLA-B27 in transfected cells, because of the increased production of IL-6, IL-8 and IL-10 and the lower production of TNFα (Ekman *et al.*, 2002; Saarinen *et al.*, 2002).

In our laboratory, we have previously found that 71.4% of patients with AS and 14.3% of healthy subjects recognized a 30 kDa band (p30) from of *S. typhimurium* ($p<0.001$) by using anti-human IgG in a western-blot analysis. Moreover, the levels of IgA and IgG against a crude extract of *S. typhimurium* were significantly higher in AS patients than in healthy subjects, though no differences in IgM levels were found. When the antibody levels against electroeluted p30 were analyzed, we found that IgG and IgA against p30 were statistically higher in AS patients than in healthy subjects; however, as in the case of the response to the crude extract of *S. typhimurium*, the absorbance obtained in IgM to this antigen showed no significant differences between groups (Zambrano-Zaragoza *et al.*, 2009).

In the sera from AS patients and controls, all four IgG subclasses were found to be involved in the recognition of the p30 from *S. typhimurium*, but the frequency of IgG3 antibodies to p30 was statistically different in AS patients compared to healthy subjects (Zambrano-Zaragoza *et al.*, 2009).

These results showed that a 30 kDa band from *S. typhimurium* is recognized by the IgG antibodies of most AS patients, compared to healthy subjects, and suggest an association between a particular antigen of *S. typhimurium* (p30) and the disease.

An association of *S. typhimurium* with AS has been reported previously (Brown & Wordsworth, 1997; Leirisalo-Repo *et al.*, 2003), but no specific antigen of this bacterium has been reported until now. Nevertheless, in association with other bacterial antigens, certain proteins have been reported to be implicated as triggers of AS (Lahesmaa *et al.*, 1991). Thus, we have reported that the 30 kDa band from *S. typhimurium* could be differentially recognized by the immune response in AS patients, and hence be involved in the immunopathogenesis of AS (Zambrano-Zaragoza *et al.*, 2009). These findings led us to ask whether antigens from *S. enteritidis* are recognized in the same way by patients with AS, or if this response is specific for *S. typhimurium.*

The interaction between HLA-B27 and *S. enteritidis* has been reported by using mouse fibroblasts transfected with HLA-B27, HLA-B7, or beta2-microglobulin only. Although *S. enteritidis* invaded all three of these transfected cells with the same efficiency, more living intracellular *Salmonella* organisms were found in the HLA-B27 transfectants than in the other transfected cell lines, suggesting that the bactericidal effect is impaired in these cells. Moreover, impaired NO production in HLA-B27-transfected cells was indicated as a possible mechanism (Virtala *et al.*, 1997).

Another study, one using transfected human monocytic U937 cell lines, demonstrated that the expression of the HLA-B27 antigen does not influence the uptake of *S. enteritidis* into U937 cells in vitro. It is interesting to note that HLA-B27 markedly impaired the elimination of *S. enteritidis* in the HLA-B27-transfected U937 cells (Laitio *et al.*, 1997).

Considering that *Salmonella typhimurium* is in fact *Salmonella enterica* serovar *typhimurium*, we asked if the antigen recognized by patients with AS (p30) is an antigen specific to *Salmonella typhimurium*, or if it can be found in another serovar of *Salmonella enterica*.

To answer this question, a group of 28 patients with AS treated with non-steroidal anti-inflammatory drugs and sulfazalasine, but without receiving tumour necrosis alpha blockers, and 28 non-AS-related healthy subjects were included to analyze the IgG and IgA humoral immune response against *Salmonella enterica* serovar *enteritidis* (*S. enteritidis)* by western-blot, using similar conditions, and protocols previously reported by us (Zambrano-Zaragoza *et al.*, 2009).

Our results show that 14/28 AS patients recognized a band with a relative molecular mass of 10 kDa (p10) from *S. enteritidis* with IgG antibodies, but that none of the subjects in the healthy group did ($p<0.001$, Figure 1). However, no differences in the recognition of *S. enteritidis* antigens were found when IgA antibodies were detected (Figure 2); suggesting that the antigenic behaviour of *S. enteritidis* and *S. typhimurium* are different, and only some antigens from each serovar could be important for the etiopathogenesis of AS. Additionally, it appear that only IgG antibodies anti- *S. enteritidis* could be important in the association with AS. These results are in agreement with Ahmadi et al, who did not find differences in the antibody levels against *S. enteritidis* in patients with AS (Ahmadi *et al.*, 1998).

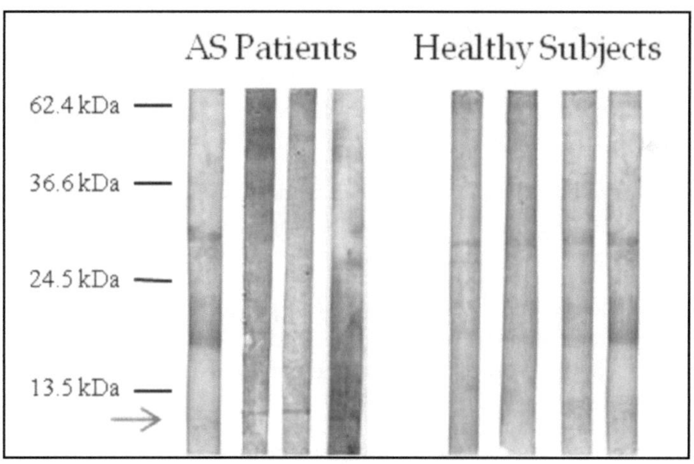

Fig. 1. Representative Western-blot strips showing antigens of *S. enteritidis* recognized by IgG antibodies in AS patients and healthy subjects. The bars on the left indicate the molecular masses of standard markers (kDa); the arrow indicates the recognized 10 kDa band.

In spite of the controversial role of bacterial antigens in the etiopathogenesis of AS, specifically the Gram negative bacterial antigens, we found a second candidate to be associated with AS, the p10 that could be a relevant antigen for patients with AS. Moreover, we also found that the humoral immune response to *S. typhimurium* is different to those for *S. enteritidis*, the antigens recognized and the antibody isotypes produced against those bacteria are different, because neither the 30 kDa band from *S. enteritidis* nor the 10 kDa band from *S. typhimurium* were recognized.

Considering that western blot is not a quantitative test, as it shows only the frequencies of recognition of some antigens, so a quantitative test must be used to determine the possible association of this antigen (p10) with AS.

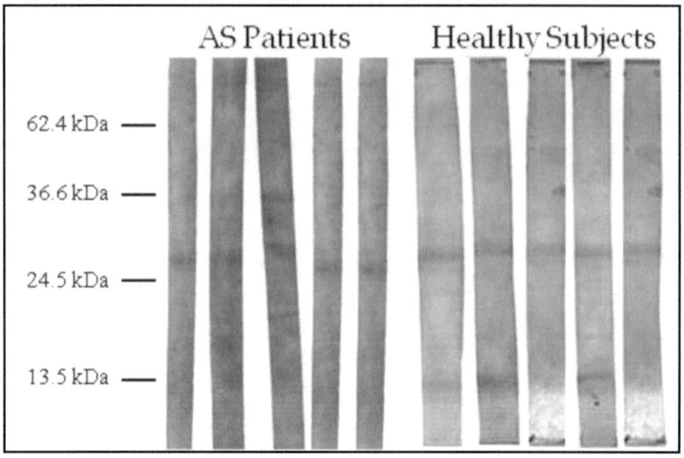

Fig. 2. Representative Western-blot strips showing antigens from *S. enteritidis* recognized by IgA antibodies in AS patients and healthy subjects. The bars on the left indicate the molecular masses of standard markers (kDa).

To do this, we analyzed the IgG and IgA antibody levels against either a crude extract or the electroeluted 10 kDa band (p10) from *S. enteritidis* using ELISA, as we have done for *S. typhymurium* (Zambrano-Zaragoza *et al.*, 2009).

We did not find any statistically significant differences in the antibody levels against either the crude extract or p10 (Figures 3 and 4), indicating that neither the total antigens nor the p10 of *S. enteritidis* are associated with AS.

Although different bacteria have been associated as possible triggers of AS, in this study we argue that the antigenic differences present in related bacteria, such as *S. typhimurium* and *S. enteritidis*, could be differentiated by the immune response of patients with AS, and thus be involved in the aetiopathogenesis of the disease.

These results indicate that not all species of *Salmonella* are associated with the disease. As has been reported, the HSP60 of *S. typhi* (Dominguez-Lopez *et al.*, 2009), and *S. typhimurium*, in particular, the p30 (Zambrano-Zaragoza *et al.*, 2009), are indeed associated with the illness. However, the relationship between the antibody levels observed and the mechanisms involved in the pathogenesis of AS has not yet been elucidated.

Considering that the differences in the IgG immune response observed could be due to a IgG subclass, we explored the IgG subclass that recognizes the p30 of *S. typhimurium* and found that patients with AS produce more IgG3 than healthy subjects (Zambrano-Zaragoza *et al.*, 2009), which suggests that the humoral immune response and, in particular, the IgG3 antibody levels, could play a role in the pathogenesis of AS.

IgG subclasses have been shown to be involved in autoimmunity, because of differences in the expression of Fc gamma receptors that explain the clearance of immune complexes from the body, and its role in the inflammatory response observed. We found that in both patients and controls recognition of the p30 of *S. typhimurium* by serum antibodies was due to all of the IgG subclasses, but that the frequency and levels of IgG3 antibodies against p30 were higher in the AS group.

These results suggest that in the humoral immune response against a microbial antigen (p30) in a susceptible individual, the IgG3 antibodies produced against this protein could be involved in the pathogenesis of AS, and that the relationship between the humoral immune response observed and the inflammatory process could be explained by differences in the expression of specific polymorphisms of receptors for the Fc of IgG. However, this suggestion must be explored much more thoroughly. In this case, the p30 antigen could cross-react with a putative auto-antigen, and the resulting antibody response could be responsible for maintaining the inflammatory process, probably through the receptors for the Fc of IgG.

Host genetics are better understood in AS compared to other types of SpAs. The strong link between AS and HLA-B27 has been known for years; the HLA-B27 is the major risk factor associated with AS, this molecule is present in many genetically diverse population, however other genes than HLA-B27 have been analyzed and associate with AS, such as endoplasmic reticulum endopeptidase I (ERAP1), interleukin 23 receptor (IL23R), and tumour necrosis factor receptor 1 (TNFR1) (Dougados & Baeten, 2011). Perhaps the definitive missing link lies in the recently discovered genetic contributions of AS and how these genes might co-localise with HLA-B27 in the presence of certain stool microflora (Carter, 2010).

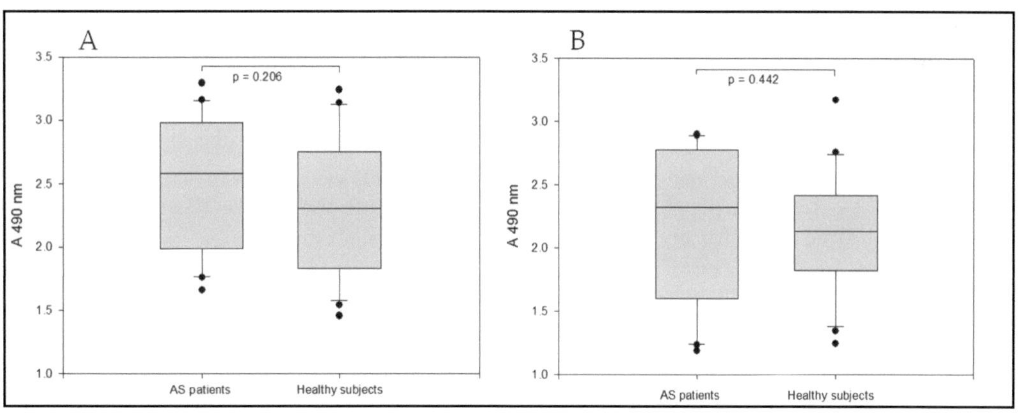

Fig. 3. Antibody levels against a crude extract of *S. enteritidis* in AS patients and healthy subjects. Levels of IgG (panel A) and IgA (panel B). The graph shows the median A490nm value for each group and the percentile at 25 and 75%. Non-statistically significant differences were found in both studies.

3. Receptors for the Fc of IgG

Specific receptors for most immunoglobulin isotypes have been described. IgG represents the dominant antibody in plasma, while the receptors for the Fc of IgG (FcγR) play important roles in the initiation and regulation of many immunological and inflammatory processes, thus providing a crucial link between humoral and cellular immune responses. Ligation of these receptors triggers a variety of signals to develop effectors of the immune response, such as macrophage phagocytosis, antibody dependent cellular cytotoxicity (ADCC), neutrophil activation, cytokine release, degranulation and the inhibition of B cell activation (Dijstelbloem *et al.*, 2001; Ravetch & Bolland, 2001; van der Pol & van de Winkel, 1998).

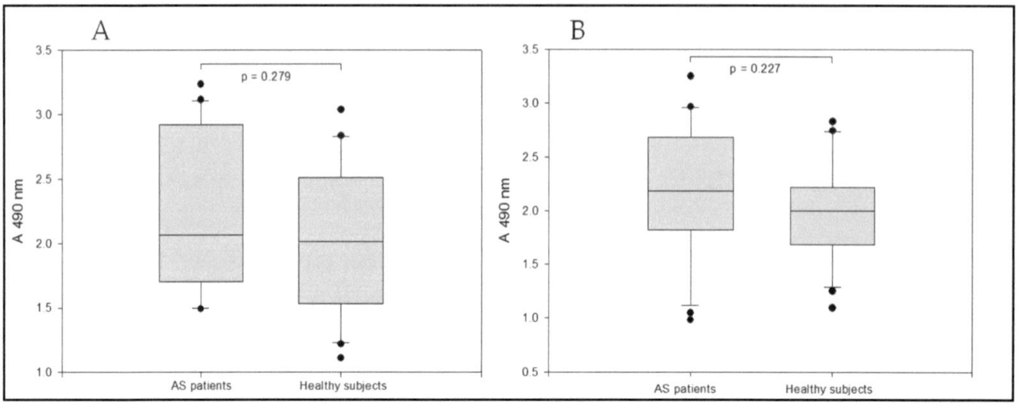

Fig. 4. Antibody levels against the p10 of *S. enteritidis* in AS patients and healthy subjects. Levels of IgG (panel A) and IgA (panel B). Antibodies determined by ELISA, assayed with 0.3 μg of antigen/well, and sera diluted to 1/400 in triplicate. The graph shows the median A490nm value for each group and the percentile at 25 and 75%. Non-statistically significant differences were found in both studies.

Three classes of FcγR have been reported on the surface of immune system cells FcγRI (CD64) that can bind to monomeric IgG, FcγRII (CD32) and FcγRIII (CD16), which then bind to immune-complexes.

These receptors can be divided into two types: activating (FcγRI, FcγRIIa and FcγRIIIa), characterized by the presence of an immunoreceptor tyrosine-based activation motif (ITAM) in the cytoplasmic domain; and inhibiting (FcγRIIb), which contain an immunoreceptor tyrosine-based inhibition motif (ITIM) in their cytoplasmic domain (Dijstelbloem *et al.*, 2001).

Most cell types express both activating and inhibitory receptors. Therefore the cellular response depends on the relative expression of activating and inhibitory receptors. This ratio is also influenced by the cytokine environment (Cohen-Solal *et al.*, 2004). Moreover, the presence of allelic variants, with different affinities for selective the antibody isotypes support their role in the regulation of the inflammatory process due to the humoral immune response.

Three polymorphisms in the FcγR genes that affect the IgG binding affinities have been described: first, a G>A point mutation in FcγRIIa (rs1801274) that causes an H-131-R substitution; second, a T>G SNP at nucleotide 559 (rs396991) in FcγRIIIa that results in a V-158-F substitution; and, third, two combinations of five nucleotides (141, 147, 227, 277 and 349) in the exon 3 of IIIb that encode two isophorms, called FcγRIIIb-NA1 and FcγRIIIb-NA2 (Willcocks *et al.*, 2009).

These haplotypes have distinct affinities for the different IgG subclasses. In this context, FcγRIIa-131H has a higher affinity for human IgG3 than FcγRIIa-131R. FcγRIIIa-158V has a higher affinity for IgG1 and IgG3 than FcγRIIIa-158-F, and FcγRIIIb-NA1 internalizes human IgG1- or IgG3-opsonized particles more efficiently than FcγRIIIb-NA2 (Dijstelbloem *et al.*, 2001).

Interest in the FcγR in the context of autoimmunity is rooted in mechanisms of immune complex handling (Salmon & Pricop, 2001), although these molecules participate in a much broader range of cell functions. In the case of rheumatic diseases such as AS, the antibody immune response has been described in several studies. However, the link between these antibodies and the pathogenesis of the diseases is still unclear.

The FcγR offer a link between the humoral and inflammatory responses because of their differences in affinity for the different IgG subclasses and cellular distribution. Hence, the hypothesis is that if AS patients develop an immune response against bacterial antigens that depends predominantly on IgG3 antibodies, as we have reported previously (Zambrano-Zaragoza *et al.*, 2009), then these antibodies will bind to a haplotype of FcγR to promote inflammation.

3.1.1 Polymorphisms in FcγR and autoimmunity

FcγR have been implicated in the pathogenesis of autoimmunity in different ways: 1) by maintaining the level of self-tolerance and increasing the activation threshold of autoreactive B cells; 2) by facilitating the elimination of some autoreactive B cells during development; 3) FcγR ligation can affect dendritic cell maturation; and, 4) FcγR are critical for the elimination of circulating IgG immune complexes (Willcocks *et al.*, 2009).

On the other hand, an allelic variant of FcγR has been reported to be present in normal populations, but without exercising any impact on the normal functions of the immune system. However, some isophorms present in certain environmental and genetic contexts can contribute to the development of autoimmune diseases.

Genetic variants of FcγR have been associated with different autoimmune and infectious diseases. Evidence supporting the role of the heterogeneity of FcγR in Systemic Lupus Erythematosus (SLE) has been controversial. SLE is the prototype of immune-complex-mediated autoimmune diseases and several studies on associations with FcγRIIa and FcγRIIIb have been published (Hong *et al.*, 2005; Michel *et al.*, 2000; Ni *et al.*, 2000).

In cases of myasthenia gravis, patients have been found to have a higher frequency of the FcγRIIIb-NA1 allele than FcγRIIb-NA2, compared to a control group (Raknes *et al.*, 1998).

In other autoimmune diseases, such as Wegener's granulomatosis, it has been reported that either FcγRIIa-131-RH or FcγRIIIa-158-VF represent an inheritable risk factor for the development of the disease (Dijstelbloem *et al.*, 1999), while other authors have reported an association with FcγRIIIb-NA1 (van der Pol & van de Winkel, 1998).

In the case of rheumatic autoimmune diseases, it has been reported that FcγRIIIa-158VV is overrepresented in RA patients, FcγRIIIa-158VF was higher in healthy controls, and FcγRIIIa-158-FF is equally distributed in both populations. However, no association between FcγRRIIIa-158-VV and clinical parameters was found (Nieto *et al.*, 2000).

3.1.2 Polymorphisms in FcγR in ankylosing spondylitis

Considering our previous findings, in which the humoral immune response against *S. typhimurium* was directed principally against p30, and the IgG subclass involved was mainly IgG3, we hypothesized that the relationship between the humoral response observed and the pathogenesis of the disease could be due (at least in part) to FcγR polymorphisms, because of the differences in IgG subclass affinity reported.

To test this hypothesis, the genotypification of FcγRIIa, FcγRIIIa and FcγRIIIb was carried out in a small cohort of 35 patients with AS and 120 non-AS-related individuals using the primers reported (Table 3) in a PCR protocol.

Receptor	Name	Sequence	Ref
FcγRIIa	EC2-131R	5'-CCA GAA TGG AAA ATC CCA GAA ATT CTC TCG-3'	(Raknes *et al.*, 1998)
	EC2-131H	5'-CCA GAA TGG AAA ATC CCA GAA ATT CTC TCA-3'	
	TM1	5'-CCA TTG GTG AAG AGC TGC CCA TGC TGG GCA-3'	
FcγRIIIa	KIM-G(V)	5'-TCT CTG AAG ACA CAT TTC TAC TCC CTA C-3'	(Van Den Berg *et al.*, 2001)
	KIM-1(F)	5'-TCT CTG AAG ACA CAT TTC TAC TCC CTA A-3'	
	A013	5'-ATA TTT ACA GAA TGG CAC AGG-3'	
FcγRIIIb	NA1	5'-CAG TGG TTT CAC AAT GTG AA-3'	(Raknes *et al.*, 1998)
	NA2	5'-CAA TGG TAC AGC GTG CTT-3'	
	NA-REV	5'-ATG GAC TTC TAG CTG CAC-3'	

Table 3. PCR primers used for genotypification of FcγR.

As internal controls, primers to either an amplified 270 bp from the TCR Vα22 (Ctrl-1 and Ctrl-2) gene, or a 439 bp fragment of the human growth hormone gene (HGH-1 and HGH-2) were used (Table 4).

Name	Sequence	Ref
HGH-1	5′-CAG TGC CTT CCC AAC CAT TCC CTT A-3′	(Raknes *et al.*, 1998)
HGH-2	5′-ATC CAC TCA CGG ATT TCT GTT GTG TTT C-3′	
Ctrl-1	5'-GAT TCA GTG ACC CAG ATG GAA GGG-3'	
Ctrl-2	5'-AGC ACA GAA GTA CAC CGC TGA GTC-3'	

Table 4. PCR primers used as internal controls.

All participants were informed as to the nature of the study and written consent was obtained in accordance with the Helsinki Declaration. Blood samples were taken by venipuncture. The study design was previously approved by the local Ethics Committee.

Genomic DNA from each individual tested was extracted from whole peripheral blood using the easy DNA kit (Invitrogen). The FcγRIIa genotypes were determined using the amplification refractory mutation system-PCR (Raknes *et al.*, 1998). For each sample, two independent PCR reactions were carried out. PCRs were performed by adding 100 ng of genomic DNA, 200 μM of each dNTPs, 3 mM $MgCl_2$, 20 ng of each control primer (Ctrl-1 and Ctrl-2), 200 ng of EC2-131-R or EC2-131-H primer and their respective reaction, and 2.0 U of *Taq* polymerase (Invitrogen) to a 50 μL solution containing PCR buffer 1X (Invitrogen). PCR conditions were as follows: Denaturation for 5 min at 94°C, 45 cycles of 94°C for 45 seconds, 63°C for 30 seconds and 72°C for 90 seconds; and a final extension step at 72°C for 10 min. A 980 bp fragment was observed in 2% agarose gels together with the 270 bp fragment of the internal control (TCR vα22 gene). Figure 5 shows a typical reaction.

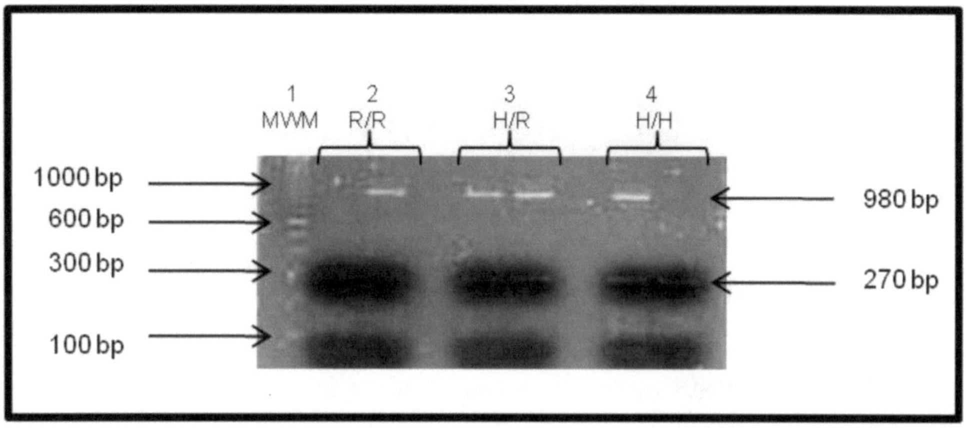

Fig. 5. A representative agarose gel (2%) of PCR products obtained from the amplification of FcγRIIa, showing the different genotypes: 1) molecular weight markers; 2) a homozygotic FcγRIIa-131RR subject; 3) a heterozygotic FcγRIIa-131HR subject; and, 4) a homozygotic FcγRIIa-131HH subject. In all cases, the 980 bp band corresponds to the fragment of FcγRIIa, and the 270 bp to the internal control.

In order to determine the FcγRIIIa genotypes, two reactions were carried out for each sample, according to the method described by Van Der Berg et al., (Van Den Berg *et al.*, 2001). PCRs were performed by adding, 100 ng of genomic DNA, 200 μM of each dNTPs, 6 mM $MgCl_2$, 20 ng of each control primer (Ctrl-1 and Ctrl-2), 200 ng of KIM-G(V) or KIM1(F) primer in their respective reaction, and 2.0 U of *Taq* polymerase (Invitrogen) to a 50 μL solution containing PCR buffer 1X (Invitrogen). PCR conditions were as follows: Denaturation for 10 min at 95°C, 37 cycles of 95°C for 30 seconds, 57°C for 20 seconds and 72°C for 25 seconds; and a final extension step at 72°C for 7 min. A 160 bp fragment was detected for the FcγRIIIa and a 270 bp fragment for the internal control used. In Figure 6 the different patterns obtained are shown.

The FcγRIIIb genotyping was done in one single reaction to amplify the 141 bp (NA1) and/or 219 bp (NA2) fragments of the receptor, and the 480 bp of the internal control (HGH, Figure 7). PCRs were performed by adding, 100 ng of genomic DNA, and 200 ng of each primer (NA1, NA2, and HGHC) to a 25 μL solution containing 1 bead of pure-taq ready to go PCR (GE healthcare). PCR conditions were: PCR conditions were as follows: Denaturation for 3 min at 94°C, 30 cycles of 94°C for 1 min, 57°C for 2 min and 72°C for 1 min; and a final extension step at 72°C for 10 min.

Genotypes and allele frequencies were obtained by direct count. Differences in genotypes and allele frequencies between patients and controls were compared using the Chi square test. Odds ratios (OR) with 95% confidence intervals (95% CI) were calculated to estimate the effect of different alleles. All analyses were carried out using the OpenEpi v 2.0 software, with $p \leq 0.05$ set as the level of statistical significance, and results are shown in Table 5.

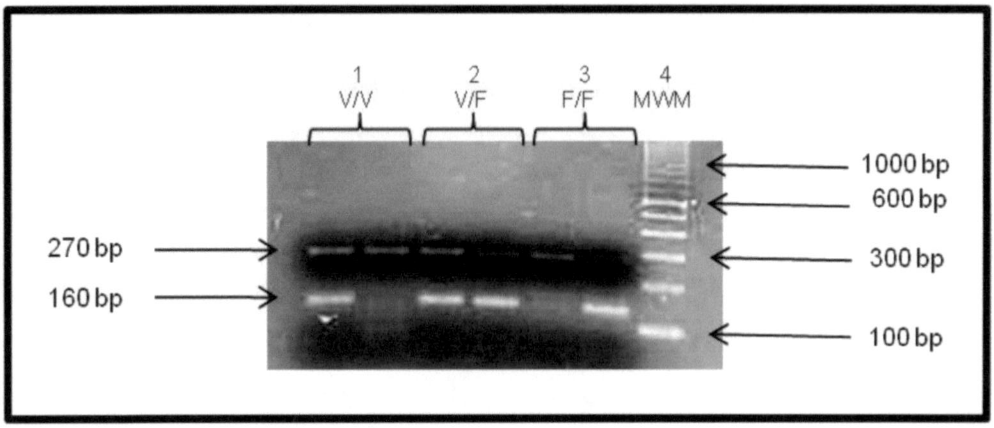

Fig. 6. A representative agarose gel (2%) of PCR products obtained from the amplification of FcγRIIIa, showing the different genotypes for: 1) a homozygotic FcγRIIIa-158VV subject; 2) a heterozygotic FcγRIIIa-158VF subject; 3) a homozygotic FcγRIIIa-158FF subject; and, 4) molecular weight markers. In all cases, the 160 bp band corresponds to the fragment of FcγRIIIa, and the 270 bp to the internal control.

For FcγRIIa polymorphisms, our results show that 16/35 patients and 29/120 healthy subjects were homozygotic 131-HH (OR = 2.642; IC= 1.205-5.796; p= 0.013); eight out of 35 patients and 42/120 healthy subjects were homozygotic 131-RR (OR=0.5503; IC=0.230-1.318; p=0.1765); and 11/35 patients and 49/120 healthy subjects were heterozygotic 131-HR (OR=0.664; IC=0.298-1.480; p= 0.3170). These results suggest that the homozygotic 131-HH of FcγRIIa allele could be associated with AS. Moreover, the frequency of allele H was significantly higher in AS patients compared to healthy controls (OR= 1.980; 95%CI= 1.149-3.412, p= 0.0138).

For FcγRIIIa, 7/35 AS patients and 5/120 healthy subjects had the 158-VV genotype (OR= 5.75; IC= 1.698-19.47; p= 0.002); 14/35 AS patients and 51/120 healthy subjects showed the 158-FF genotype (OR= 0.902; IC= 0.419-1.942; p=0.792); and 14/35 and 64/120 showed the 158-VF genotype (OR= 0.737; IC = 0.364-1.569; p= 0.0427). Our results suggest that the homocygotic 158-V of FcγRIIIa could be associated with AS.

In the case of FcγRIIIb, we found that 9 out of 35 AS patients and 16/120 healthy subjects had NA1/NA1 genotype (OR=2.25; IC=0.894-5.662; p= 0.080); 15/35 AS patients and 64/120 healthy subjects had the NA2/NA2 genotype (OR=0.656; IC=0.307-1.402; p= 0.275); and 11/35 AS patients and 40/120 healthy subjects were NA1/NA2 (OR= 0.917; IC=0.408-2.057; p=0.833). No significant association was found between the NA1 and NA2 haplotypes of FcγRIIIb and AS.

In spite of the statistical differences among groups, it is important to emphasize that the study population is small and, therefore, the results must be taken as only indicative of the possible role of these polymorphisms in the pathogenesis of AS; they are by no means conclusive.

FcγRIIa which is expressed in most immune cells has two allelic variants with different affinities for IgG subclasses. The mutation is G519A that results in an amino acid

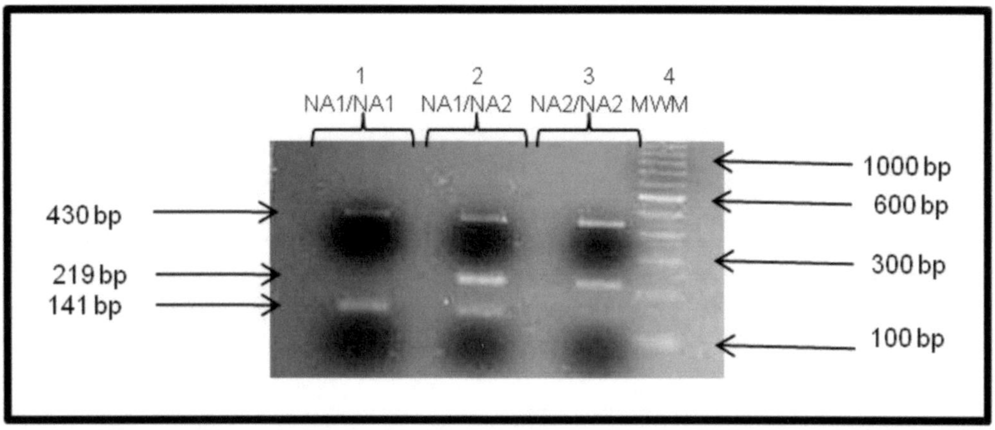

Fig. 7. A representative agarose gel (2%) of PCR products obtained from the amplification of FcγRIIIa, showing the different genotypes: 1) a homozygotic FcγRIIIb-NA1 subject; 2) a heterozygotic FcγRIIIb-NA1/NA2 subject; 3) a homozygotic FcγRIIIb-NA2 subject; and, 4) molecular weight markers. In all cases, the 141 and 219 bp bands correspond to the NA1 and NA2 amplification products, respectively, while the 439 bp indicates the internal control.

substitution at position 131. The 131-H variant has higher affinity for IgG3 than 131R. FcγRIIIa, which is expressed on mononuclear phagocytes and natural killer cells, also has two co-dominantly expressed alleles, which differ at amino acid position 158 in the extracellular domain (valine or phenylalanine, respectively). FcγRIIIa allelic variants differ in IgG1 and IgG3 binding; VV homozygotes bind to IgG1 and IgG3 more avidly than do FF homozygotes, and here we report that AS patients show mostly the VV genotype, compared to the control group (Dijstelbloem *et al.*, 2001).

As we have reported, all IgG subclasses anti-p30 are produced by AS patients, with higher levels compared to healthy controls (Zambrano-Zaragoza *et al.*, 2009). These data altogether with those of FcγR polymorphisms suggest that IgG3 could be important in maintenance of the inflammatory process observed in AS, because of the presence of the allelic variants FcγRIIa-131-HH and FcγRIIIa-158-VV in the group of AS patients, and then could contribute to the pathogenesis of the disease. Additionally IgG2 anti-p30, that is also produced by AS patients (Zambrano-Zaragoza *et al.*, 2009), could have a synergic action with IgG3 in the FcγRIIa, because the higher affinity of the 131-HH allelic variant for IgG2.

It has been reported that mononuclear cells infiltrate the cartilaginous structures of sacroiliac joints and inter-vertebral discs, leading to destruction and ankylosis (Braun & Sieper, 2007). Thus, inflammation and the cellular immune response could be modulated through the FcγR. Therefore, we propose that one link between the humoral immune response against an environmental antigen such as p30 and AS could be through the FcγR and, more specifically, the 131-HH genotype of FcγRIIa, and the 158-VV genotype of FcγRIIIa, which is involved in inflammation mediated by immune complexes.

There is convincing evidence that imbalanced immune responses are responsible for autoimmune diseases such as arthritis, multiple sclerosis, and systemic lupus erythematosus (SLE). It is also widely accepted that many factors, including genetic and environmental components, are involved in the initiation and severity of autoimmune symptoms. Thus,

Polymorphisms	AS (n=35)	Controls (n=120)	p	OR	95% CI
FcγRIIa					
- Genotype					
HH	16 (45.7%)	29 (24.2%)	0.01347	2.642	1.205-5.796
RR	8 (22.9%)	42 (35%)	0.176	0.550	0.223-1.318
HR	11 (31.4%)	49 (40.8%)	0.317	0.664	0.298-1.480
- Allele					
H	43 (61.4%)	107(44.6%)	0.0138	1.980	1.149-3.412
R	27 (38.6%)	133 (55.4%)			
FcγRIIIa					
- Genotype					
VV	7(20%)	5 (4.2%)	0.002	5.75	1.698-19.47
FF	14(40%)	51 (42.5%)	0.792	0.902	0.419-1.942
VF	14 (40%)	64 (53.3%)	0.427	0.737	0.364-1.569
- Allele					
V	28(40%)	74 (30.8%)	0.151	1.495	0.862-2.595
F	42 (60%)	166 69.2%)			
FcγRIIIb					
- Genotype					
NA1/NA1	9 (25.7%)	16 (13.33%)	0.080	2.25	0.894-5.662
NA2/NA2	15 (42.9%)	64 (53.33%)	0.275	0.656	0.307-1.402
NA1/NA2	11 (31.4%)	40 (33.33%)	0.833	0.917	0.408-2.057
- Allele					
NA1	29 (41.4%)	72(30%)	0.073	1.650	0.952-2.860
NA2	41 (58.6%)	168 (70%)			

Table 5. Genotype and allele frequencies of FcγRIIa, FcγRIIIa and FcγRIIIb polymorphisms in patients with AS and controls.

identifying these components could prove helpful in gaining further insight into these diseases and developing novel immunotherapeutic strategies to interfere with chronic inflammation.

On the basis of these findings, we proposed a hypothetical model of interaction between two factors: one environmental, the other genetic (Figure 8). In this model, the immune response against *S. typhimurium* in a susceptible subject leads to the recognition of p30 and the production of IgG3 antibodies. p30 should cross-react with a putative auto-antigen, such that the humoral immune response is maintained by this putative auto-antigen, and it is responsible of the maintenance of the antibody levels.

Then, in the susceptible subject, the FcγRIIa-131-HH and FcγRIIIa-158-VV polymorphism, which have a higher affinity for IgG3, promote and maintain (at least in part) the inflammatory response observed, as well as the ankylosis that is due mainly to the inflammatory response that trigger new bone formation (Braun & Sieper, 2007). However, it is necessary to enlarge the study population in order to confirm both the genetic data and the association of this polymorphism with AS.

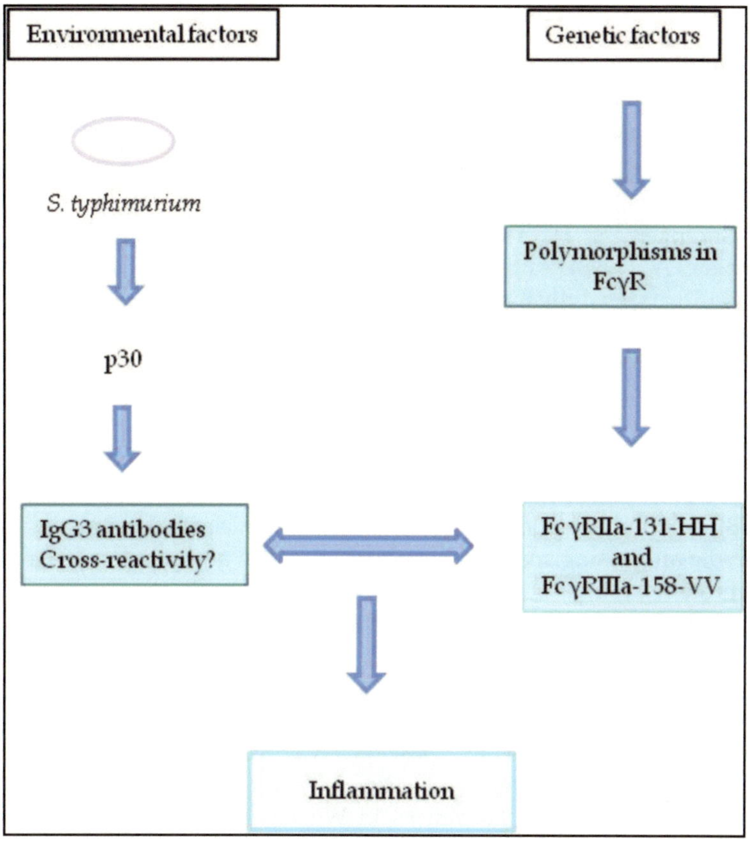

Fig. 8. A hypothetical model of the interaction between the environmental (the p30 from *S. typhimurium*), and the genetic (allelic variants FcγRIIA-131-HH, and FcγRIIIa-158-VV) factor in the inflammatory process observed in AS.

4. Conclusion

In this chapter, we proposed a link between the humoral immune response in a susceptible individual and a genetic factor, FcγRIIa-131-HH, and FcγRIIIa-158-VV.

The immune response against *S. typihumium* appears to be strain-specific, because of the difference observed with the humoral immune response against *S. enteritidis*. Patients with AS produce IgG3 antibodies against the p30 of *S. typhimurium,* in contrast to healthy controls. Moreover, patients with AS have higher frequencies of FcγRIIa-131-HH and FcγRIIIa-158-VV, which suggests a link between these environmental and genetic factors.

5. Acknowledgments

This work was supported in part by the *Programa Integral de Fortalecimiento Institucional* (PIFI)-2001, 2003, 2008 and 2010.

The authors would like to thank Georgina Nataly Ibarra Muro and Alma Senorina de Jesús Ornelas Muñoz for their technical assistance.

6. References

Ahmadi, K., Wilson, C., Tiwana, H., Binder, A. & Ebringer, A. (1998). Antibodies to Klebsiella pneumoniae lipopolysaccharide in patients with ankylosing spondylitis. *Br J Rheumatol* 37(12): 1330-1333.

Amor, B., Dougados, M. & Mijiyawa, M. (1990). [Criteria of the classification of spondylarthropathies]. *Rev Rhum Mal Osteoartic* 57(2): 85-89.

Blankenberg-Sprenkels, S. H., Fielder, M., Feltkamp, T. E., Tiwana, H., Wilson, C. & Ebringer, A. (1998). Antibodies to Klebsiella pneumoniae in Dutch patients with ankylosing spondylitis and acute anterior uveitis and to Proteus mirabilis in rheumatoid arthritis. *J Rheumatol* 25(4): 743-747.

Braun, J. & Sieper, J. (2007). Ankylosing spondylitis. *Lancet* 369(9570): 1379-1390.

Brown, M. & Wordsworth, P. (1997). Predisposing factors to spondyloarthropathies. *Curr Opin Rheumatol* 9(4): 308-314.

Cancino-Diaz, M. E., Perez-Salazar, J. E., Dominguez-Lopez, L., Escobar-Gutierrez, A., Granados-Arreola, J., Jimenez-Zamudio, L., Burgos-Vargas, R. & Garcia-Latorre, E. (1998). Antibody response to Klebsiella pneumoniae 60 kDa protein in familial and sporadic ankylosing spondylitis: role of HLA-B27 and characterization as a GroEL-like protein. *J Rheumatol* 25(9): 1756-1764.

Carter, J. D. (2010). Bacterial agents in spondyloarthritis: a destiny from diversity? *Best Pract Res Clin Rheumatol* 24(5): 701-714.

Cohen-Solal, J. F., Cassard, L., Fridman, W. H. & Sautes-Fridman, C. (2004). Fc gamma receptors. *Immunol Lett* 92(3): 199-205.

Dijstelbloem, H. M., Scheepers, R. H., Oost, W. W., Stegeman, C. A., van der Pol, W. L., Sluiter, W. J., Kallenberg, C. G., van de Winkel, J. G. & Tervaert, J. W. (1999). Fcgamma receptor polymorphisms in Wegener's granulomatosis: risk factors for disease relapse. *Arthritis Rheum* 42(9): 1823-1827.

Dijstelbloem, H. M., van de Winkel, J. G. & Kallenberg, C. G. (2001). Inflammation in autoimmunity: receptors for IgG revisited. *Trends Immunol* 22(9): 510-516.

Dominguez-Lopez, M. L., Burgos-Vargas, R., Galicia-Serrano, H., Bonilla-Sanchez, M. T., Rangel-Acosta, H. H., Cancino-Diaz, M. E., Jimenez-Zamudio, L., Granados, J. & Garcia-Latorre, E. (2002). IgG antibodies to enterobacteria 60 kDa heat shock proteins in the sera of HLA-B27 positive ankylosing spondylitis patients. *Scand J Rheumatol* 31(5): 260-265.

Dominguez-Lopez, M. L., Cancino-Diaz, M. E., Jimenez-Zamudio, L., Granados-Arreola, J., Burgos-Vargas, R. & Garcia-Latorre, E. (2000). Cellular immune response to Klebsiella pneumoniae antigens in patients with HLA-B27+ ankylosing spondylitis. *J Rheumatol* 27(6): 1453-1460.

Dougados, M. & Baeten, D. (2011). Spondyloarthritis. *Lancet* 377(9783): 2127-2137.

Dougados, M., van der Linden, S., Juhlin, R., Huitfeldt, B., Amor, B., Calin, A., Cats, A., Dijkmans, B., Olivieri, I., Pasero, G. & et al. (1991). The European Spondylarthropathy Study Group preliminary criteria for the classification of spondylarthropathy. *Arthritis Rheum* 34(10): 1218-1227.

Ebringer, A. & Wilson, C. (2000). HLA molecules, bacteria and autoimmunity. *J Med Microbiol* 49(4): 305-311.

Ekman, P., Saarinen, M., He, Q., Gripenberg-Lerche, C., Gronberg, A., Arvilommi, H. & Granfors, K. (2002). HLA-B27-transfected (Salmonella permissive) and HLA-A2-

transfected (Salmonella nonpermissive) human monocytic U937 cells differ in their production of cytokines. *Infect Immun* 70(3): 1609-1614.

Feldtkeller, E., Khan, M. A., van der Heijde, D., van der Linden, S. & Braun, J. (2003). Age at disease onset and diagnosis delay in HLA-B27 negative vs. positive patients with ankylosing spondylitis. *Rheumatol Int* 23(2): 61-66.

Hong, C. H., Lee, J. S., Lee, H. S., Bae, S. C. & Yoo, D. H. (2005). The association between fcgammaRIIIB polymorphisms and systemic lupus erythematosus in Korea. *Lupus* 14(5): 346-350.

Lahesmaa, R., Skurnik, M., Vaara, M., Leirisalo-Repo, M., Nissila, M., Granfors, K. & Toivanen, P. (1991). Molecular mimickry between HLA B27 and Yersinia, Salmonella, Shigella and Klebsiella within the same region of HLA alpha 1-helix. *Clin Exp Immunol* 86(3): 399-404.

Laitio, P., Virtala, M., Salmi, M., Pelliniemi, L. J., Yu, D. T. & Granfors, K. (1997). HLA-B27 modulates intracellular survival of Salmonella enteritidis in human monocytic cells. *Eur J Immunol* 27(6): 1331-1338.

Leirisalo-Repo, M., Hannu, T. & Mattila, L. (2003). Microbial factors in spondyloarthropathies: insights from population studies. *Curr Opin Rheumatol* 15(4): 408-412.

Michel, M., Piette, J. C., Roullet, E., Duron, F., Frances, C., Nahum, L., Pelletier, N., Crassard, I., Nunez, S., Michel, C., Bach, J. & Tournier-Lasserve, E. (2000). The R131 low-affinity allele of the Fc gamma RIIA receptor is associated with systemic lupus erythematosus but not with other autoimmune diseases in French Caucasians. *Am J Med* 108(7): 580-583.

Ni, P., Shen, F., Meng, W., Jiang, F. & Feng, S. (2000). [The association and linkage analysis between the FcgammaR II a-131 and system lupus erythematosus]. *Zhonghua Yi Xue Yi Chuan Xue Za Zhi* 17(6): 409-412.

Nieto, A., Caliz, R., Pascual, M., Mataran, L., Garcia, S. & Martin, J. (2000). Involvement of Fcgamma receptor IIIA genotypes in susceptibility to rheumatoid arthritis. *Arthritis Rheum* 43(4): 735-739.

Pacheco-Tena, C., Alvarado De La Barrera, C., Lopez-Vidal, Y., Vazquez-Mellado, J., Richaud-Patin, Y., Amieva, R. I., Llorente, L., Martinez, A., Zuniga, J., Cifuentes-Alvarado, M. & Burgos-Vargas, R. (2001). Bacterial DNA in synovial fluid cells of patients with juvenile onset spondyloarthropathies. *Rheumatology (Oxford)* 40(8): 920-927.

Parra-Campos, V., Escobar-Gutierrez, A., Dominguez-Lopez, M. L., Cancino-Diaz, M., Burgos-Vargas, R., Granados-Arreola, J., Jimenez-Zamudio, L. & Garcia-Latorre, E. (1996). Antibody response to nitrogenase-positive and -negative Klebsiella pneumoniae strains in juvenile-onset ankylosing spondylitis patients and their first degree relatives: lack of differential recognition of the bacterial nitrogenase. *Rev Latinoam Microbiol* 38(2): 121-127.

Raknes, G., Skeie, G. O., Gilhus, N. E., Aadland, S. & Vedeler, C. (1998). FcgammaRIIA and FcgammaRIIIB polymorphisms in myasthenia gravis. *J Neuroimmunol* 81(1-2): 173-176.

Rashid, T. & Ebringer, A. (2007). Ankylosing spondylitis is linked to Klebsiella--the evidence. *Clin Rheumatol* 26(6): 858-864.

Ravetch, J. V. & Bolland, S. (2001). IgG Fc receptors. *Annu Rev Immunol* 19: 275-290.

Reveille, J. D. & Arnett, F. C. (2005). Spondyloarthritis: update on pathogenesis and management. *Am J Med* 118(6): 592-603.

Saarinen, M., Ekman, P., Ikeda, M., Virtala, M., Gronberg, A., Yu, D. T., Arvilommi, H. & Granfors, K. (2002). Invasion of Salmonella into human intestinal epithelial cells is modulated by HLA-B27. *Rheumatology (Oxford)* 41(6): 651-657.

Salmon, J. E. & Pricop, L. (2001). Human receptors for immunoglobulin G: key elements in the pathogenesis of rheumatic disease. *Arthritis Rheum* 44(4): 739-750.

Tani, Y., Tiwana, H., Hukuda, S., Nishioka, J., Fielder, M., Wilson, C., Bansal, S. & Ebringer, A. (1997). Antibodies to Klebsiella, Proteus, and HLA-B27 peptides in Japanese patients with ankylosing spondylitis and rheumatoid arthritis. *J Rheumatol* 24(1): 109-114.

Van Den Berg, L., Myhr, K. M., Kluge, B. & Vedeler, C. A. (2001). Fcgamma receptor polymorphisms in populations in Ethiopia and Norway. *Immunology* 104(1): 87-91.

van der Linden, S., Valkenburg, H. A. & Cats, A. (1984). Evaluation of diagnostic criteria for ankylosing spondylitis. A proposal for modification of the New York criteria. *Arthritis Rheum* 27(4): 361-368.

van der Pol, W. & van de Winkel, J. G. (1998). IgG receptor polymorphisms: risk factors for disease. *Immunogenetics* 48(3): 222-232.

Virtala, M., Kirveskari, J. & Granfors, K. (1997). HLA-B27 modulates the survival of Salmonella enteritidis in transfected L cells, possibly by impaired nitric oxide production. *Infect Immun* 65(10): 4236-4242.

Willcocks, L. C., Smith, K. G. & Clatworthy, M. R. (2009). Low-affinity Fcgamma receptors, autoimmunity and infection. *Expert Rev Mol Med* 11: e24.

Zambrano-Zaragoza, J. F., de Jesus Duran-Avelar, M., Rodriguez-Ocampo, A. N., Garcia-Latorre, E., Burgos-Vargas, R., Dominguez-Lopez, M. L., Pena-Virgen, S. & Vibanco-Perez, N. (2009). The 30-kDa band from Salmonella typhimurium: IgM, IgA and IgG antibody response in patients with ankylosing spondylitis. *Rheumatology (Oxford)* 48(7): 748-754.

7

Genetics in Ankylosing Spondylitis – Beyond HLA-B*27

Bruno Filipe Bettencourt[1,3], Iris Foroni[1,3], Ana Rita Couto[1,3], Manuela Lima[2,3] and Jácome Bruges-Armas[1,3]
[1]*Serviço Especializado de Epidemiologia e Biologia Molecular, Hospital de Santo Espírito de Angra do Heroísmo*
[2]*Grupo de Epidemiologia e Genética Humana do Departamento de Biologia da Universidade dos Açores*
[3]*Genetic and Arthritis Research Group (GARG), Institute for Molecular and Cell Biology (IBMC), University of Porto*
Portugal

1. Introduction

The association between HLA-B27 and ankylosing spondylitis (AS) has lead to intense research over the last 4 decades. In the course of this research, it was possible to obtain the best example of an association between a disease and a genetic marker. Genetic factors contribute with more than 90% for the susceptibility risk to AS being the MHC region, in particularly HLA-B27, the main contributor (Brown, et al., 1996). This evidence is supported by studies using familial cohorts; segregation and twin studies (Brown, et al., 1997; Jarvinen, 1995; Rubin, et al., 1994).

The advent of genotyping technologies, in particular the use of genome-wide linkage studies (GWLS) and whole-genome association studies (WGAS), allowed a wider view of the genetic factors related to AS and supported the presence of non-MHC genetic AS susceptibility factors. The first whole genome wide linkage study identified numerous loci in linkage with the disease, on chromosomes 1p, 2q, 6p, 9q, 10q, 16q, and 19q (Laval, et al., 2001). These results prompted to an even more intense research on AS and, consequently, the investigation of other areas outside MHC. Later, three other major studies tried to narrow down the chromosome areas first identified (Consortium TASC, 2010; Consortium TASC/WTCCC2, 2011; Consortium WTCCC/TASC, 2007). This way it was possible to identify specific gene regions that would lead to new insights in the mechanisms underlying the disease susceptibility (Table 1). In this chapter we intend to provide an overview of the main genes, other than HLA-B*27, which were identified as been associated to AS during the last decade.

2. Genes with consistent association to ankylosing spondylitis

2.1 Major histocompatibility complex

At this moment, over 80 subtypes of HLA-B27 (coding and non-coding) are known (http://hla.alleles.org/alleles/class1.html). All variants were originated from the parental

B*27:05 as a result of different mechanisms, such as point mutation, gene conversion, reciprocal recombination and interlocus gene conversion (Reveille, J D & Maganti, 2009). The data obtained from studies within same ethnic groups allowed the perception that there are differences in the rank of association of each B27 subtype and AS. The allele HLA-B*27:05 is the most frequent variant of B27 worldwide, although the frequencies of all the known subtypes diverge when different ethnic groups are compared (Reveille, J D, 2011). For that reason, it has been very difficult to establish a clear ranking of B27 variants and association with AS, that could be applied to all groups (Brown, 2010).

Among European Caucasians, B*27:05 and B*27:02 are suggested to be the strongest disease associated variants (Brown, et al., 1996; MacLean, et al., 1993; Reveille, J D, 2011). In Asian cohorts, HLA-B*27:04 was found to be more strongly associated with AS than B*27:05 (Hou, et al., 2007; Liu, et al., 2010; Lopez-Larrea, C, et al., 1995). Other B*27 alleles were already reported in AS cases, namely B*27:01 (Ball & Khan, 2001), *27:03 (Gonzalez-Roces, et al., 1997), *27:07, *27:08 (Armas, et al., 1999), *27:10 (Garcia, et al., 1998), *27:14, *27:15 (Garcia-Fernandez, et al., 2001), and *27:19 (Tamouza, et al., 2001).

The information obtained in studies with B27 subtypes confirm this allele as a critical factor on AS susceptibility. However, since it is known that less than 8% of B27 individuals develop AS (van der Linden, et al., 1984), it is difficult to exclude another gene nearby B27 as the one responsible for the AS susceptibility. The high level of linkage disequilibrium (LD) in the MHC region is a major barrier to the identification of any other possible gene directly involved.

New insights were reached inside MHC, despite all the complexity involving this region. HLA-B60 (B*40:01) was identified as the first non-HLA-B*27 gene strongly associated to AS susceptibility. The first report of this association stated that HLA-B60 was increased among AS patients HLA-B27 positive, in five independent data sets. On the other hand, the studied variant was not increased in HLA-B27 negative patients with AS. A whole view of the obtained data show that the susceptibility to AS is threefold higher in individuals both B27/B60 positive (Robinson, et al., 1989). These findings were later supported by other studies using different cohorts. In a group of UK patients with AS, not only the association strength of B27/B60 positive was confirmed. The presence of HLA-B60 was observed in HLA-B27 negative patients, suggesting that, despite having a much weaker effect, it may function as an AS susceptibility gene independent of HLA-B27 (Brown, et al., 1996). Moreover, in a group of Taiwan Chinese it was confirmed the association of B60 with AS and also, for the first time, an independent association of B61 was found. Both alleles were strongly increased in HLA-B27 negative patients (Wei, et al., 2004). Although all this replications confirming the relationship between HLA-B60 and AS, the same was not seen in Mexican Mestizos where, instead, HLA-B49 was identified as significantly increased in patients with AS (Vargas-Alarcón, et al., 1994).

Another allele, HLA-B*39, has been reported to be increased in HLA-B27 negative White Caucasian and Japanese AS patients (Khan, et al., 1980; Yamaguchi, et al., 1995). The studies that provided this data used small cohorts and consequently it is not possible to state if this is an effective association neither the level of its power. Even so, it was formulated a parallelism between B27 and B*39 components of the peptide-anchoring B pocket as well as peptide-ligand motifs, supporting some potential explanation for the HLA-B27 influence in the development of AS (Yamaguchi, et al., 1995). This results were not confirmed in a cohort composed by White Caucasians and Mexican Mestizos (Maksymowych, W P, et al., 2000). The prevalence of AS in Sub-Saharan black Africans is very low, a fact that has been related to the low frequency of HLA-B27 in that region. The allele HLA-B*1403, found exclusively in African or Afro-American populations, was reported in four out of eight AS Togolese patients, a population where HLA-B27 is considered to be virtually absent (Lopez-Larrea, C, et al., 2002). It was the first time that a variant of B*14 was found to be present in AS patients. However, a confirmation is needed and a mandatory replication of this study in other sub-Saharan populations is still missing. These findings in HLA-B alleles, other than HLA-B27, are not clear enough to understand if there is a direct association with AS or if this is the result of LD with another MHC gene.

Data derived from GWAS for susceptibility loci in AS extended the HLA association in the MHC region between markers D6S276 and DRB1 (Brown, et al., 1998b). This finding has been supported by the results obtained in different ethnic groups (Brown, et al., 1998a; Jaakkola, et al., 2006; Kchir, et al., 2010; Mahfoudh, et al., 2011; Ploski, et al., 1995; Said-Nahal, et al., 2002; Sims, A M, et al., 2007). HLA-DRB1 was found to have a strong association with AS. In British patients the level of this association was increased in DR1 homozygotes, a fact that may suggest a B27-independent association, excluding a possible LD effect (Brown, et al., 1998a; Sims, A M, et al., 2007). On the other hand, in French families the association between DR1 and AS seems to be a consequence of LD with HLA-B27 (Said-Nahal, et al., 2002). Here, it was reported an excess of transmission of HLA-DR4 to patients, independently of its LD with B27. Together with the lack of transmission of DR4 to HLA-B27 positive siblings, this report suggests that the presence of DR4 may contribute to AS simultaneously with B27. The HLA-DR1 is associated to SpA in Mexican patients, however, this finding was not confirmed when only AS patients were analysed (Vargas-Alarcon, et al., 2002). The sample size and the high prevalence of peripheral enthesopathy and arthropathy in the studied group may explain this result, different from the results obtained in the British population.

Consistent results, on the association of DRB1 alleles with AS, have been difficult to ascertain in different ethnic groups. A Finnish report proposed that, in this specific population, the HLA-DRB1 alleles do not seem to play a strong role in AS susceptibility , but may influence the age of symptom onset (Jaakkola, et al., 2006). The results, in this case-control study, are limited due to the sample size. Still, a strong association of DRB1*08, both independent and as part of a HLA-B27 haplotype, was suggested. HLA-DRB1*08 had been already reported in juvenile-AS B27-positive individuals, in Norwegian population (Ploski, et al., 1995). Two haplotypes were identified in a British case-control study: B*27positive /DRB1*07positive and B*27negative /DRB1*03positive (Sims, A M, et al., 2007). The frequency of HLA-DRB1*15 was found to be increased, in Tunisian AS patients, but this allele was in LD with B27 (Mahfoudh, et al., 2011). Within the same population, a case-control study reported a significant increase in HLA-DRB1*11 frequency among patients. It was also found a possible protective effect of HLA-DRB1*13 (Kchir, et al., 2010).

Recently, in a Spanish/Portuguese cohort, it was reported the association between HLA-DPA1 and HLA-DPB1 alleles and AS (Díaz-Peña, et al., 2011). The study was focused on these two MHC genes that lay on a region unrelated to B27. Both AS patients and controls were HLA-B27 positive. This way it was possible to achieve results from an HLA-B27 neutral point of view. The data showed significant results between AS and DPA1*01:03,

DPA1*02:01, DPB1*13:01. It was also found an association between two haplotypes and AS, namely: DPA1*02:01-DPB1*11:01:01 and DPA1*02:01-DPB1*13:01. This was the first study to show an association between this region of MHC and susceptibility to AS. Consequently, further replicates are needed to confirm these results.

Genes with consistent association to ankylosing spondylitis			
Gene	Locus	Mechanism	Population origin
HLA-B27	6p21.3	Presents endogenously processed antigens to T cells	Caucasian and non-Caucasian
HLA-B60 (*4001)	6p21.3	Presents endogenously processed antigens to T cells	Caucasian and non-Caucasian
ERAP1/ARTS1	5q15	Peptide trimming prior to HLA Class I presentation and cleaving cytokine receptors from cell surface	Caucasian and Han-Chinese
IL23R	1p31.3	Differentiation of naive CD4 T cells into helper Th17 T cells	Caucasian and Han-Chinese
KIF21B	1p32	Transport of essential cellular components along axonal and dendritic microtubules	Caucasian
-	2p15	Unknown	Caucasian
-	21q22	Unknown	Caucasian
Genes with suggestive association to ankylosing spondylitis			
Gene	Locus	Mechanism	Population origin
IL1R2	2q11	Interference in the binding of IL-1 to IL-1R1	Caucasian and non-Caucasian
IL12B	5q31	Heterodimerises with the IL23 p19 subunit, to form IL23R	Caucasian
CYP2D6	22q13.1	Metabolism of xenobiotics	Caucasian (North European)
TNFR1	12p13	Influence on TNF signaling	Caucasian
TNFSF15	9q32	Differentiation of naive CD4 T cells into helper Th17 T cells	Caucasian
ANTRX2	4q21	Binds to collagen IV and laminin, possibly involved in extracellular matrix adhesion	Caucasian and Han-Chinese
Other genes			
Gene	Locus	Mechanism	Population origin
ANKH	5p15.2	Exports inorganic pyrophosphate from intracellular to extracellular compartments. Regulates tissue calcification	Caucasian and Japanese (small cohorts)
KIR	19q13.4	Regulates activation of NK cells via recognition of HLA class I molecules on target cells	Caucasian and Han-Chinese (small cohorts)
TGFB1	19q13	Mediates inflammation, fibrosis and bone remodelling	Caucasian (one study)
TNAP	1p36.1	Receptor on monocytes important in apoptosis, binds lipopolysaccharide	Caucasian (one study)
CD14	5q31.1	A phosphoethanolamine and pyridoxal-5'-PO4 actingectophosphatase. Degrades PPi	Caucasian (Finnish small cohort)

Table 1. Genes associated to AS - adapted from (Brown, 2010; Reveille, J D, 2011).

2.2 Non-major histocompatibility complex genes

2.2.1 ERAP1/ARTS1

The association between Endoplasmic Reticulum Aminopeptidase 1 (ERAP1) and AS was first reported in Caucasians, together with IL23R (Consortium WTCCC/TASC, 2007). Contrarily to the IL23R, the association of *ERAP1* was later confirmed in other ethnic groups (Chen, R., et al., 2011). ERAP1 molecules are encoded by the oxytocinase subfamily, a group of three genes located on the chromosome 5 (5q15) (Brionez & Reveille, 2008), and are located in the endoplasmatic reticulum lumen (Saric, et al., 2002).

The involvement between *ERAP1* and MHC class I presentation was the first suggested and confirmed function attributed to this aminopeptidase (Saric, et al., 2002; Saveanu, et al., 2005). ERAP1 is MHC class I dependent and play a major role on peptide trimming, processing it to optimal length, for presentation at cell surface (Saveanu, et al., 2005), having an important connection to the immune recognition mechanism related to CD8+ T cells. However, it is proposed that the referred importance varies depending both on the antigen and the cell physiological state. It was shown that, contrarily to other peptidases, ERAP1 cleaves NH_2-terminal from peptides longer than ten residues and, consequently, is able to produce peptides containing eight to nine residues from longer precursors (York, et al., 2002). This fact support the relation with MHC class I molecules and indicates a possible co-evolution between these 2 groups of molecules, since MHC class I require eight to nine residues peptides for a stable binding (York, et al., 2002). Due to the involvement between ERAP1 and MHC class I, these molecules and their trimming mechanisms are consequently involved with HLA-B27, an MHC class I variant (Campbell, et al., 2011). For some years, it was stated that a deeper understanding about *ERAP1* function and its relation with B27, at peptide production level, would lead to new insights on the paths that support the well known association between HLA-B27 and AS.. This aspiration was recently fulfilled by the latest GWAS on AS (Consortium TASC/WTCCC2, 2011). It was shown that HLA-B27 positive and negative AS cases differ in association with *ERAP1*. This fact provided the first reliable replicated example of a gene-gene interaction in AS, indicating that the mechanism by which HLA-B27 induces AS involves aberrant presentation or handling of peptides (Consortium TASC/WTCCC2, 2011).

The cleavage of cytokine cell surface receptors is another function documented to *ERAP1*. The shedding of IL-1R2, promoted by ERAP1, was already reported in co-immunoprecipitation experiments (Cui, et al., 2003a). Through the use of cell lines, it was possible to achieve a correspondence between *ERAP1* overexpression, the increase of IL1-R2 shedding and the decrease of membrane-associated IL1-R2. It was also found that ERAP1 is necessary for constitutive IL1-R2 shedding, as basal IL1-R2 shedding is absent from *ERAP1* knockout cell lines (Cui, et al., 2003a). The exact same correlations were already observed in reports regarding TNFR1 (Cui, et al., 2002) and IL6R (Cui, et al., 2003b). These findings were not confirmed when was measured the appearance of those receptors in cell culture supernatants from single-cell suspensions, stimulated with plate-bound anti-CD3 (Clone 145-2C11) and phorbol 12-myristate 13-acetate (PMA), prepared from mouse spleens. No difference in the levels of these receptors was observed over time, indicating that ERAP1 does not have a major influence on cytokine receptor trimming, at least in mice (Consortium TASC/WTCCC2, 2011). Further tests may contribute to the clarification of the mechanisms underlying the association between ERAP1 and AS. An abnormal increase or decrease in the amount of those cytokine cell surface receptors is an expected outcome of ERAP1 malfunctioning. Thus, the susceptibility to AS can emerge as a consequence of pro-inflammatory effects related to that amount variation (Chen, R., et al., 2011; Consortium WTCCC/TASC, 2007).

Since the confirmed association between ERAP1 and AS reported in 2007(Consortium WTCCC/TASC, 2007), some replications occurred in studies involving Caucasian (Consortium TASC, 2010; Harvey, et al., 2009a; Maksymowych, W. P., et al., 2009; Pazar, et al., 2010; Pimentel-Santos, et al., 2009; Tsui, F. W., et al., 2010) and Han Chinese cohorts (Bang, et al., 2011; Choi, et al., 2010; Davidson, et al., 2009). The Wellcome Trust Case-Control consortium and Australo-Anglo-American Spondyloarthritis Consortium first described the association of five *ERAP1* single nucleotide polymorphisms (SNPs) and AS (Consortium WTCCC/TASC, 2007), namely rs27044, rs17482078, rs10050860, rs30187 and rs2287987. Two of these SNPs, rs27044 and rs30187, gathered more consistent results in the subsequent reports and were the only markers that showed significant association both in Caucasian and in Han Chinese groups (Choi, et al., 2010; Harvey, et al., 2009a; Maksymowych, W. P., et al., 2009; Pazar, et al., 2010; Pimentel-Santos, et al., 2009). The significant relation between rs27044 and AS was not confirmed in Canadian, contrarily to all other replicates involving this SNP and Caucasian groups. However, in that same cohort, it was found an *ERAP1* haplotype, containing rs27044, which increased the risk of AS: rs2044/10060860/30187-CCT (Maksymowych, W. P., et al., 2009). The other mentioned SNP, rs30187, did not show a significant association with AS in a group from Hungary (Pazar, et al., 2010). However, this result has low impact compared to the other studies performed, since the obtained P-value was 0.051 and the sample was the smallest of all the mentioned cohorts. The rs30187 (Arg528Lys) is the only coding marker within a SNP block recently identified in GWAS (Consortium TASC, 2010). This variant showed a really strong significant association in another GWAS using a large Caucasian cohort ($P=1.8x10^{-27}$) (Consortium TASC/WTCCC2, 2011). It was shown that this marker originates a significant decrease in aminopeptidase activity toward a synthetic peptide substrate. Moreover, modeling of ERAP1 protein points out to the presence of Arg528 at the mouth of the putative enzyme substrate pocket. This location can explain the reduction of the aminopeptidase activity of the molecules that contain this variation (Goto, et al., 2008; Kochan, et al., 2011). These results and reported data from family based studies (Tsui, F. W., et al., 2010) support this SNP as one of the *ERAP1* variants with strongest association to AS.

The remaining SNPs found by The Australo-Anglo-American Spondyloarthritis Consortium (TASC) & Wellcome Trust Case Control Consortium (WTCCC) didn't show consistent results in other sudies. The first published study, after WTCCC/TASC report, was not able to identify a significant association between rs2287987, rs17482078 or rs10050860 and AS in a Portuguese group (Pimentel-Santos, et al., 2009). The same result was obtained in a Han Chinese group (Choi, et al., 2010). The rs17482078 significant association (Consortium WTCCC/TASC, 2007) was not confirmed also in already mentioned Hungary group (Pazar, et al., 2010). Other replications using Caucasian cohorts were able to find significant associations between rs2287987, rs10050860 and AS (Harvey, et al., 2009a; Maksymowych, W. P., et al., 2009; Pazar, et al., 2010). Recently, a meta-analysis that included all the *ERAP1* association studies, confirmed the presence of a significant association between the SNPs reported by the Consortium WTCCC/TASC and AS (Chen, R., et al., 2011). Moreover, it was proposed that the contradictory results, obtained in some replications, can be an effect of the clinical heterogeneity, ethnic differences or real genetic heterogeneity, the small sample size of the studies or their low statistical power (Chen, R., et al., 2011).

The Consortium TASC included *ERAP1* in the first GWAS for AS, already mentioned above. This work included a large Caucasian cohort and narrowed down the ERAP1 region, associated to AS, to a block of SNPs lying in a 4.6-kb region between rs27529 (exon 9) and rs469758 (intron 12) (Consortium TASC, 2010). The identified region showed an association 50 times more significant than any other imputed SNP ($P<10^{-11}$). The overall results showed strong association of two SNPs that were not reported in previous Caucasian studies, rs27037 and rs27434. The data obtained in a Han Chinese group, published before TASC GWAS showed moderate association of rs27037 (P=0.012) and did not observe the association of rs27434 (P=0.14) (Davidson, et al., 2009). The same result was attained by the recent meta-analysis already cited (Chen, R., et al., 2011). On the other hand, the strong association of both markers was recently confirmed in a Korean group (Bang, et al., 2011). Once more, together with ethnic differences, the results seem to be influenced by the effect genetic heterogeneity.

The data concerning *ERAP1* haplotypes is limited; however the available results seem to point out to some haplotypes that influence the risk of disease. The rs2044/10060860/30187-CCT haplotypes increased the risk of disease in 3 Canadian case-control cohorts. This haplotype is in one of the two strongly significant haplotypes, out of four, that were identified among Koreans: rs27044/rs17482078/rs10050860/rs30187-GCCT and rs27044/rs17482078/rs10050860/rs30187-CCCC (Choi, et al., 2010). All these four SNPs formed an LD block with almost complete LD (95<D'<100) (Choi, et al., 2010; Tsui, F. W., et al., 2010). The Canadian study reported a protection effect of rs30187/26618/26653-CTG ERAP1 haplotype (Maksymowych, W. P., et al., 2009). A family-based study was not able to support the significant association of rs2044/10060860/30187 haplotype, but here a relatively small sample was used (Tsui, F. W., et al., 2010). Moreover, the results are probably an underestimate since some of the studied families had more than two affected individuals (3-5) and the method used by the authors for power estimation took into account only two affected family members. Despite this lack of confirmation, it was possible to identify significant association between rs27044/rs2549782-GT and rs30187/rs2549782-TT haplotypes and AS. In addition, a novel finding showing that rs27044/rs30187/rs2549782-GTT haplotype in the ERAP1-ERAP2 loci was significantly associated with disease susceptibility for both models used (Tsui, F. W., et al., 2010).

2.2.2 IL23R

The association between Interleukin 23 receptor (IL23R) and AS has been confirmed throughout the last few years, since the first association evidence, reported by the WTCCC/TASC study (Consortium WTCCC/TASC, 2007) .

IL23R is a member of heamopoietin receptor family, which binds to IL-23 mediating its activity. This hemopoietic cytokine receptor is encoded on chromosome 1 (1p31.3), by a gene located 150kb far from the gene for IL-12Rβ2 (Parham, C., et al., 2002). IL23 is a heterodimeric cytokine consisting of two subunits: p40, which is shared with IL-12, and p19 (Oppmann, et al., 2000). IL-23 has also other biological connections with IL-12; activated human PHA blast T cells, when induced by IL-23, register a better proliferation and IFN-γ production, like when they are induced by IL-12. However, IFN-γ levels produced in cells stimulated by IL-23 are always lower than those induced by IL-12. In the presence of IL-23, naive T cells only increase the producing of IFN-γ after a long stimulation. In contrast, memory T cells - human and mouse – and NKL cells register a strong response to IL-23, enhancing IFN-γ production (Oppmann, et al., 2000; Parham, C., et al., 2002). The cells response to either IL-12 or IL-23 is linked to the level of IL-12Rβ2 or IL23R expression, respectively (Parham, C., et al., 2002).

IL23R is one of the two subunits of IL-23 receptor complex, present on IL-23-responsive cells. The other component is IL-12Rβ1 and is shared with IL-12 receptor. Despite the similarities in the structure of both receptors, in the presence of IL23R subunit, cells respond to IL-23 and not to IL-12 (Parham, C., et al., 2002). Human *IL23R* is expressed on T cells, Natural-Killer (NK) cells, monocytes and DCs, all cells that are able to respond to IL-23 (Belladonna, et al., 2002; Parham, C., et al., 2002). The IL23R has an important role in CD4 T-cell differentiation, since it encodes a critical cytokine receptor in the TH17 lymphocyte subset. The TH17 cells were already identified as mediators of inflammatory process in several models of autoimmunity (Cua, et al., 2003; Murphy, et al., 2003). Furthermore, they are considered as a distinct subset of T-cells, expressing high levels of IL-17 in response to stimulation (Park, et al., 2005) and are associated to tissue damage in brain, joints, heart, lungs and intestines (Steinman, 2007). Genetic variants of IL23R have also been related with susceptibility to several autoimmune diseases, namely inflammatory bowel disease (IBD) (Duerr, et al., 2006), psoriasis (Cargill, et al., 2007), multiple sclerosis (Nunez, et al., 2008) and AS (Consortium WTCCC/TASC, 2007). A significant association between *IL-12Rβ1* and AS (rs6556416; $P=1.9 \times 10^{-8}$), which encodes one of IL23R and IL-12R subunits, was reported recently by the Consortium WTCCC2/TASC (Consortium TASC/WTCCC2, 2011).

The Consortium WTCCC/TASC reported the strong association ($p \leq 0.008$) of eight *IL23R* SNPs and AS, rs11209026, rs1004819, rs10489629, rs11465804, rs1343151, rs10889677, rs11209032, rs1495965 (Consortium WTCCC/TASC, 2007). The strongest association reported was with SNP rs11209032 ($p= 7.5 \times 10^{-9}$) with an attributable risk of 9%. The power of this association was consistent, even when only AS cases, without IBD. were considered. It was stated that this fact could be the result of a primary association with AS, and thus, not related to the presence of IBD (Consortium WTCCC/TASC, 2007). These findings were replicated in several studies; however, there are some conflicting results, especially when analyzing different ethnic groups. A recent GWAS used the same British cohort, and included a new sample composed by Australian, British and North American individuals. In this large cohort a strong AS association to SNP rs11209026 ($p= 2.3 \times 10^{-9}$) was identified (Consortium TASC, 2010). This association was soon after confirmed by the most recent GWAS reported by the TASC/WTCCC2 consortia (Consortium TASC/WTCCC2, 2011).

Closely after the WTCCC/TASC report, a Canadian and a Spanish study were able to replicate some of the already studied *IL23R* SNPs (Rahman, et al., 2008; Rueda, et al., 2008). The Canadian study encompassed 3 cohorts and tested the association of 10 *IL23R* SNPs: rs7517847 and rs2201841, plus the SNPs reported by WTCCC/TASC. Significant associations, to the SNPs rs1004819 and rs11209032, were also found in a Portuguese cohort (Pimentel-Santos, et al., 2009), and in the Alberta population, respectively. The SNPs rs11209026 (Arg381Gln) and rs11465804 revealed association with AS in both Newfoundland and Toronto groups. The last SNP, revealed the strongest protective effect in these two cohorts and it was in LD with rs11209026. The Toronto population also registered significant differences in rs7517847 (Rahman, et al., 2008).

In the Spanish group, the obtained results were able to corroborate the previous findings for rs1343151, rs11209026 and rs10889677. In this cohort the SNPs revealed a protective effect. The association of the remaining SNPs, reported by the consortium WTCCC/TASC, was not confirmed. The involvement of rs11465804 was not tested, on the other hand, like in the Canadian study, it was included the SNP rs7517847 but no significant result was found for this variation (Rueda, et al., 2008). In this population, rs1343151 showed a stronger association ($P=2x10^{-4}$). This findings, together with the Canadian study results previously mentioned (Rahman, et al., 2008), points out to a protection effect of the Arg381Gln non-synonymous polymorphism. The changing of Arg381 for Gln381 may modify the interaction between IL23R and its associated JAK2 kinase (Parham, C., et al., 2002). The authors proposed that this variation can interfere with the IL23R transducing pathway leading to a reduction in cellular response to IL-23, explaining this way the protective effect of Gln381 allele (Rahman, et al., 2008; Rueda, et al., 2008).

A Portuguese study was not able to confirm all this findings (Pimentel-Santos, et al., 2009). The modest power of the study can explain the results. However, as it was already mentioned, a significant association was found for rs1004819. The minor allele frequencies observed in this study were similar to those reported in British and North Americans. Furthermore, this association had a similar magnitude of effect to the one already reported in those populations. The attributable risk for rs1004819 in Portuguese cohort, is very similar to the one reported to rs11209032 in the British/North American populations (Consortium WTCCC/TASC, 2007; Pimentel-Santos, et al., 2009). Using the obtained results, the authors performed a meta-analysis study combining the Portuguese data and the previously published Spanish data (Rueda, et al., 2008). Considering fixed effects, three *IL23R* SNPs revealed significant association rs1004819, rs1343151 and rs11209026. When random effects were considered for the analysis of combined data, only rs1004819 was found to have significant association, confirming the result found when only the Portuguese cohort was analyzed (Pimentel-Santos, et al., 2009).

The results obtained for rs1004819 in the Iberian population were confirmed in the Hungarian population (Pimentel-Santos, et al., 2009; Safrany, et al., 2009). This study was performed with a small number of samples; even so, it was possible to register some significant associations. It was shown that the presence of rs1004819 allele A increases the risk for AS in more than two-fold. The same increase was registered when rs10889677 was considered. Significant results were also found for rs11209026. Besides the SNPs reported in the initial association study (Consortium WTCCC/TASC, 2007), the authors also included rs11805303, which was significantly increased in patients with AS. The minor allele of this SNP conferred a 1.6-fold risk for the development of the disease in the studied cohort (Safrany, et al., 2009). The presence of rs11209026 revealed no significant difference between patients and controls when only HLA-B27 positive AS patients were included in the statistical analysis. Thus, the association found for rs11805303 and rs10889677 had a marginal significance when comparing controls with the HLA-B27 patients. Nevertheless, all the other variants kept their significant results, showing that HLA-B27 status has no real effect on the effect of IL23R (Safrany, et al., 2009).

A meta-analysis, reported at the same year, included the first United Kingdom and United States cohort published (Consortium WTCCC/TASC, 2007), the Canadian groups (Alberta, Newfoundland and Toronto) (Rahman, et al., 2008), the Spanish results (Rueda, et al., 2008) plus a new British group (Karaderi, et al., 2009). Just like stated by WTCCC/TASC, the results of this study confirmed the association between AS and all the eight IL23R SPNs analyzed. Once more, the strongest associations were seen with rs11209026 (P<10-10) and rs11209032 (P=4.06x10-9) (Karaderi, et al., 2009). The last variant had the same order of magnitude reported by the WTCCC/TASC study (Consortium WTCCC/TASC, 2007). This meta-analysis confirmed the connection of IL23R and AS susceptibility in Caucasians.

The first replication, performed in a group with a different ethnic background, did not confirm the association of IL23R and AS in Han Chinese (Davidson, et al., 2009; Sung, et al., 2009). These findings may indicate a difference in the mechanism of disease pathogenesis between Caucasian and Han Chinese populations. The authors proposed that the development of AS developing Chinese can result from a mechanism independent of any *IL23R* polymorphism. This difference could be the result of the association with a different gene also involved in the *IL23R* signaling pathway (Davidson, et al., 2009). Other explanation to this lack of association is the absence of polymorphism of rs11209026 in Chinese. This variant, as described above, is pointed out as one of the causative SNP for disease susceptibility in Europeans. However, recent published data reported association of some *IL23R* SNPs and AS in a Chinese cohort (Wang, et al., 2010). In this group it was found, for the first time, a significant association between rs6677188, located in the intergenic region, and AS susceptibility. The previously reported association of rs11209032 in Caucasians was confirmed also in Chinese. Through the analysis of paiwised LD, it was found that rs11209032 and rs6677188 were in strong LD, in this population (Wang, et al., 2010).

2.2.3 KIF21B

The gene *KIF21B* (Kinesin Family 21B) is one of the most recent loci with confirmed association to AS. This gene belongs to a family of kinesin motor proteins that are involved in the transport of essential components along axonal and denditric microtubules by neurons. A GWS found strong association for rs11584383 (1q32) ($P = 1.6x10^{-10}$), a SNP located downstream of and flanked by *KIF21B* (Danoy, et al., 2010). This strong association was corroborated by WTCCC2/TASC. Here, the SNP rs2297909 showed the strongest association with AS ($P=5.2 \times 10^{-12}$) (Consortium TASC/WTCCC2, 2011). Both studies were conducted with Caucasian cohorts. Despite the confirmed association in this ethnic group, further replications in other ethnic groups are mandatory.

2.3 Intergenic regions - 2p15 and 21q22

It has been estimated that approximately 25% of the human genome consists of gene deserts defined as generally long regions, ranging from a few base pairs to 5.1 Mb, containing no protein-coding sequences and with no obvious biological functions (Venter, et al., 2001). Ovcharenko *et al.* found that conservation clearly separates two distinct categories of gene deserts: weakly conserved variable gene deserts and more conserved stable gene deserts (Ovcharenko, et al., 2005). Moreover, it has already been shown that some human gene deserts harbour distant regulatory elements that are deeply conserved in vertebrate species

(Kimura-Yoshida, et al., 2004; Nobrega, et al., 2003). Several diseases have been associated with these particular areas of the genome; possible explanations to elucidate the mechanisms underlying these associations include: 1) epigenetic effects, 2) unknown protein-coding transcripts, 3) effects of long range transcriptional regulatory elements and 4) effects of non-coding RNA that can influence gene expression (Brown, 2010).

A GWAS has recently identified the new association of two narrow intergenic regions, in chromosomes 2 (23kb) and 21 (11kb), with AS. This study found, in each intergenic region, a block of SNPs in tight linkage disequilibrium encompassing areas that likely contain the causative variants responsible for the observed association (Consortium TASC, 2010). Another GWAS recent study replicated this association and has shown that SNPs at these intergenic regions are independent of the HLA-B27 presence, since it is associated with AS in both HLA-B27 positive and HLA-B27-negative patients (Consortium TASC/WTCCC2, 2011).

The intergenic area 2p15 does not contain any known gene and, until now, this has been the only association to a disease (Reveille, J. D., et al., 2010). The association to AS was already been replicated in a small study in the Spanish population. The SNP rs10865331 was typed in four hundred and fifty six AS patients and 300 healthy donors, and the result was a significant association with AS, while no association was found for rs2242944, in 21q22 (Consortium TASC/WTCCC2, 2011).

The other intergenic AS associated area, at chromosome 21q22, has already been associated with a closely related condition: paediatric-onset inflammatory bowel disease (IBD) (Kugathasan, et al., 2008). Remarkably, the most strongly IBD associated SNP is in strong linkage disequilibrium with the strongest ankylosing spondylitis-associated marker (Consortium TASC, 2010). The nearest gene, to this region, lies at 82kb distance (PSMG1) and encodes for a proteasome assembly chaperone 1 (Consortium TASC, 2010). According to the authors' opinion, it is unlikely that *PSMG1* is a candidate gene directly involved in AS susceptibility since 1) this gene was not differentially expressed in peripheral blood mononuclear cells from cases with active AS when compared with healthy controls, 2) the large distance to the associated locus and 3) the lack of evidence of a relevant biological function.

It is suggested that both these regions at chromosomes 2p15 and 21q22, contain long mRNA-like noncoding RNA species or until now unreported protein-coding genes that may be involved in AS susceptibility (Consortium TASC, 2010).

3. Genes suggestively associated with ankylosing spondylitis

3.1 IL1 gene cluster

Interleukin-1 (IL-1) and its related family members are key cytokines in autoimmune and inflammatory diseases produced by monocytes, macrophages, and dendritic cells. They are cell surface associated proteins and stimulate the expression of several genes, affecting both the innate and acquired immune systems (Dinarello, 2002). IL1-F1, IL1-F2, IL1-F3, and IL1-F4 are the primary members of the family. IL1-F1, IL1-F2, and IL1-F4 are each agonist while IL1-F3 is a receptor antagonist for IL1-F1, IL1-F2 (Dinarello, 2002). When the antagonist occupies the receptor, there is no signal transduction as the IL1-F1 and IL1-F2 can not bind the specific receptor. All *IL-1* genes are located on the long arm of chromosome 2 except IL-18 and IL-18 binding protein (IL-18BP) which are located on chromosome 11. Some member of the family as IL1-F5, IL1-F7, and IL1-F9 are gene duplications and they are very closely related to IL1-F3 (Mulero, et al., 1999). The exact function of these genes is still unclear.

The IL-1 receptor family is composed of nine genes. IL1-R1, IL1-R2, and IL1-R3 are the bona fide receptors while the rest are called 'orphan' receptors as they lack of specific ligand Anyway, some gene regulation studies found non-specific proteins binding to orphan receptors (Gayle, et al., 1996; Moritz, et al., 1998; Parnet, et al., 1996; Torigoe, et al., 1997). The most studied receptor of the family is the IL1-R2 (Symons, et al., 1991). IL1-R2 receptor acts as a decoy receptor. It has a high affinity for IL1-F1 and IL1-F2 and a lower affinity for IL1-F3. After the cleavage from cell membrane by ERAP1, IL1-R2 binds IL1-F1 interfering with IL1-F1 / IL1-R1 binding. Its extracellular domain is homologue of the IL1-R1 but the intracellular domain is shorter and lacks of TIR domain (Dunne & O'Neill, 2003). Therefore when activated, IL-R2 is unable to initiate any biological response.

Positive association between AS and *IL1-F3* gene was observed in earlier studies with high frequency of the allele 2 of *IL1-F3* variable nucleotide tandem repeat (VNTR) in AS patients (Dunne & O'Neill, 2003; van der Paardt, et al., 2002). The result was further confirmed through a recent study on meta-analysis of *IL-1* gene cluster (Wu & Gu, 2007). A significant association between two *IL1-F3* intronic SNPs and AS susceptibility was also found at position 30735 and 30017 in exon 6 (Chou, et al., 2006; Maksymowych, W. P., et al., 2003). A significant difference of the distribution of haplotypes was found between the AS affected and healthy individuals. On the contrary, in earlier studies no association between AS and *IL1-F3* gene was found (Djouadi, et al., 2001; Jin, et al., 2004; Kim, et al., 2005; Maksymowych, W. P., et al., 2006; Timms, A. E., et al., 2004). These findings were also observed in the genome scan carried out by North American Spondylitis Consortium (NASC) (Jin, et al., 2004). In this work, six exons and introns in 102 white patients and 50 controls were sequenced and no association was revealed. Moreover, other genes in the *IL-1* cluster have been analyzed. In nine *IL-1* genes, were identified SNPs showing significant association with AS (Timms, A. E., et al., 2004). Maksymowych et al. identified 14 SNPs with high association in at least one cohort (Maksymowych, W. P., et al., 2006). The most significant cohorts were in IL1-F1 and IL1-F2. In a more recent meta-analysis nine SNPs were analyzed and a strong association was observed in three IL1-F1 loci (Sims, A. M., et al., 2008).

3.2 ANTXR2

The *ANTXR2* gene encodes for a transmembrane protein which serves as receptor of anthrax toxin (Thomas & Brown, 2010). Also known as capillary morphogenesis protein 2 (CMP2), the receptor recognises and binds the toxin, allowing anthrax to attach the cells and triggering the disease process. It is widely expressed in human tissue including in the hearth, lung, liver, placenta, small intestine, kidney, colon, and skeletal muscles. Expressed primarily in macrofages, it is involved in capillary formation and extracellular matrix adhesion (Reveille, J D, 2011). Recessive mutations in ANTXR2 gene are associated to two autosomal diseases, infantile systemic hyalinosis (ISH; MIM#237490) and juvenile hyaline fibromatosis (JHF; MIM#228600) (Consortium TASC, 2010).

In a recent study on unrelated cases of AS among Australian, British, and North American individuals of European descent, carried out by TASC, a strong association between polymorphism in *ANTXR2* gene and AS was found (Consortium TASC, 2010). In the same year, investigating on AS susceptibility in 1164 Korean patients, Bang et al. confirmed the differentially expression of *ANTXR2* gene in AS (Bang, et al., 2011). In contrast no association was observed between *ANTXR2* polymorphism and AS in Chinese Han population (Chen, C., et al., 2010). With these divergent results, it is still not clear if ANTXR2 influences the disease and how it is involved in the pathogenesis. IT has been suggested that it can act at intestinal permeability level given its function in epithelial barriers (Thomas & Brown, 2010). The previous results reported by TASC were confirmed by another GWS that also found significant association in the ANTXR2 area ($P = 9.4 \times 10^{-8}$) (Consortium TASC/WTCCC2, 2011).

3.3 TNFSF15

The Tumor Necrosis Factor Ligand Superfamily, Member 15 (TNFSF15, also known as TNF superfamily ligand A, TL1A or vascular endothelial cell growth inhibitor, VEGI) is a TNF-like factor encoded on the chromosome 9 (9q32). The molecules are primarily expressed in endothelial cells and its expression is highly inducible by TNF and IL-1A (Migone, et al., 2002; Yue, et al., 1999). Strong evidences point to a significant genetic association between the TNFSF15 gene and inflammatory bowel disease (IBD). The data was obtained in populations from different ethnic backgrounds, namely Caucasians and Japanese (Yamazaki, et al., 2005). A WGAS for AS in Caucasians reported the existence of linkage on chromosome 9q (Laval, et al., 2001). This was supported by another WGS for spondyloarthropathies (SpA) susceptibility genes, performed on multiplex families, which detected a significant linkage on chromosome 9q31-34, including the TNFSF15 encoding region (Miceli-Richard, et al., 2004). However, this region was not identified in a recent GWAS (Consortium TASC, 2010).

Recently, comprehensive linkage and association analyses reported, for the first time, an association between several SNPs near the *TNFSF15* gene and SpA (Zinovieva, et al., 2009). The authors aimed to narrow down the susceptibility region for SpA found on the first GWAS reported by the same authors (Miceli-Richard, et al., 2004). The obtained data showed two areas of statistically significance linkage. The highest linkage peak was located on the marker D9S1824 at 115.9 Mb from the p-telomere. The second significant area was located near D9S1682, a suggestive linkage peak reported in WGS for AS (Laval, et al., 2001). This finding supports the validity of linkage between this region and SpA.

The analysis of combined data from family-based and case/control studies showed a strong association ($P<0.001$) of 7 SNPs: rs4979459, rs7849556, rs10817669, rs10759734, rs6478105, rs10982396 and rs10733612 (Zinovieva, et al., 2009). The SNP rs4246905 also showed a significant result but with a lower level ($P=0.01$). Six of this SNPs compose a 40.3 Kb block with a high degree of LD, found in the same study. This LD block included two genes, *LOC389786* and *TNFSF15* (Zinovieva, et al., 2009). The rs6478105 revealed to be the strongest individual associated SNP in the overall dataset ($P=3x10^{-5}$). The SNPs associated with Crohn's disease were not associated with SpA in this study. Haplotypes research also confirmed this tendency and showed that haplotypes composed of markers of this block were significantly associated with the disease. Two significant individual haplotypes were found in family-based study: rs7849556/ rs10817669/ rs10759734/ rs6478105/ rs10982396/ rs10733612 - AAAACC and rs7849556/ rs10817669/ rs10759734/ rs6478105/ rs10982396/ rs10733612 - CGGACT. The pooled case/control investigation revealed a significant strong association of the individual haplotype rs7849556/ rs10817669/ rs10759734/ rs6478105/ rs10982396/ rs10733612 - CGGGGT (Zinovieva, et al., 2009).

TNFSF15 is a ligand for the receptors DR3 (death domain receptor 3, also known as TNFRSF25 (tumor necrosis factor receptor super-family, member 25) and TR6/DcR3 (decoy receptor 3, also called TNFRSF6B - tumor necrosis factor receptor super-family, member 6b) (Migone, et al., 2002). The ligand-receptor pairing of TNFSF15-DR3 was already pointed as a regulator of Th17 differentiation and activation (Pappu, et al., 2008; Takedatsu, et al., 2008). An increased level of Th17 cells in AS patients, when compared to healthy controls, was already reported (Jandus, et al., 2008). Therefore, targeting the TNFSF15-DR3 pathway could provide new insights in the role of TNFS15 in AS development.

3.4 TNFRSF1A and TRADD

The TNFRSF1A (Tumor necrosis factor receptor superfamily member 1A, also known as tumor necrosis factor receptor 1 - TNFR1) association with AS was reported by the TASC GWAS. Several *TNFRSF1A* SNPs showed moderate levels of association in the discovery set and, among them, rs1800693 showed the strongest association (P=6.9x10-5) (Consortium TASC, 2010). It was hypothasized that TNF1, encoded by *TNFRSF1A*, was cleaved by ERAP1. The data suggested that ERAP1 extracellular domain binds to the TNFR1 extracellular domain and acts as an extracellular TNFR1 regulatory protein that would promote TNFR1 shedding (Cui, et al., 2002). However, as already mentioned in ERAP1 section, no correlation between presence of ERAP1 and decrease of TNFR1 levels was observed in cultured cells from mice (Consortium TASC/WTCCC2, 2011).

TNF antagonists are highly effective in suppressing inflammation in AS. Thus, some data obtained from studies with mice showed that mesenchymal cells are common primary targets for TNF in the development of AS, and that selective expression of *TNFRSF1A* on those cells is enough to cause the complete development of AS, as well as inflammatory polyarthritis and inflammatory bowel disease (IBD) (Armaka, et al., 2008). The determination of the polymorphisms involved on that action would allow a better understanding of the relation between *TNFRSF1A* gene and AS. TRADD (TNF receptor type 1-associated death domain) is located on chromosome 16q, a region already reported in linkage studies (Laval, et al., 2001). TRADD registered moderate levels of association and lies between the SNPs rs9033 and rs868213, which already showed strong association with AS (Pointon, et al., 2010). This gene is a key component of the TNFR1-signaling cascade and is involved in TLR3, TLR4 and D3 signaling (Chen, N. J., et al., 2008; Chinnaiyan, et al., 1996; Hsu, H., et al., 1995).

Recently it was found an AS associated SNP at chromosome 12p13 between LTBR (lymphotoxin beta receptor) and TNFRSF1A (rs11616188; $P = 4.1 \times 10{-}12$). The authors also found an association at chromosome 17q21 near *TBKBP1* (encoding TBK binding protein 1), a component of the TNFR signaling pathway (rs8070463, $P = 5.3 \times 10{-}8$). Here, TRADD also showed suggestive association with AS in this study, namely SNP rs9033 ($P = 4.9 \times 10{-}5$) (Consortium TASC/WTCCC2, 2011). Once more, it is mandatory to continue research at this level to determine the precise mechanism underlying these associations.

3.5 CYP2D6

The cytochrome P450 enzymes are responsible for the majority of oxidative (phase I) drug metabolism (1)(Gonzalez, 1992); they are polymorphic although 5-10% of Europeans lack this activity (described as poor metabolisers) (Cholerton, et al., 1992). At least 15 allelic variants of *CYP2D6*, that is inherited as an autosomal recessive trait, can cause poor metaboliser phenotype, but 75% of these are CYP2D6*4 (Brown, et al., 2000). The *CYP2D6* genotype was found to be associated with other chronic inflammatory disease and with cancer (Baer, et al., 1986; Daly, et al., 1994).

Beyeler et al. (Beyeler, et al., 1996) first reported a relationship between this gene and the susceptibility to AS, investigating 54 patients and 662 healthy volunteers. The association was modest between AS and CYP2D6 genotype and the effect was greatest for the *CYP2D6B* allele.

Brown et al. (Brown, et al., 2000) studied linkage of the *CYP2D6* gene and association of the main poor metabolizer genotype in 617 unrelated AS patients, 402 healthy controls, and in 361 families with AS. Significant association was observed between homozygosity for CYP2D6*4 and AS, but heterozygosity for allele 4 was not disease associated, and weak linkage of the *CYP2D6* polymorphism and AS was found with a LOD score of 0.9. The authors suggested that dysfunction of the *CYP2D6* gene increases the risk of AS, although only contributing a small proportion of the overall risk of the disease.

A more recent Turkish study, investigating 100 unrelated AS patients and 52 healthy controls, found no significant risk of AS development for patients with one or two CYP2D6*4 alleles (Erden, et al., 2009).

In conclusion, the cytochrome P450 gene debrisoquine 4-hydroxilase (*CYP2D6*), encoded at 22q13.1, may have a moderate support for involvement in susceptibility to AS. The mechanisms for susceptibility are unknown but it is possible that the ubiquitous environmental trigger of AS is a natural toxin and reducing its metabolism could increase susceptibility to disease (Brown, 2006).

4. Other genes

4.1 KIR

The Killer immunoglobulin-like receptor (KIR) genes are a polymorphic group of genes located on chromosome 19q13.4, and they span 150Kb of the leucocyte receptor complex (LCR) (Hsu, K. C., et al., 2002). They express a family of proteins which are activating and inhibitory receptors expressed on natural killer (NK) cells and on a subset of T cells (CD8+). They have been classified in two types: Activating KIRs (KIR2DS and KIR3DS), which have a short (S) cytoplasmic tail with the capacity to interact with activating adaptor proteins such as DAP12 (Lanier, et al., 1998), and inhibitory *KIR* (KIR2DL and KIR3DL), which has one or two immunoreceptor tyrosine-based inhibition motifs in their long (L) cytoplasmic tail. Further to the allelic polymorphism, haplotypic variability is also described and according to gene content, haplotypes were divided in two basic groups: Haplotype A contains only one activating KIR gene, 2DS4, whereas Haplotype B contains various combinations of activating *KIR* genes, KIR2DS1, -2DS2, -2DS3, -2DS5, - 3DS1, and -2DS4, exhibiting extreme diversity, resulting in different signaling potentials to NK and T cells (Hsu, K. C., et al., 2002).

The precise function of some KIRs is controversial but it was demonstrated that mature class I complexes act as ligands for immunomodulatary receptors, and it is known that KIR proteins recognize subsets of HLA-A, -B, or –C alleles (Parham, P., 2005). It is possible that KIRs may synergise with HLAs to generate activating or inhibitory compound genotypes that provide different levels of activation and inhibition for NK or T cells, which may be associated with differing susceptibility to or protection against a range of diseases.

A study in Caucasian populations demonstrated genetic evidence for the implication of KIR3DL1 and the activating counterpart, KIR3DS1 in AS (Lopez-Larrea, C., et al., 2006). In this study the inhibitory allele was decreased in AS patients compared with B27-positive healthy controls, whereas KIR3DS1 was increased in AS patients. Another study by the same group in two Asian B27-positive populations (China and Thailand), reported some KIR associations with AS susceptibility (Diaz-Pena, et al., 2008). The authors hypothesized that AS patients could possess more activating *KIR* genes than the healthy control subjects, which could create a genetic imbalance between inhibitory and activating *KIR* genes that could have influence on the AS pathogenesis.

Another study genotyped 200 UK AS patients and 405 healthy controls for 14 *KIR* genes. Additionally, sequence-specific oligonucleotide probes were used to subtype 368 cases with AS and 366 controls for 12 KIR3DL2 alleles. The authors concluded that neither the *KIR* gene content of particular KIR haplotypes nor KIR3DL2 polymorphisms contribute to AS (Harvey, et al., 2009b).

Two more recent studies, one from China and another one from Spain investigated the association of KIR and AS susceptibility. The Chinese study investigated 115 unrelated HLA-B27-positive AS patients and 119 HLA-B27-positive healthy controls, and concluded that the frequencies of KIR2DL1 and KIR2DL5 were significantly higher in the AS patient group although they did not reach statistical significance. Furthermore, the investigators also concluded that HLA-Cw*08 was present more frequently in AS patients than in healthy B27 controls, raising the possibility that HLA-Cw*08 recognized KIRs through the Asp80, thereby contributing to the immune regulation in AS (Jiao, et al., 2010). In the Spanish study 270 AS patients and 435 healthy HLA-B27-positive controls from Spain were genotyped for KIR3DL1/S1 alleles. The authors found that the KIR3DS1*013 allele frequency was increased in patients with AS, and that the null allele KIR3DL1*004 was a unique inhibitory KIR3DL1 allele that showed a negative association with AS (Diaz-Pena, et al., 2010).

Genome-wide scans have implicated regions on chromosomes 2q, 6q, 10q, 11q, 16q, 17q, and 19q in AS. The *KIR* genes are located on chromosome 19q13.4 in the LCR, and obviously are good candidates for AS susceptibility (Carter, et al., 2007). More recent investigations using different approaches like the report of the TASC/WTCCC2, did not identify this chromosome region as involved in AS susceptibility (Consortium TASC/WTCCC2, 2011). The influence of KIR/HLA genotypes in AS susceptibility may be mediated by a general imbalance between the protective/inhibitory and the risk/activating allotypes. Further studies in other populations are needed to confirm the role of KIR genes in AS susceptibility.

4.2 ANKH

The *ANKH* gene maps to human chromosome 5 (5p15.1) and encodes a 492 amino acid multiple-pass transmembrane protein (ANK) which transports the inorganic pyrophosphate (PPi) across the plasma membrane into the extracellular compartment (Gurley, K.A., et al., 2006b). ANK function is essential in joints to inhibit mineral formation in joints and maintain mobility (Gurley, K. A., et al., 2006a). Mutations in the *ANKH* gene have been consistently associated with two autosomal dominant skeletal disorders: familial chondrocalcinosis (MIM #118600) and craniometaphyseal dysplasia (MIM #123000).

In the last decade, a very small number of reports suggested an association of AN*KH* with AS. In 2003, two polymorphisms - ANKH-OR and ANKH-TR - in complete linkage disequilibrium, located in the 5'-noncoding region and in the promoter region of this gene, respectively, were found to be significantly associated with AS. After linkage analysis and family-based association studies the authors concluded that *ANKH* could be among the most important non-MHC loci for AS susceptibility (Tsui, F W, et al., 2003). In a follow-up study, with 201 multiplex AS families, it was reported that the region associated with AS in women only showed significance in the test of interaction among the subset of families with affected individuals of both genders. These findings supported the concept that *ANKH* plays a role in genetic susceptibility to AS revealing a gender-genotype specificity in this interaction (Tsui, H W, et al., 2005). Contradicting these results, a small study performed in a cohort of 233 patients and 478 controls, revealed no association between *ANKH* locus and either susceptibility to AS or its clinical manifestations (Timms, A E, et al., 2003).

In another study, the authors examined a total of 45 SNPs in 15 genes by a sequential screening. 170 Japanese AS patients and 896 controls for the SNPs were first genotyped. Then, eight SNPs with $P < 0.05$ in the first screen were genotyped for 108 additional Japanese patients. The replication of the association of the most significant SNP was checked by genotyping 219 Taiwanese AS patients and 185 controls. After combining the first and second screens, four SNPs showed nominal significance of $P < 0.05$. One synonymous SNP in *ANKH*, c.963T > G, showed a marginal association in the Japanese population ($P = 0.045$) (Furuichi, et al., 2008). This association is not consistent and was not replicated in recent GWAS studies with large cohorts.

4.3 TGFB1

The *TGFB1* gene codifies for the human transforming growth factor β1 (TGFβ1) (van der Paardt, et al., 2005b) located on chromosome 19q21.1. It is a multifunctional cytokine involved in inflammation, fibrosis and bone remodelling (Reveille, J D, 2011). The concentration of TGFβ1 in cartilage and bone is 100 times superior to other tissues (Centrella, et al., 1991). It was demonstrate that injections of TGFβ1 into young rat bone induce formation of cartilaginous mass and subsequently bone tissue (Joyce, et al., 1990). Whether the effect is positive with growing bones or negative with damaged bones depends on the concentration of TGFβ1 and the presence of other hormones (Archer & Keat, 1999). Therefore, TGFβ1 represent a good candidate for a key cytokine in a disease characterized by chronic inflammation of the sacroiliac joints.

A marginal association between TGFB1 and AS was observed in a study of Finnish and British families (Jaakkola, et al., 2004) and in a Scottish case study (McGarry, et al., 2002).

The Scottish genotype showed a strong correlation with high concentration of TGFβ1. On the other side, no significant association with AS susceptibility was reported in two following studies in Dutch and Southern Chinese populations (Howe, et al., 2005; van der Paardt, et al., 2005b); although, in the Dutch study, the frequency of mutated allele was greater in AS patients than in the healthy individuals. The TGFB1 polymorphism might be implicated to the AS disease at bone formation level but further studies are necessary. Understanding the role of TGFβ1 in AS could be interesting especially to develop new pharmacological approaches in order to prevent the disorder (van der Paardt, et al., 2005b).

4.4 CD14

The Cluster of differentiation 14 (CD14) gene maps to chromosome 5 (5q22-q3215q31.1) and encodes 2 protein forms: a 50 to 55 kD glycosylphosphatidylinositol-anchored membrane protein (mCD14) and a monocyte or liver-derived soluble serum protein (sCD14) that lacks the anchor. Both molecules are essential for lipopolysaccharide (LPS)-dependent signal transduction. Increased sCD14 levels are associated with inflammatory infectious diseases and high mortality in gram-negative shock (LeVan, et al., 2001).

A putative role of *CD14* in the pathogenesis of AS was investigated due to its significant role on the innate immune system. The polymorphism C-260T was studied in genomic DNA from 113 unrelated Dutch AS patients and 170 healthy controls. No significant differences were found between the frequency of this allele in patients and controls suggesting that this polymorphism is not involved in the susceptibility to AS (van der Paardt, et al., 2005a). On the other hand, evidence of association was identified between this allele and AS in a small cohort of Finnish families (Pointon, et al., 2008). No other studies about CD14 and its association with AS have been published suggesting that this association is not established.

4.5 TNAP

Tissue-Nonspecific Alkaline Phosphatase (TNAP) is an isozyme of a family of four homologous human alkaline phosphatase genes. It is present in the matrix vesicles and has the ability of hydrolyze PPi. In humans, this enzyme is enconded by the gene *TNAP*, that maps in chromosome 1, containing 12 exons. Deactivating mutations in the *TNAP* gene cause hypophosphatasia [MIM#241500 (Infantile form), MIM#146300 (Adult type)], characterized by poorly mineralized cartilage and bones, spontaneous bone fractures, chondrocalcinosis by calcium pyrophosphate deposition and elevated concentrations of pyrophosphate (PPi) (Mornet, et al., 1998).

One study has shown the significant association of the *TNAP* haplotype rs3767155(G) / rs3738099 (G) / rs1780329 (T) with AS but in men only (Tsui, H. W., et al., 2007). This association was later investigated in a case control study involving a cohort of 353 AS patients and 514 unrelated healthy controls, and a family-based association study with 57 pedigrees, of the Chinese Han population. Two intronic SNPs (rs3767155 and rs1780329) were genotyped; the results showed no significant difference in allele, genotype or haplotype frequencies between AS patients and controls (Cheng, et al., 2009). No other studies have replicated the association of TNAP to AS.

5. Conclusion

AS susceptibility is no longer an HLA-B27 exclusive. The association of AS and ERAP1, IL23R and the intergenic regions 2p15 and 21q22 has been confirmed in large cohort studies. This knowledge increased the complexity of genes involved in AS susceptibility; however, it is shortening the way to a better understanding about AS immunopathogenesis.

The identification of associated genetic regions outside MHC will require a large number of replicates in populations with different ethnic backgrounds. The consistent data already obtained, and the results that will come up from new replicates, should provide a solid basis to new research that may unravel the mechanisms underlying all these associations. Consequently, the AS pathway will start to present an even more conclusive and consistent shape, providing new tools to clinicians and allowing an improvement in the disease diagnosis and treatment. More, the identified and confirmed markers could be used to create a complete diagnosis testing panel, along with HLA-B27.

6. References

Archer, J. R. & A. C. Keat. (1999). Ankylosing spondylitis: time to focus on ankylosis. *J Rheumatol*,Vol. 26, No. 4, (Apr), pp. (761-4), 0315-162X

Armaka, M., M. Apostolaki, P. Jacques, D. L. Kontoyiannis, D. Elewaut & G. Kollias. (2008). Mesenchymal cell targeting by TNF as a common pathogenic principle in chronic inflammatory joint and intestinal diseases. *J Exp Med*,Vol. 205, No. 2, (Feb 18), pp. (331-7), 1540-9538 (Electronic), 0022-1007 (Linking)

Armas, J. B., S. Gonzalez, J. Martinez-Borra, F. Laranjeira, E. Ribeiro, J. Correia, M. L. Ferreira, M. Toste, A. Lopez-Vazquez & C. Lopez-Larrea. (1999). Susceptibility to ankylosing spondylitis is independent of the Bw4 and Bw6 epitopes of HLA-B27 alleles. *Tissue Antigens*,Vol. 53, No. 3, pp. (237-43),

Baer, A. N., C. B. McAllister, G. R. Wilkinson, R. L. Woosley & T. Pincus. (1986). Altered distribution of debrisoquine oxidation phenotypes in patients with systemic lupus erythematosus. *Arthritis Rheum*,Vol. 29, No. 7, (Jul), pp. (843-50), 0004-3591 (Print), 0004-3591 (Linking)

Ball, E. J. & M. A. Khan. (2001). HLA-B27 polymorphism. *Joint Bone Spine*,Vol. 68, No. 5, (October 2001), pp. (378-382),

Bang, S. Y., T. H. Kim, B. Lee, E. Kwon, S. H. Choi, K. S. Lee, S. C. Shim, A. Pope, P. Rahman, J. D. Reveille & R. D. Inman. (2011). Genetic studies of ankylosing spondylitis in Koreans confirm associations with ERAP1 and 2p15 reported in white patients. *J Rheumatol*,Vol. 38, No. 2, (Feb), pp. (322-4), 0315-162X

Belladonna, M. L., J. C. Renauld, R. Bianchi, C. Vacca, F. Fallarino, C. Orabona, M. C. Fioretti, U. Grohmann & P. Puccetti. (2002). IL-23 and IL-12 have overlapping, but distinct, effects on murine dendritic cells. *J Immunol*,Vol. 168, No. 11, (Jun 1), pp. (5448-54), 0022-1767

Beyeler, C., M. Armstrong, H. A. Bird, J. R. Idle & A. K. Daly. (1996). Relationship between genotype for the cytochrome P450 CYP2D6 and susceptibility to ankylosing spondylitis and rheumatoid arthritis. *Ann Rheum Dis*,Vol. 55, No. 1, (Jan), pp. (66-8), 0003-4967 (Print)

Brionez, T. F. & J. D. Reveille. (2008). The contribution of genes outside the major histocompatibility complex to susceptibility to ankylosing spondylitis. *Curr Opin Rheumatol*,Vol. 20, No. 4, (Jul), pp. (384-91), 1040-8711

Brown, M. A., K. D. Pile, L. G. Kennedy, A. Calin, C. Darke, J. Bell, B. P. Wordsworth & F. Cornelis. (1996). HLA class I associations of ankylosing spondylitis in the white population in the United Kingdom. *Annals of the Rheumatic Diseases*,Vol. 55, No. 4, (April 1996), pp. (268-70),

Brown, M. A., L. G. Kennedy, A. J. MacGregor, C. Darke, E. Duncan, J. L. Shatford, A. Taylor, A. Calin & P. Wordsworth. (1997). Susceptibility to ankylosing spondylitis in twins: the role of genes, HLA, and the environment. *Arthritis Rheum*,Vol. 40, No. 10, (October 1997), pp. (1823-1828),

Brown, M. A., L. G. Kennedy, C. Darke, K. Gibson, K. D. Pile, J. L. Shatford, A. Calin & B. P. Wordsworth. (1998a). The effect of HLA-DR genes on susceptibility to and severity of ankylosing spondylitis. *Arthritis Rheum*,Vol. 41, No. 3, (March 1998), pp. (460-465),

Brown, M. A., K. D. Pile, L. G. Kennedy, D. Campbell, L. Andrew, R. March, J. L. Shatford, D. E. Weeks, A. Calin & B. P. Wordsworth. (1998b). A genome wide-screen for susceptibility loci in ankylosing spondylitis. *Arthritis Rheum*,Vol. 41, No. 4, (April 1998), pp. (588-595),

Brown, M. A., S. Edwards, E. Hoyle, S. Campbell, S. Laval, A. K. Daly, K. D. Pile, A. Calin, A. Ebringer, D. E. Weeks & B. P. Wordsworth. (2000). Polymorphisms of the CYP2D6 gene increase susceptibility to ankylosing spondylitis. *Hum Mol Genet*,Vol. 9, No. 11, (Jul 1), pp. (1563-6), 0964-6906 (Print), 0964-6906 (Linking)

Brown, M. A. (2006). Non-major-histocompatibility-complex genetics of ankylosing spondylitis. *Best Pract Res Clin Rheumatol*,Vol. 20, No. 3, (Jun), pp. (611-21), 1521-6942 (Print), 1521-6942 (Linking)

Brown, M. A. (2010). Genetics of ankylosing spondylitis. *Curr Opin Rheumatol*,Vol. 22, No. 2, (March 2010), pp. (126-132), 1531-6963 (Electronic)

Campbell, E. C., F. Fettke, S. Bhat, K. D. Morley & S. J. Powis. (2011). Expression of MHC class I dimers and ERAP1 in an ankylosing spondylitis patient cohort. *Immunology*,Vol. 133, No. 3, (Jul), pp. (379-85), 1365-2567 (Electronic), 0019-2805 (Linking)

Cargill, M., S. J. Schrodi, M. Chang, V. E. Garcia, R. Brandon, K. P. Callis, N. Matsunami, K. G. Ardlie, D. Civello, J. J. Catanese, D. U. Leong, J. M. Panko, L. B. McAllister, C. B. Hansen, J. Papenfuss, S. M. Prescott, T. J. White, M. F. Leppert, G. G. Krueger & A. B. Begovich. (2007). A large-scale genetic association study confirms IL12B and leads to the identification of IL23R as psoriasis-risk genes. *Am J Hum Genet*,Vol. 80, No. 2, (Feb), pp. (273-90), 0002-9297 (Print), 0002-9297 (Linking)

Carter, K. W., A. Pluzhnikov, A. E. Timms, C. Miceli-Richard, C. Bourgain, B. P. Wordsworth, H. Jean-Pierre, N. J. Cox, L. J. Palmer, M. Breban, J. D. Reveille & M. A. Brown. (2007). Combined analysis of three whole genome linkage scans for Ankylosing Spondylitis. *Rheumatology (Oxford)*,Vol. 46, No. 5, (May), pp. (763-71), 1462-0324

Centrella, M., T. L. McCarthy & E. Canalis. (1991). Transforming growth factor-beta and remodeling of bone. *J Bone Joint Surg Am*,Vol. 73, No. 9, (Oct), pp. (1418-28), 0021-9355

Chen, C., X. Zhang & Y. Wang. (2010). ANTXR2 and IL-1R2 polymorphisms are not associated with ankylosing spondylitis in Chinese Han population. *Rheumatol Int*,Vol. (Jul 21), 1437-160X (Electronic), 0172-8172 (Linking)

Chen, N. J., Chio, II, W. J. Lin, G. Duncan, H. Chau, D. Katz, H. L. Huang, K. A. Pike, Z. Hao, Y. W. Su, K. Yamamoto, R. F. de Pooter, J. C. Zuniga-Pflucker, A. Wakeham, W. C. Yeh & T. W. Mak. (2008). Beyond tumor necrosis factor receptor: TRADD signaling in toll-like receptors. *Proc Natl Acad Sci U S A*,Vol. 105, No. 34, (Aug 26), pp. (12429-34), 1091-6490 (Electronic), 0027-8424 (Linking)

Chen, R., L. Yao, T. Meng & W. Xu. (2011). The association between seven ERAP1 polymorphisms and ankylosing spondylitis susceptibility: a meta-analysis involving 8,530 cases and 12,449 controls. *Rheumatol Int*,Vol. (Jan 13), pp. 1437-160X (Electronic), 0172-8172 (Linking)

Cheng, N., Q. Cai, M. Fang, S. Duan, J. Lin, J. Hu, R. Chen & S. Sun. (2009). No significant association between genetic polymorphisms in the TNAP gene and ankylosing spondylitis in the Chinese Han population. *Rheumatol Int*,Vol. 29, No. 3, (Jan), pp. (305-10), 0172-8172 (Print), 0172-8172 (Linking)

Chinnaiyan, A. M., K. O'Rourke, G. L. Yu, R. H. Lyons, M. Garg, D. R. Duan, L. Xing, R. Gentz, J. Ni & V. M. Dixit. (1996). Signal transduction by DR3, a death domain-containing receptor related to TNFR-1 and CD95. *Science*,Vol. 274, No. 5289, (Nov 8), pp. (990-2), 0036-8075 (Print), 0036-8075 (Linking)

Choi, C. B., T. H. Kim, J. B. Jun, H. S. Lee, S. C. Shim, B. Lee, A. Pope, M. Uddin, P. Rahman & R. D. Inman. (2010). ARTS1 polymorphisms are associated with ankylosing spondylitis in Koreans. *Ann Rheum Dis*,Vol. 69, No. 3, (Mar), pp. (582-4), 1468-2060 (Electronic), 0003-4967 (Linking)

Cholerton, S., A. K. Daly & J. R. Idle. (1992). The role of individual human cytochromes P450 in drug metabolism and clinical response. *Trends Pharmacol Sci*,Vol. 13, No. 12, (Dec), pp. (434-9), 0165-6147 (Print), 0165-6147 (Linking)

Chou, C. T., A. E. Timms, J. C. Wei, W. C. Tsai, B. P. Wordsworth & M. A. Brown. (2006). Replication of association of IL1 gene complex members with ankylosing spondylitis in Taiwanese Chinese. *Ann Rheum Dis*,Vol. 65, No. 8, (Aug), pp. (1106-9), 0003-4967 (Print), 0003-4967 (Linking)

Consortium TASC. (2010). Genome-wide association study of ankylosing spondylitis identifies non-MHC susceptibility loci. *Nat Genet*,Vol. 42, No. 2, (Feb), pp. (123-7), 1546-1718 (Electronic), 1061-4036 (Linking)

Consortium TASC/WTCCC2. (2011). Interaction between ERAP1 and HLA-B27 in ankylosing spondylitis implicates peptide handling in the mechanism for HLA-B27 in disease susceptibility. *Nat Genet*,Vol. (Jul 10 - [Epub]), pp. 1546-1718 (Electronic), 1061-4036 (Linking)

Consortium WTCCC/TASC. (2007). Association scan of 14,500 nonsynonymous SNPs in four diseases identifies autoimmunity variants. *Nat Genet*,Vol. 39, No. 11, (Nov), pp. (1329-37), 1546-1718 (Electronic), 1061-4036 (Linking)

Cua, D. J., J. Sherlock, Y. Chen, C. A. Murphy, B. Joyce, B. Seymour, L. Lucian, W. To, S. Kwan, T. Churakova, S. Zurawski, M. Wiekowski, S. A. Lira, D. Gorman, R. A. Kastelein & J. D. Sedgwick. (2003). Interleukin-23 rather than interleukin-12 is the critical cytokine for autoimmune inflammation of the brain. *Nature*,Vol. 421, No. 6924, (Feb 13), pp. (744-8), 0028-0836 (Print), 0028-0836 (Linking)

Cui, X., F. Hawari, S. Alsaaty, M. Lawrence, C. A. Combs, W. Geng, F. N. Rouhani, D. Miskinis & S. J. Levine. (2002). Identification of ARTS-1 as a novel TNFR1-binding protein that promotes TNFR1 ectodomain shedding. *J Clin Invest*,Vol. 110, No. 4, (Aug), pp. (515-26), 0021-9738 (Print), 0021-9738 (Linking)

Cui, X., F. N. Rouhani, F. Hawari & S. J. Levine. (2003a). Shedding of the type II IL-1 decoy receptor requires a multifunctional aminopeptidase, aminopeptidase regulator of TNF receptor type 1 shedding. *J Immunol*,Vol. 171, No. 12, (Dec 15), pp. (6814-9), 0022-1767 (Print), 0022-1767 (Linking)

Cui, X., F. N. Rouhani, F. Hawari & S. J. Levine. (2003b). An aminopeptidase, ARTS-1, is required for interleukin-6 receptor shedding. *J Biol Chem*,Vol. 278, No. 31, (Aug 1), pp. (28677-85), 0021-9258 (Print), 0021-9258 (Linking)

Daly, A. K., S. Cholerton, M. Armstrong & J. R. Idle. (1994). Genotyping for polymorphisms in xenobiotic metabolism as a predictor of disease susceptibility. *Environ Health Perspect*,Vol. 102 Suppl 9, (Nov), pp. (55-61), 0091-6765 (Print), 0091-6765 (Linking)

Danoy, P., K. Pryce, J. Hadler, L. A. Bradbury, C. Farrar, J. Pointon, M. Ward, M. Weisman, J. D. Reveille, B. P. Wordsworth, M. A. Stone, W. P. Maksymowych, P. Rahman, D. Gladman, R. D. Inman & M. A. Brown. (2010). Association of variants at 1q32 and STAT3 with ankylosing spondylitis suggests genetic overlap with Crohn's disease. *PLoS Genet*,Vol. 6, No. 12, pp. (e1001195), 1553-7404 (Electronic), 1553-7390 (Linking)

Davidson, S. I., X. Wu, Y. Liu, M. Wei, P. A. Danoy, G. Thomas, Q. Cai, L. Sun, E. Duncan, N. Wang, Q. Yu, A. Xu, Y. Fu, M. A. Brown & H. Xu. (2009). Association of ERAP1, but not IL23R, with ankylosing spondylitis in a Han Chinese population. *Arthritis Rheum*,Vol. 60, No. 11, (Nov), pp. (3263-8), 0004-3591 (Print), 0004-3591 (Linking)

Diaz-Pena, R., M. A. Blanco-Gelaz, B. Suarez-Alvarez, J. Martinez-Borra, A. Lopez-Vazquez, R. Alonso-Arias, J. Bruges-Armas, J. R. Vidal-Castineira & C. Lopez-Larrea. (2008). Activating KIR genes are associated with ankylosing spondylitis in Asian populations. *Hum Immunol*,Vol. 69, No. 7, (Jul), pp. (437-42), 0198-8859 (Print), 0198-8859 (Linking)

Diaz-Pena, R., J. R. Vidal-Castineira, R. Alonso-Arias, B. Suarez-Alvarez, J. L. Vicario, R. Solana, E. Collantes, A. Lopez-Vazquez, J. Martinez-Borra & C. Lopez-Larrea. (2010). Association of the KIR3DS1*013 and KIR3DL1*004 alleles with susceptibility to ankylosing spondylitis. *Arthritis Rheum*,Vol. 62, No. 4, (Apr), pp. (1000-6), 1529-0131 (Electronic), 0004-3591 (Linking)

Díaz-Peña, R., A. M. Aransay, J. Bruges-Armas, A. López-Vázquez, R.-E. N, I. Mendibil, A. Sánchez, T.-A. J. C, B. F. Bettencourt, J. Mulero, E. Collantes & C. López-Larrea. (2011). Fine Mapping of Major Histocompatibility Complex in Ankylosing Spondylitis: Association od HLA-DPA1 and HLA-DPB1 region. *In press*,Vol. pp.

Dinarello, C. A. (2002). The IL-1 family and inflammatory diseases. *Clin Exp Rheumatol*,Vol. 20, No. 5 Suppl 27, (Sep-Oct), pp. (S1-13), 0392-856X (Print), 0392-856X (Linking)

Djouadi, K., B. Nedelec, R. Tamouza, E. Genin, R. Ramasawmy, D. Charron, M. Delpech & S. Laoussadi. (2001). Interleukin 1 gene cluster polymorphisms in multiplex families with spondylarthropathies. *Cytokine*,Vol. 13, No. 2, (Jan 21), pp. (98-103), 1043-4666 (Print), 1043-4666 (Linking)

Duerr, R. H., K. D. Taylor, S. R. Brant, J. D. Rioux, M. S. Silverberg, M. J. Daly, A. H. Steinhart, C. Abraham, M. Regueiro, A. Griffiths, T. Dassopoulos, A. Bitton, H. Yang, S. Targan, L. W. Datta, E. O. Kistner, L. P. Schumm, A. T. Lee, P. K. Gregersen, M. M. Barmada, J. I. Rotter, D. L. Nicolae & J. H. Cho. (2006). A genome-wide association study identifies IL23R as an inflammatory bowel disease gene.

Science,Vol. 314, No. 5804, (Dec 1), pp. (1461-3), 1095-9203 (Electronic), 0036-8075 (Linking)

Dunne, A. & L. A. O'Neill. (2003). The interleukin-1 receptor/Toll-like receptor superfamily: signal transduction during inflammation and host defense. *Sci STKE*,Vol. 2003, No. 171, (Feb 25), pp. (re3), 1525-8882 (Electronic), 1525-8882 (Linking)

Erden, G., F. S. Acar, E. E. Inal, A. O. Soydas, K. Ozoran, H. Bodur & M. M. Yildirimkaya. (2009). Frequency of mutated allele CYP2D6*4 in the Turkish ankylosing spondylitis patients and healthy controls. *Rheumatol Int*,Vol. 29, No. 12, (Oct), pp. (1431-4), 1437-160X (Electronic), 0172-8172 (Linking)

Furuichi, T., K. Maeda, C. T. Chou, Y. F. Liu, T. C. Liu, Y. Miyamoto, A. Takahashi, K. Mori, K. Ikari, N. Kamatani, H. Kurosawa, H. Inoue, S. F. Tsai & S. Ikegawa. (2008). Association of the MSX2 gene polymorphisms with ankylosing spondylitis in Japanese. *J Hum Genet*,Vol. 53, No. 5, pp. (419-24), 1434-5161 (Print), 1434-5161 (Linking)

Garcia-Fernandez, S., S. Gonzalez, J. Martinez-Borra, M. Blanco-Gelaz, A. Lopez-Vazquez & C. Lopéz-Larrea. (2001). New insights regarding HLA-B27 diversity in the Asian population. *Tissue Antigenes*,Vol. 58, No. 4, (October 2001), pp. (259-262),

Garcia, F., D. Rognan, J. R. Lamas, A. Marina & L. d. C. J. A. (1998). An HLA-B27 polymorphism (B*2710) that is critical for T-cell recognition has limited effects on peptide specificity. *Tissue Antigens*,Vol. 51, No. 1, (January 1998), pp. (1-9),

Gayle, M. A., J. L. Slack, T. P. Bonnert, B. R. Renshaw, G. Sonoda, T. Taguchi, J. R. Testa, S. K. Dower & J. E. Sims. (1996). Cloning of a putative ligand for the T1/ST2 receptor. *J Biol Chem*,Vol. 271, No. 10, (Mar 8), pp. (5784-9), 0021-9258 (Print), 0021-9258 (Linking)

Gonzalez-Roces, S., M. V. Alvarez, S. Gonzalez, A. Dieye, H. Makni, D. G. Woodfield, L. Housan, V. Konenkov, M. C. Abbadi, N. Grunnet, E. Coto & C. Lopez-Larrea. (1997). HLA-B27 polymorphism and worldwide susceptibility to ankylosing spondylitis. *Tissue Antigens*,Vol. 49, No. 2, (February 1997), pp. (116-123),

Gonzalez, F. J. (1992). Human cytochromes P450: problems and prospects. *Trends Pharmacol Sci*,Vol. 13, No. 9, (Sep), pp. (346-52), 0165-6147 (Print), 0165-6147 (Linking)

Goto, Y., H. Tanji, A. Hattori & M. Tsujimoto. (2008). Glutamine-181 is crucial in the enzymatic activity and substrate specificity of human endoplasmic-reticulum aminopeptidase-1. *Biochem J*,Vol. 416, No. 1, (Nov 15), pp. (109-16), 1470-8728 (Electronic), 0264-6021 (Linking)

Gurley, K. A., H. Chen, C. Guenther, E. T. Nguyen, R. B. Rountree, M. Schoor & D. M. Kingsley. (2006a). Mineral formation in joints caused by complete or joint-specific loss of ANK function. *J Bone Miner Res*,Vol. 21, No. 8, (Aug), pp. (1238-47), 0884-0431 (Print)

Gurley, K. A., R. J. Reimer & D. M. Kingsley. (2006b). Biochemical and Genetic Analysis of *ANK* in Arthritis and Bone Disease. *Am. J. Hum. Genet.*,Vol. 79, pp. (1017-1029),

Harvey, D., J. J. Pointon, D. M. Evans, T. Karaderi, C. Farrar, L. H. Appleton, R. D. Sturrock, M. A. Stone, U. Oppermann, M. A. Brown & B. P. Wordsworth. (2009a). Investigating the genetic association between ERAP1 and ankylosing spondylitis. *Hum Mol Genet*,Vol. 18, No. 21, (Nov 1), pp. (4204-12), 1460-2083 (Electronic), 0964-6906 (Linking)

Harvey, D., J. J. Pointon, C. Sleator, A. Meenagh, C. Farrar, J. Y. Sun, D. Senitzer, D. Middleton, M. A. Brown & B. P. Wordsworth. (2009b). Analysis of killer immunoglobulin-like receptor genes in ankylosing spondylitis. *Ann Rheum Dis*,Vol. 68, No. 4, (Apr), pp. (595-8), 1468-2060 (Electronic), 0003-4967 (Linking)

Hou, T. Y., H. C. Chen, C. H. Chen, D. M. Chang, F. C. Liu & J. H. Lai. (2007). Usefulness of human leucocyte antigen-B27 subtypes in predicting ankylosing spondylitis: Taiwan experience. *Intern Med J.*,Vol. 37, No. 11, (November 2007), pp. (749-752),

Howe, H. S., P. L. Cheung, K. O. Kong, H. Badsha, B. Y. Thong, K. P. Leong, E. T. Koh, T. Y. Lian, Y. K. Cheng, S. Lam, D. Teo, T. C. Lau & B. P. Leung. (2005). Transforming growth factor beta-1 and gene polymorphisms in oriental ankylosing spondylitis. *Rheumatology (Oxford)*,Vol. 44, No. 1, (Jan), pp. (51-4), 1462-0324 (Print), 1462-0324 (Linking)

Hsu, H., J. Xiong & D. V. Goeddel. (1995). The TNF receptor 1-associated protein TRADD signals cell death and NF-kappa B activation. *Cell*,Vol. 81, No. 4, (May 19), pp. (495-504), 0092-8674 (Print), 0092-8674 (Linking)

Hsu, K. C., S. Chida, D. E. Geraghty & B. Dupont. (2002). The killer cell immunoglobulin-like receptor (KIR) genomic region: gene-order, haplotypes and allelic polymorphism. *Immunol Rev*,Vol. 190, (Dec), pp. (40-52), 0105-2896 (Print), 0105-2896 (Linking)

Jaakkola, E., A. M. Crane, K. Laiho, I. Herzberg, A. M. Sims, L. Bradbury, A. Calin, S. Brophy, M. Kauppi, K. Kaarela, B. P. Wordsworth, J. Tuomilehto & M. A. Brown. (2004). The effect of transforming growth factor beta1 gene polymorphisms in ankylosing spondylitis. *Rheumatology (Oxford)*,Vol. 43, No. 1, (Jan), pp. (32-8), 1462-0324 (Print), 1462-0324 (Linking)

Jaakkola, E., I. Herzberg, K. Laiho, M. C. Barnardo, J. J. Pointon, M. Kauppi, K. Kaarela, E. Tuomilehto-Wolf, J. Tuomilehto, B. P. Wordsworth & M. A. Brown. (2006). Finnish HLA studies confirm the increased risk conferred by HLA-B27 homozygosity in ankylosing spondylitis. *Ann Rheum Dis*,Vol. 65, No. 6, (Jun), pp. (775-80), 0003-4967 (Print), 0003-4967 (Linking)

Jandus, C., G. Bioley, J. P. Rivals, J. Dudler, D. Speiser & P. Romero. (2008). Increased numbers of circulating polyfunctional Th17 memory cells in patients with seronegative spondylarthritides. *Arthritis Rheum*,Vol. 58, No. 8, (Aug), pp. (2307-17), 0004-3591 (Print), 0004-3591 (Linking)

Jarvinen, P. (1995). Occurrence of ankylosing spondylitis in a nationwide series of twins. *Arthritis Rheum*,Vol. 38, No. 3, (March 1995), pp. (381-383),

Jiao, Y. L., B. C. Zhang, L. You, J. F. Li, J. Zhang, C. Y. Ma, B. Cui, L. C. Wang, Z. J. Chen & Y. R. Zhao. (2010). Polymorphisms of KIR gene and HLA-C alleles: possible association with susceptibility to HLA-B27-positive patients with ankylosing spondylitis. *J Clin Immunol*,Vol. 30, No. 6, (Nov), pp. (840-4), 1573-2592 (Electronic), 0271-9142 (Linking)

Jin, L., G. Zhang, J. M. Akey, J. Luo, J. Lee, M. H. Weisman, J. Bruckel, R. D. Inman, M. A. Stone, M. A. Khan, H. R. Schumacher, W. P. Maksymowych, M. L. Mahowald, A. D. Sawitzke, F. B. Vasey, D. T. Yu & J. D. Reveille. (2004). Lack of linkage of IL1RN genotypes with ankylosing spondylitis susceptibility. *Arthritis Rheum*,Vol. 50, No. 9, (Sep), pp. (3047-8), 0004-3591 (Print), 0004-3591 (Linking)

Joyce, M. E., S. Jingushi & M. E. Bolander. (1990). Transforming growth factor-beta in the regulation of fracture repair. *Orthop Clin North Am*,Vol. 21, No. 1, (Jan), pp. (199-209), 0030-5898 (Print), 0030-5898 (Linking)

Karaderi, T., D. Harvey, C. Farrar, L. H. Appleton, M. A. Stone, R. D. Sturrock, M. A. Brown, P. Wordsworth & J. J. Pointon. (2009). Association between the interleukin 23 receptor and ankylosing spondylitis is confirmed by a new UK case-control study and meta-analysis of published series. *Rheumatology (Oxford)*,Vol. 48, No. 4, (Apr), pp. (386-9), 1462-0332 (Electronic), 1462-0324 (Linking)

Kchir, M. M., W. Hamdi, L. Laadhar, S. Kochbati, D. Kaffel, K. Saadellaoui, H. Lahmar, M. M. Ghannouchi, D. Azzouz, L. Daoud, A. Ben Hamida, B. Zouari, M. Zitouni & S. Makni. (2010). HLA-B, DR and DQ antigens polymorphism in Tunisian patients with ankylosing spondylitis (a case-control study). *Rheumatol Int*,Vol. 30, No. 7, (May), pp. (933-939), 1437-160X (Electronic), 0172-8172 (Linking)

Khan, M. A., I. Kushner & W. E. Braun. (1980). Genetic heterogeneity in primary ankylosing sondylitis. *J Rheumatol*,Vol. 7, No. 3, (May 1980), pp. (383- 386),

Kim, T. H., M. A. Stone, P. Rahman, D. H. Yoo, Y. W. Park, U. Payne, D. Hallett & R. D. Inman. (2005). Interleukin 1 and nuclear factor-kappaB polymorphisms in ankylosing spondylitis in Canada and Korea. *J Rheumatol*,Vol. 32, No. 10, (Oct), pp. (1907-10), 0315-162X (Print), 0315-162X (Linking)

Kimura-Yoshida, C., K. Kitajima, I. Oda-Ishii, E. Tian, M. Suzuki, M. Yamamoto, T. Suzuki, M. Kobayashi, S. Aizawa & I. Matsuo. (2004). Characterization of the pufferfish Otx2 cis-regulators reveals evolutionarily conserved genetic mechanisms for vertebrate head specification. *Development*,Vol. 131, No. 1, (Jan), pp. (57-71), 0950-1991 (Print), 0950-1991 (Linking)

Kochan, G., T. Krojer, D. Harvey, R. Fischer, L. Chen, M. Vollmar, F. von Delft, K. L. Kavanagh, M. A. Brown, P. Bowness, P. Wordsworth, B. M. Kessler & U. Oppermann. (2011). Crystal structures of the endoplasmic reticulum aminopeptidase-1 (ERAP1) reveal the molecular basis for N-terminal peptide trimming. *Proc Natl Acad Sci U S A*,Vol. 108, No. 19, (May 10), pp. (7745-50), 1091-6490 (Electronic), 0027-8424 (Linking)

Kugathasan, S., R. N. Baldassano, J. P. Bradfield, P. M. Sleiman, M. Imielinski, S. L. Guthery, S. Cucchiara, C. E. Kim, E. C. Frackelton, K. Annaiah, J. T. Glessner, E. Santa, T. Willson, A. W. Eckert, E. Bonkowski, J. L. Shaner, R. M. Smith, F. G. Otieno, N. Peterson, D. J. Abrams, R. M. Chiavacci, R. Grundmeier, P. Mamula, G. Tomer, D. A. Piccoli, D. S. Monos, V. Annese, L. A. Denson, S. F. Grant & H. Hakonarson. (2008). Loci on 20q13 and 21q22 are associated with pediatric-onset inflammatory bowel disease. *Nat Genet*,Vol. 40, No. 10, (Oct), pp. (1211-5), 1546-1718 (Electronic), 1061-4036 (Linking)

Lanier, L. L., B. C. Corliss, J. Wu, C. Leong & J. H. Phillips. (1998). Immunoreceptor DAP12 bearing a tyrosine-based activation motif is involved in activating NK cells. *Nature*,Vol. 391, No. 6668, (Feb 12), pp. (703-7), 0028-0836 (Print), 0028-0836 (Linking)

Laval, S. H., A. Timms, S. Edwards, L. Bradbury, S. Brophy, A. Milicic, L. Rubin, K. A. Siminovitch, D. E. Weeks, A. Calin, B. P. Wordsworth & M. A. Brown. (2001). Whole-genome screening in ankylosing spondylitis: evidence of non-MHC genetic-susceptibility loci. *Am J Hum Genet*,Vol. 68, No. 4, (Apr), pp. (918-26), 0002-9297 (Print), 0002-9297 (Linking)

LeVan, T. D., J. W. Bloom, T. J. Bailey, C. L. Karp, M. Halonen, F. D. Martinez & D. Vercelli. (2001). A common single nucleotide polymorphism in the CD14 promoter decreases the affinity of Sp protein binding and enhances transcriptional activity. *J Immunol*,Vol. 167, No. 10, (Nov 15), pp. (5838-44), 0022-1767 (Print), 0022-1767 (Linking)

Liu, Y., L. Jiang, Q. Cai, P. Danoy, M. C. Barnardo, M. A. Brown & H. Xu. (2010). Predominant association of HLA-B*2704 with ankylosing spondylitis in Chinese Han patients. *Tissue Antigens*,Vol. 75, No. 1, (January 2010), pp. (61-64),

Lopez-Larrea, C., K. Sujirachato, N. K. Mehra, P. Chiewsilp, D. Isarangkura, U. Kanga, O. Dominguez, E. Coto, M. Pena & F. Setien. (1995). HLA-B27 subtypes in Asian patients with ankylosing spondylitis. Evidence for new associations. *Tissue Antigens*,Vol. 45, No. 3, (March 1995), pp. (1698- 76),

Lopez-Larrea, C., M. Mijiyawa, S. Gonzalez, J. L. Fernandez-Morera, M. A. Blanco-Gelaz, J. Martinez-Borra & A. Lopez-Vazquez. (2002). Association of Ankylosing Spondylitis with HLA-B*1403 in a West African population. *Arthritis Rheum*,Vol. 46, No. 11, (November 2002), pp. (2968- 2971),

Lopez-Larrea, C., M. A. Blanco-Gelaz, J. C. Torre-Alonso, J. Bruges Armas, B. Suarez-Alvarez, L. Pruneda, A. R. Couto, S. Gonzalez, A. Lopez-Vazquez & J. Martinez-Borra. (2006). Contribution of KIR3DL1/3DS1 to ankylosing spondylitis in human leukocyte antigen-B27 Caucasian populations. *Arthritis Res Ther*,Vol. 8, No. 4, pp. (R101), 1478-6362 (Electronic), 1478-6354 (Linking)

MacLean, I. L., S. Iqball, P. Woo, A. C. Keat, R. A. Hughes, G. H. Kingsley & S. C. Knight. (1993). HLA-B27 subtypes in the spondarthropathies. *Clin Exp Immunol*,Vol. 91, pp. (214 -9),

Mahfoudh, N., M. Siala, M. Rihl, A. Kammoun, F. Frikha, H. Fourati, M. Younes, R. Gdoura, L. Gaddour, F. Hakim, Z. Bahloul, S. Baklouti, N. Bargaoui, S. Sellami, A. Hammami & H. Makni. (2011). Association and frequency of HLA-A, B and HLA-DR genes in south Tunisian patients with spondyloarthritis (SpA). *Clin Rheumatol*,Vol. (Mar 1), pp. 1434-9949 (Electronic), 0770-3198 (Linking)

Maksymowych, W. P., S. Tao, J. Vaile, M. Suarez-Almazor, C. Ramos-Remus & A. S. Russell. (2000). LMP2 polymorphism is associated with extraspinal disease in HLA-B27 negative Caucasian and Mexican Mestizo patients with ankylosing spondylitis. *J Rheumatol.*,Vol. 27, No. 1, (January 2000), pp. (183-189),

Maksymowych, W. P., J. P. Reeve, J. D. Reveille, J. M. Akey, H. Buenviaje, L. O'Brien, P. M. Peloso, G. T. Thomson, L. Jin & A. S. Russell. (2003). High-throughput single-nucleotide polymorphism analysis of the IL1RN locus in patients with ankylosing spondylitis by matrix-assisted laser desorption ionization-time-of-flight mass spectrometry. *Arthritis Rheum*,Vol. 48, No. 7, (Jul), pp. (2011-8), 0004-3591 (Print), 0004-3591 (Linking)

Maksymowych, W. P., P. Rahman, J. P. Reeve, D. D. Gladman, L. Peddle & R. D. Inman. (2006). Association of the IL1 gene cluster with susceptibility to ankylosing spondylitis: an analysis of three Canadian populations. *Arthritis Rheum*,Vol. 54, No. 3, (Mar), pp. (974-85), 0004-3591 (Print), 0004-3591 (Linking)

Maksymowych, W. P., R. D. Inman, D. D. Gladman, J. P. Reeve, A. Pope & P. Rahman. (2009). Association of a specific ERAP1/ARTS1 haplotype with disease susceptibility in ankylosing spondylitis. *Arthritis Rheum*,Vol. 60, No. 5, (May), pp. (1317-23), 0004-3591 (Print), 0004-3591 (Linking)

McGarry, F., L. Cousins, R. D. Sturrock & M. Field. (2002). A polymorphism within the Transforming Growth Factor β1 gene is associated with ankylosing spondylitis (AS). *Arthritis Res*,Vol. 4, No. Suppl 1, (Feb 2002), pp. (22),

Miceli-Richard, C., H. Zouali, R. Said-Nahal, S. Lesage, F. Merlin, C. De Toma, H. Blanche, M. Sahbatou, M. Dougados, G. Thomas, M. Breban & J. P. Hugot. (2004). Significant linkage to spondyloarthropathy on 9q31-34. *Hum Mol Genet*,Vol. 13, No. 15, (Aug 1), pp. (1641-8), 0964-6906 (Print), 0964-6906 (Linking)

Migone, T. S., J. Zhang, X. Luo, L. Zhuang, C. Chen, B. Hu, J. S. Hong, J. W. Perry, S. F. Chen, J. X. Zhou, Y. H. Cho, S. Ullrich, P. Kanakaraj, J. Carrell, E. Boyd, H. S. Olsen, G. Hu, L. Pukac, D. Liu, J. Ni, S. Kim, R. Gentz, P. Feng, P. A. Moore, S. M. Ruben & P. Wei. (2002). TL1A is a TNF-like ligand for DR3 and TR6/DcR3 and functions as a T cell costimulator. *Immunity*,Vol. 16, No. 3, (Mar), pp. (479-92), 1074-7613 (Print), 1074-7613 (Linking)

Moritz, D. R., H. R. Rodewald, J. Gheyselinck & R. Klemenz. (1998). The IL-1 receptor-related T1 antigen is expressed on immature and mature mast cells and on fetal blood mast cell progenitors. *J Immunol*,Vol. 161, No. 9, (Nov 1), pp. (4866-74), 0022-1767 (Print), 0022-1767 (Linking)

Mornet, E., A. Taillandier, S. Peyramaure, F. Kaper, F. Muller, R. Brenner, P. Bussière, P. Freisinger, J. Godard, M. Le Merrer, J. F. Oury, H. Plauchu, R. Puddu, J. M. Rival, A. Superti-Furga, R. L. Touraine, J. L. Serre & B. Simon-Bouy. (1998). Identification of fifteen nvel mutations in the tissue-nonspecific alkaline phosphatase (TNSALP) gene in European patients with severe hypophosphatasia. *Eur J Hum Genet*,Vol. 6, pp. (308-314),

Mulero, J. J., A. M. Pace, S. T. Nelken, D. B. Loeb, T. R. Correa, R. Drmanac & J. E. Ford. (1999). IL1HY1: A novel interleukin-1 receptor antagonist gene. *Biochem Biophys Res Commun*,Vol. 263, No. 3, (Oct 5), pp. (702-6), 0006-291X (Print), 0006-291X (Linking)

Murphy, C. A., C. L. Langrish, Y. Chen, W. Blumenschein, T. McClanahan, R. A. Kastelein, J. D. Sedgwick & D. J. Cua. (2003). Divergent pro- and antiinflammatory roles for IL-23 and IL-12 in joint autoimmune inflammation. *J Exp Med*,Vol. 198, No. 12, (Dec 15), pp. (1951-7), 0022-1007 (Print), 0022-1007 (Linking)

Nobrega, M. A., I. Ovcharenko, V. Afzal & E. M. Rubin. (2003). Scanning human gene deserts for long-range enhancers. *Science*,Vol. 302, No. 5644, (Oct 17), pp. (413), 1095-9203 (Electronic), 0036-8075 (Linking)

Nunez, C., B. Dema, M. C. Cenit, I. Polanco, C. Maluenda, R. Arroyo, V. de las Heras, M. Bartolome, E. G. de la Concha, E. Urcelay & A. Martinez. (2008). IL23R: a susceptibility locus for celiac disease and multiple sclerosis? *Genes Immun*,Vol. 9, No. 4, (Jun), pp. (289-93), 1476-5470 (Electronic), 1466-4879 (Linking)

Oppmann, B., R. Lesley, B. Blom, J. C. Timans, Y. Xu, B. Hunte, F. Vega, N. Yu, J. Wang, K. Singh, F. Zonin, E. Vaisberg, T. Churakova, M. Liu, D. Gorman, J. Wagner, S. Zurawski, Y. Liu, J. S. Abrams, K. W. Moore, D. Rennick, R. de Waal-Malefyt, C. Hannum, J. F. Bazan & R. A. Kastelein. (2000). Novel p19 protein engages IL-12p40 to form a cytokine, IL-23, with biological activities similar as well as distinct from IL-12. *Immunity*,Vol. 13, No. 5, (Nov), pp. (715-25), 1074-7613 (Print), 1074-7613 (Linking)

Ovcharenko, I., G. G. Loots, M. A. Nobrega, R. C. Hardison, W. Miller & L. Stubbs. (2005). Evolution and functional classification of vertebrate gene deserts. *Genome Res*,Vol. 15, No. 1, (Jan), pp. (137-45), 1088-9051 (Print), 1088-9051 (Linking)

Pappu, B. P., A. Borodovsky, T. S. Zheng, X. Yang, P. Wu, X. Dong, S. Weng, B. Browning, M. L. Scott, L. Ma, L. Su, Q. Tian, P. Schneider, R. A. Flavell, C. Dong & L. C. Burkly. (2008). TL1A-DR3 interaction regulates Th17 cell function and Th17-mediated autoimmune disease. *J Exp Med*,Vol. 205, No. 5, (May 12), pp. (1049-62), 1540-9538 (Electronic), 0022-1007 (Linking)

Parham, C., M. Chirica, J. Timans, E. Vaisberg, M. Travis, J. Cheung, S. Pflanz, R. Zhang, K. P. Singh, F. Vega, W. To, J. Wagner, A. M. O'Farrell, T. McClanahan, S. Zurawski, C. Hannum, D. Gorman, D. M. Rennick, R. A. Kastelein, R. de Waal Malefyt & K. W. Moore. (2002). A receptor for the heterodimeric cytokine IL-23 is composed of IL-12Rbeta1 and a novel cytokine receptor subunit, IL-23R. *J Immunol*,Vol. 168, No. 11, (Jun 1), pp. (5699-708), 0022-1767 (Print), 0022-1767 (Linking)

Parham, P. (2005). MHC class I molecules and KIRs in human history, health and survival. *Nat Rev Immunol*,Vol. 5, No. 3, (Mar), pp. (201-14), 1474-1733 (Print), 1474-1733 (Linking)

Park, H., Z. Li, X. O. Yang, S. H. Chang, R. Nurieva, Y. H. Wang, Y. Wang, L. Hood, Z. Zhu, Q. Tian & C. Dong. (2005). A distinct lineage of CD4 T cells regulates tissue inflammation by producing interleukin 17. *Nat Immunol*,Vol. 6, No. 11, (Nov), pp. (1133-41), 1529-2908 (Print), 1529-2908 (Linking)

Parnet, P., K. E. Garka, T. P. Bonnert, S. K. Dower & J. E. Sims. (1996). IL-1Rrp is a novel receptor-like molecule similar to the type I interleukin-1 receptor and its homologues T1/ST2 and IL-1R AcP. *J Biol Chem*,Vol. 271, No. 8, (Feb 23), pp. (3967-70), 0021-9258 (Print), 0021-9258 (Linking)

Pazar, B., E. Safrany, P. Gergely, S. Szanto, Z. Szekanecz & G. Poor. (2010). Association of ARTS1 gene polymorphisms with ankylosing spondylitis in the Hungarian population: the rs27044 variant is associated with HLA-B*2705 subtype in Hungarian patients with ankylosing spondylitis. *J Rheumatol*,Vol. 37, No. 2, (Feb), pp. (379-84), 0315-162X (Print), 0315-162X (Linking)

Pimentel-Santos, F. M., D. Ligeiro, M. Matos, A. F. Mourao, E. Sousa, P. Pinto, A. Ribeiro, M. Sousa, A. Barcelos, F. Godinho, M. Cruz, J. E. Fonseca, H. Guedes-Pinto, H. Trindade, D. M. Evans, M. A. Brown & J. C. Branco. (2009). Association of IL23R and ERAP1 genes with ankylosing spondylitis in a Portuguese population. *Clin Exp Rheumatol*,Vol. 27, No. 5, (Sep-Oct), pp. (800-6), 0392-856X (Print), 0392-856X (Linking)

Ploski, R., B. Flato, O. Vinje, W. Maksymowych, O. Forre & E. Thorsby. (1995). Association to HLA-DRB1*08, HLA-DPB1*0301 and homozygosity for an HLA-linked proteasome gene in juvenile ankylosing spondylitis. *Hum Immunol*,Vol. 44, No. 2, (Oct), pp. (88-96), 0198-8859 (Print), 0198-8859 (Linking)

Pointon, J. J., K. Chapman, D. Harvey, A. M. Sims, L. Bradbury, K. Laiho, M. Kauppi, K. Kaarela, J. Tuomilehto, M. A. Brown & B. P. Wordsworth. (2008). Toll-like receptor 4 and CD14 polymorphisms in ankylosing spondylitis: evidence of a weak association in Finns. *J Rheumatol*,Vol. 35, No. 8, (Aug), pp. (1609-12), 0315-162X (Print), 0315-162X (Linking)

Pointon, J. J., D. Harvey, T. Karaderi, L. H. Appleton, C. Farrar, M. A. Stone, R. D. Sturrock, J. D. Reveille, M. H. Weisman, M. M. Ward, M. A. Brown & B. P. Wordsworth. (2010). The chromosome 16q region associated with ankylosing spondylitis includes the candidate gene tumour necrosis factor receptor type 1-associated death domain (TRADD). *Ann Rheum Dis*,Vol. 69, No. 6, (Jun), pp. (1243-6), 1468-2060 (Electronic), 0003-4967 (Linking)

Rahman, P., R. D. Inman, D. D. Gladman, J. P. Reeve, L. Peddle & W. P. Maksymowych. (2008). Association of interleukin-23 receptor variants with ankylosing spondylitis. *Arthritis Rheum*,Vol. 58, No. 4, (Apr), pp. (1020-5), 0004-3591 (Print), 0004-3591 (Linking)

Reveille, J. D. & R. M. Maganti. (2009). Subtypes of HLA-B27: history and implications in the pathogenesis of ankylosing spondylitis. *Adv Exp Med Bio*,Vol. 649, pp. (159-176),

Reveille, J. D., A. M. Sims, P. Danoy, D. M. Evans, P. Leo, J. J. Pointon, R. Jin, X. Zhou, L. A. Bradbury, L. H. Appleton, J. C. Davis, L. Diekman, T. Doan, A. Dowling, R. Duan, E. L. Duncan, C. Farrar, J. Hadler, D. Harvey, T. Karaderi, R. Mogg, E. Pomeroy, K. Pryce, J. Taylor, L. Savage, P. Deloukas, V. Kumanduri, L. Peltonen, S. M. Ring, P. Whittaker, E. Glazov, G. P. Thomas, W. P. Maksymowych, R. D. Inman, M. M. Ward, M. A. Stone, M. H. Weisman, B. P. Wordsworth & M. A. Brown. (2010). Genome-wide association study of ankylosing spondylitis identifies non-MHC susceptibility loci. *Nat Genet*,Vol. 42, No. 2, (Feb), pp. (123-7), 1546-1718 (Electronic), 1061-4036 (Linking)

Reveille, J. D. (2011). The genetic basis of spondyloarthritis. *Ann Rheum Dis*,Vol. 70, No. Suppl 1, (March 2011), pp. (i44-50),

Robinson, W. P., S. M. van der Linden, M. A. Khan, H. U. Rentsch, A. Cats, A. Russell & G. Thomson. (1989). HLA-Bw60 increases susceptibility to ankylosing spondylitis in HLA-B27 + patients. *Arthritis Rheum*,Vol. 32, No. 9, (September 1989), pp. (1135-1141),

Rubin, L. A., C. I. Amos, J. A. Wade, J. R. Martin, S. J. Bale, A. H. Little, D. D. Gladman, G. E. Bonney, J. D. Rubenstein & K. A. Siminovitch. (1994). Investigating the genetic basis for ankylosing spondylitis. Linkage studies with the major histocompatibility complex region. *Arthritis Rheum*,Vol. 37, No. 8, (August 1994), pp. (1212-1220),

Rueda, B., G. Orozco, E. Raya, J. L. Fernandez-Sueiro, J. Mulero, F. J. Blanco, C. Vilches, M. A. Gonzalez-Gay & J. Martin. (2008). The IL23R Arg381Gln non-synonymous polymorphism confers susceptibility to ankylosing spondylitis. *Ann Rheum Dis*,Vol. 67, No. 10, (Oct), pp. (1451-4), 1468-2060 (Electronic), 0003-4967 (Linking)

Safrany, E., B. Pazar, V. Csongei, L. Jaromi, N. Polgar, C. Sipeky, I. F. Horvath, M. Zeher, G. Poor & B. Melegh. (2009). Variants of the IL23R gene are associated with ankylosing spondylitis but not with Sjogren syndrome in Hungarian population samples. *Scand J Immunol*,Vol. 70, No. 1, (Jul), pp. (68-74), 1365-3083 (Electronic), 0300-9475 (Linking)

Said-Nahal, R., C. Miceli-Richard, C. Gautreau, R. Tamouza, N. Borot, R. Porcher, D. Charron, M. Dougados & M. Breban. (2002). The role of HLA genes in familial spondyloarthropathy: a comprehensive study of 70 multiplex families. *Ann Rheum Dis*,Vol. 61, No. 3, (Mar), pp. (201-206), 0003-4967 (Print), 0003-4967 (Linking)

Saric, T., S. C. Chang, A. Hattori, I. A. York, S. Markant, K. L. Rock, M. Tsujimoto & A. L. Goldberg. (2002). An IFN-gamma-induced aminopeptidase in the ER, ERAP1, trims precursors to MHC class I-presented peptides. *Nat Immunol*,Vol. 3, No. 12, (Dec), pp. (1169-76), 1529-2908 (Print), 1529-2908 (Linking)

Saveanu, L., O. Carroll, V. Lindo, M. Del Val, D. Lopez, Y. Lepelletier, F. Greer, L. Schomburg, D. Fruci, G. Niedermann & P. M. van Endert. (2005). Concerted peptide trimming by human ERAP1 and ERAP2 aminopeptidase complexes in the endoplasmic reticulum. *Nat Immunol*,Vol. 6, No. 7, (Jul), pp. (689-97), 1529-2908 (Print), 1529-2908 (Linking)

Sims, A. M., M. Barnardo, I. Herzberg, L. Bradbury, A. Calin, B. P. Wordsworth, C. Darke & M. A. Brown. (2007). Non-B27 MHC associations of ankylosing spondylitis. *Genes Immun*,Vol. 8, No. 2, (March 2007), pp. (115-123),

Sims, A. M., A. E. Timms, J. Bruges-Armas, R. Burgos-Vargas, C. T. Chou, T. Doan, A. Dowling, R. N. Fialho, P. Gergely, D. D. Gladman, R. Inman, M. Kauppi, K.

Kaarela, K. Laiho, W. Maksymowych, J. J. Pointon, P. Rahman, J. D. Reveille, R. Sorrentino, J. Tuomilehto, G. Vargas-Alarcon, B. P. Wordsworth, H. Xu & M. A. Brown. (2008). Prospective meta-analysis of interleukin 1 gene complex polymorphisms confirms associations with ankylosing spondylitis. *Ann Rheum Dis*,Vol. 67, No. 9, (Sep), pp. (1305-9), 1468-2060 (Electronic), 0003-4967 (Linking)

Steinman, L. (2007). A brief history of T(H)17, the first major revision in the T(H)1/T(H)2 hypothesis of T cell-mediated tissue damage. *Nat Med*,Vol. 13, No. 2, (Feb), pp. (139-45), 1078-8956 (Print), 1078-8956 (Linking)

Sung, I. H., T. H. Kim, S. Y. Bang, T. J. Kim, B. Lee, L. Peddle, P. Rahman, C. M. Greenwood, P. Hu & R. D. Inman. (2009). IL-23R polymorphisms in patients with ankylosing spondylitis in Korea. *J Rheumatol*,Vol. 36, No. 5, (May), pp. (1003-5), 0315-162X (Print), 0315-162X (Linking)

Symons, J. A., J. A. Eastgate & G. W. Duff. (1991). Purification and characterization of a novel soluble receptor for interleukin 1. *J Exp Med*,Vol. 174, No. 5, (Nov 1), pp. (1251-4), 0022-1007 (Print), 0022-1007 (Linking)

Takedatsu, H., K. S. Michelsen, B. Wei, C. J. Landers, L. S. Thomas, D. Dhall, J. Braun & S. R. Targan. (2008). TL1A (TNFSF15) regulates the development of chronic colitis by modulating both T-helper 1 and T-helper 17 activation. *Gastroenterology*,Vol. 135, No. 2, (Aug), pp. (552-67), 1528-0012 (Electronic), 0016-5085 (Linking)

Tamouza, R., I. Mansour, N. Bouguacha, S. Klayme, K. Djouadi, S. Laoussadi, M. Azoury, N. Dulphy, R. Ramasawmy, R. Krishnamoorthy, A. Toubert, R. Naman & D. Charron. (2001). A new HLA-B*27 allele (B*2719) identified in a Lebanese patient affected with ankylosing spondylitis. *Tissue Antigens*,Vol. 58, No. 1, (July 2001), pp. (30-3),

Thomas, G. P. & M. A. Brown. (2010). Genetics and genomics of ankylosing spondylitis. *Immunol Rev*,Vol. 233, No. 1, (Jan), pp. (162-80), 1600-065X (Electronic), 0105-2896 (Linking)

Timms, A. E., Y. Zhang, L. Bradbury, B. P. Wordsworth & M. A. Brown. (2003). Investigation of the role of ANKH in ankylosing spondylitis. *Arthritis Rheum*,Vol. 48, No. 10, pp. (2898-902),

Timms, A. E., A. M. Crane, A. M. Sims, H. J. Cordell, L. A. Bradbury, A. Abbott, M. R. Coyne, O. Beynon, I. Herzberg, G. W. Duff, A. Calin, L. R. Cardon, B. P. Wordsworth & M. A. Brown. (2004). The interleukin 1 gene cluster contains a major susceptibility locus for ankylosing spondylitis. *Am J Hum Genet*,Vol. 75, No. 4, (Oct), pp. (587-95), 0002-9297 (Print), 0002-9297 (Linking)

Torigoe, K., S. Ushio, T. Okura, S. Kobayashi, M. Taniai, T. Kunikata, T. Murakami, O. Sanou, H. Kojima, M. Fujii, T. Ohta, M. Ikeda, H. Ikegami & M. Kurimoto. (1997). Purification and characterization of the human interleukin-18 receptor. *J Biol Chem*,Vol. 272, No. 41, (Oct 10), pp. (25737-42), 0021-9258 (Print), 0021-9258 (Linking)

Tsui, F. W., H. W. Tsui, E. Y. Cheng, M. Stone, U. Payne, J. D. Reveille, M. J. Shulman & A. D. I. Paterson, R D. (2003). Novel genetic markers in the 5'-flanking region of ANKH are associated with ankylosing spondylitis. *Arthritis Rheum*,Vol. 48, No. 3, pp. (791-7),

Tsui, F. W., N. Haroon, J. D. Reveille, P. Rahman, B. Chiu, H. W. Tsui & R. D. Inman. (2010). Association of an ERAP1 ERAP2 haplotype with familial ankylosing spondylitis. *Ann Rheum Dis*,Vol. 69, No. 4, (Apr), pp. (733-6), 1468-2060 (Electronic), 0003-4967 (Linking)

Tsui, H. W., R. D. Inman, A. D. Paterson, J. D. Reveille & T. FW. (2005). ANKH variants associated with ankylosing spondylitis: gender differences. *Arthritis Res Ther*,Vol. 7, No. 3, pp. (513-25),

Tsui, H. W., R. D. Inman, J. D. Reveille & F. W. Tsui. (2007). Association of a TNAP haplotype with ankylosing spondylitis. *Arthritis Rheum*,Vol. 56, No. 1, (Jan), pp. (234-43), 0004-3591 (Print), 0004-3591 (Linking)

van der Linden, S. M., H. A. Valkenburg, B. M. de Jongh & A. Cats. (1984). The risk of developing ankylosing spondylitis in HLA-B27 positive individuals. A comparison of relatives of spondylitis patients with the general population. *Arthritis Rheum.* ,Vol. 27, No. 3, (March 1984), pp. (241-249),

van der Paardt, M., J. B. Crusius, M. A. Garcia-Gonzalez, P. Baudoin, P. J. Kostense, B. Z. Alizadeh, B. A. Dijkmans, A. S. Pena & I. E. van der Horst-Bruinsma. (2002). Interleukin-1beta and interleukin-1 receptor antagonist gene polymorphisms in ankylosing spondylitis. *Rheumatology (Oxford)*,Vol. 41, No. 12, (Dec), pp. (1419-23), 1462-0324 (Print), 1462-0324 (Linking)

van der Paardt, M., J. B. Crusius, M. H. de Koning, S. A. Morre, R. J. van de Stadt, B. A. Dijkmans, A. S. Pena & I. E. van der Horst-Bruinsma. (2005a). No evidence for involvement of the Toll-like receptor 4 (TLR4) A896G and CD14-C260T polymorphisms in susceptibility to ankylosing spondylitis. *Ann Rheum Dis*,Vol. 64, No. 2, (Feb), pp. (235-8), 0003-4967 (Print), 0003-4967 (Linking)

van der Paardt, M., J. B. Crusius, M. A. Garcia-Gonzalez, B. A. Dijkmans, A. S. Pena & I. E. van der Horst-Bruinsma. (2005b). Susceptibility to ankylosing spondylitis: no evidence for the involvement of transforming growth factor beta 1 (TGFB1) gene polymorphisms. *Ann Rheum Dis*,Vol. 64, No. 4, (Apr), pp. (616-9), 0003-4967 (Print), 0003-4967 (Linking)

Vargas-Alarcon, G., J. D. Londono, G. Hernandez-Pacheco, C. Pacheco-Tena, E. Castillo, M. H. Cardiel, J. Granados & R. Burgos-Vargas. (2002). Effect of HLA-B and HLA-DR genes on susceptibility to and severity of spondyloarthropathies in Mexican patients. *Ann Rheum Dis*,Vol. 61, No. 8, (Aug), pp. (714-717), 0003-4967 (Print), 0003-4967 (Linking)

Vargas-Alarcón, G., A. Garcia, S. Bahena, H. Melin-Aldana, F. Andrade, G. Ibañez-de-Kasep, J. Alcocer-Varela, D. Alarcón-Segovia & J. Granados. (1994). HLA-B alleles and complotypes in Mexican patients with seronegative spondyloarthropathies. *Ann Rheum Dis*,Vol. 53, No. 11, (November 1994), pp. (755-758),

Venter, J. C., M. D. Adams, E. W. Myers, P. W. Li, R. J. Mural, G. G. Sutton, H. O. Smith, M. Yandell, C. A. Evans, R. A. Holt, J. D. Gocayne, P. Amanatides, R. M. Ballew, D. H. Huson, J. R. Wortman, Q. Zhang, C. D. Kodira, X. H. Zheng, L. Chen, M. Skupski, G. Subramanian, P. D. Thomas, J. Zhang, G. L. Gabor Miklos, C. Nelson, S. Broder, A. G. Clark, J. Nadeau, V. A. McKusick, N. Zinder, A. J. Levine, R. J. Roberts, M. Simon, C. Slayman, M. Hunkapiller, R. Bolanos, A. Delcher, I. Dew, D. Fasulo, M. Flanigan, L. Florea, A. Halpern, S. Hannenhalli, S. Kravitz, S. Levy, C. Mobarry, K. Reinert, K. Remington, J. Abu-Threideh, E. Beasley, K. Biddick, V. Bonazzi, R. Brandon, M. Cargill, I. Chandramouliswaran, R. Charlab, K. Chaturvedi, Z. Deng, V. Di Francesco, P. Dunn, K. Eilbeck, C. Evangelista, A. E. Gabrielian, W. Gan, W. Ge, F. Gong, Z. Gu, P. Guan, T. J. Heiman, M. E. Higgins, R. R. Ji, Z. Ke, K. A. Ketchum, Z. Lai, Y. Lei, Z. Li, J. Li, Y. Liang, X. Lin, F. Lu, G. V. Merkulov, N. Milshina, H. M. Moore, A. K. Naik, V. A. Narayan, B. Neelam, D. Nusskern, D. B. Rusch, S. Salzberg, W. Shao, B. Shue, J. Sun, Z. Wang, A. Wang, X. Wang, J. Wang,

M. Wei, R. Wides, C. Xiao, C. Yan, et al. (2001). The sequence of the human genome. *Science*,Vol. 291, No. 5507, (Feb 16), pp. (1304-51), 0036-8075 (Print), 0036-8075 (Linking)

Wang, X., J. Huang, Z. Lin, Z. Liao, C. Li, Q. Wei, Y. Jiang, L. Zhao & J. Gu. (2010). Single-nucleotide polymorphisms and expression of IL23R in Chinese ankylosing spondylitis patients. *Rheumatol Int*,Vol. 30, No. 7, (May), pp. (955-9), 1437-160X (Electronic), 0172-8172 (Linking)

Wei, J. C., W. C. Tsai, H. S. Lin, C. Y. Tsai & C. T. Chou. (2004). HLA-B60 and B61 are strongly associated with ankylosing spondylitis in HLA-B27-negative Taiwan Chinese patients. *Rheumatology*,Vol. 43, No. 7, (Jun 2004), pp. (839-42),

Wu, Z. & J. R. Gu. (2007). A meta-analysis on interleukin-1 gene cluster polymorphism and genetic susceptibility for ankylosing spondylitis. *Zhonghua Yi Xue Za Zhi*,Vol. 87, No. 7, (Feb 13), pp. (433-7), 0376-2491 (Print), 0376-2491 (Linking)

Yamaguchi, A., N. Tsuchiya, H. Mitsui, M. Shiota, A. Ogawa, K. Tokunaga, S. Yoshinoya, T. Juji & K. Ito. (1995). Association of HLA-B39 with HLA-B27-negative ankylosing spondylitis and pauciarticular juvenile rheumatoid arthritis in Japanese patients. Evidence for a role of the peptide-anchoring B pocket. *Arthritis Rheum*,Vol. 38, No. 11, (November 1995), pp. (1672-1677),

Yamazaki, K., D. McGovern, J. Ragoussis, M. Paolucci, H. Butler, D. Jewell, L. Cardon, M. Takazoe, T. Tanaka, T. Ichimori, S. Saito, A. Sekine, A. Iida, A. Takahashi, T. Tsunoda, M. Lathrop & Y. Nakamura. (2005). Single nucleotide polymorphisms in TNFSF15 confer susceptibility to Crohn's disease. *Hum Mol Genet*,Vol. 14, No. 22, (Nov 15), pp. (3499-506), 0964-6906 (Print), 0964-6906 (Linking)

York, I. A., S. C. Chang, T. Saric, J. A. Keys, J. M. Favreau, A. L. Goldberg & K. L. Rock. (2002). The ER aminopeptidase ERAP1 enhances or limits antigen presentation by trimming epitopes to 8-9 residues. *Nat Immunol*,Vol. 3, No. 12, (Dec), pp. (1177-84), 1529-2908 (Print), 1529-2908 (Linking)

Yue, T. L., J. Ni, A. M. Romanic, J. L. Gu, P. Keller, C. Wang, S. Kumar, G. L. Yu, T. K. Hart, X. Wang, Z. Xia, W. E. DeWolf, Jr. & G. Z. Feuerstein. (1999). TL1, a novel tumor necrosis factor-like cytokine, induces apoptosis in endothelial cells. Involvement of activation of stress protein kinases (stress-activated protein kinase and p38 mitogen-activated protein kinase) and caspase-3-like protease. *J Biol Chem*,Vol. 274, No. 3, (Jan 15), pp. (1479-86), 0021-9258

Zinovieva, E., C. Bourgain, A. Kadi, F. Letourneur, B. Izac, R. Said-Nahal, N. Lebrun, N. Cagnard, A. Vigier, S. Jacques, C. Miceli-Richard, H. J. Garchon, S. Heath, C. Charon, D. Bacq, A. Boland, D. Zelenika, G. Chiocchia & M. Breban. (2009). Comprehensive linkage and association analyses identify haplotype, near to the TNFSF15 gene, significantly associated with spondyloarthritis. *PLoS Genet*,Vol. 5, No. 6, (Jun), 1553-7390

8

Lessons from Genomic Profiling in AS

Fernando M. Pimentel-Santos[1], Jaime C. Branco[1] and Gethin Thomas[2]
[1]*Universidade Nova de Lisboa, Faculdade de Ciências Médicas, Chronic Diseases Research Center (CEDOC), Lisboa,*
[2]*University of Queensland Diamantina Institute, Princess Alexandra Hospital, Brisbane,*
[1]*Portugal*
[2]*Australia*

1. Introduction

Ankylosing Spondylitis (AS) is a common cause of chronic inflammatory arthritis worldwide, with a prevalence of 0.2-0.9% in white European populations (Braun *et al.*, 1998), with unknown etiology. The progressive ankylosis of affected joints is currently irreversible and it is, therefore, logical that early diagnosis and treatment offers the best opportunity to improve its prognosis. Several studies have shown a delay of more than 8 years between the onset of symptoms and diagnosis, with consequent delay in starting an effective therapy (Feldtkeller *et al.*, 2003; Hamilton *et al.*, 2011). This is a critical period clinically, with diagnosis frequently occurring after significant irreversible radiological damage has already occurred. Currently, diagnosis of AS relies on a combination of clinical and imaging parameters (van der Linden *et al.*, 1984 and Boonen *et al.*, 2010) with no single blood derived biomarker that by itself is sufficiently sensitive and specific to identify AS cases or to be useful in disease management.

In this context, recent advances in molecular biology, in particular, the completion of the genome human sequence, the improvement in computational tools and the rapid access to large databases, allow an integrated understanding of biological systems, through "omic" approaches. The main challenge, however, is to extract relevant knowledge from the huge amount of data provided by these technologies for the development of biomarkers for diagnosis, prognosis, therapy monitoring and both prediction and monitoring of treatment response. Such technological advances represent the beginning of patient-specific personalized medicine (Kandpal *et al.*, 2009).

In contrast to traditional DNA-based diagnostic tests that largely focus on single genes associated with rare conditions, microarray-based genotyping and expression assays are ideal for the study of diseases with underlying complex genetic causes (Li *et al.*, 2008). Microarray gene expression technology can be used for the detection and quantification of differentially expressed genes. Its ability to study expression of several thousand genes or even all of the genes of the entire genome in a single experiment has changed biomedical research. Gene-expression profiling confers a "snapshot" of cellular activity providing information on the mechanisms mediating stress responses of human cells (Belcher *et al.*, 2000; Guillemin *et al.*, 2002), identification of signaling cascades (Shaffer *et al.*, 2000; Diehn *et al.*, 2002), disease changes, or mechanisms underlying therapy responses (Raetz & Moos, 2004). It represents an advance to the traditional molecular genomic techniques that have been previously applied in a large broad of clinical research as cancer, infections, metabolic, genetics and more recently, in rheumatic diseases.

1.1 Microarray fundamentals

Gene expression techniques, based on measuring mRNA levels, have greatly evolved since the development of the Northern Blot, in 1975 (Southern, 1975) to microarrays, in the mid 1990s (Shalon *et al.*, 1996). From a single labeled mRNA (probe), hybridized on a membrane (Northern Blot), to multiple probes hybridized on a membrane (macroarrays) or on glass (microarrays), the improvement was tremendous. Today several platforms, with pre-designed and custom arrays are available in the market (Hardiman, 2004) from Affymetrix, Agilent and Illumina. Table 1 summarizes similarities and differences between the most widely used platforms.

	Platforms		
	Affymetrix	**Agilent**	**Illumina**
Array format	25-mer	60-mer	50-mer
Starting RNA requirement	5µg total RNA	**Fluorescent Direct Label Kit (cDNA labeling):** 10µg total RNA, or200ng polyA+ RNA **Low input RNA Fluorescent Linear Amplification kit (Amplified cDNA labeling):** 50ng total RNA **Low input RNA Fluorescent Linear Amplification kit (Amplified cRNA labeling):** 50ng total RNA	50-500ng total RNA
Hybridization time	16h	**Fluorescent Direct Label Kit:** 3-4 hours **Low input RNA Fluorescent Linear Amplification kit Amplified cDNA labeling**: 10 hours **Amplified cRNA labeling:** 6 hours	16h
Hybridization temperature	45ºC	60ºC	55ºC
Detection method	Streptavidin-phycoerythrin	Cyanine 3 (Cy3) and cyanine 5 (Cy5) fluorescent labeling	Streptavidin-Cy3
Advantages	Reproducibility; Full genome coverage; Mature platform; Customization; More probes per gene.	Reproducibility; content; mature platform; sensitivity; customization	Reproducibility; Full genome coverage; Sensitivity; Low background; Mature platform; Low cost/sample; Low starting material required
Disadvantages	Short oligonucleotides; Less sensitive; High cost/sample.	Two-color dye bias and ozone-related degradation	Currently only available for human, rat and mouse studies; Less probes per gene; not so sensitive to detect splice variants.

Table 1. Microarray platform comparison.

Despite minor differences between platforms, the basic steps involved in a microarrays experiment are similar (Fig. 1) (Repsilber *et al.*, 2005). Key points in undertaking an expression profiling study are:

1. Establish your research question.
2. Selection of the tissue/cell most relevant to the question and the selection of the control group.
3. Total mRNA is extracted from the chosen tissue/cell, and reverse transcribed generating cDNA which is labelled with radioactive or fluorescent markers.
4. Labeled transcripts are hybridized onto the microarray.
5. Bound probes are detected and quantified by imaging tools and every gene/probe assigned a signal intensity.
6. Signals are corrected for common bias i.e. normalized. For each mRNA, the signal intensity difference between the disease and the control sample correlates to the change in gene expression (genes up- or down-regulated) that might be associated with the studied condition. Several methods have been implemented to reduce variability in DNA microarray experiments (Workman *et al.*, 2002). A critical step in the whole procedure is an appropriate analysis of the large volumes of data generated using sophisticated software. Bioconductor (www.bioconductor.org) or BRB ArrayTools (Simon *et al.*, 2007), examples of bioinformatic platforms, provide tools for analysis and comprehension of genomic data.
7. Candidate genes are validated through another technology. Usually quantitative reverse-transcription PCR (qPCR) is the preferred method.
8. Data is integrated and applied to the initial question.

1.2 Microarray challenges and concerns

Large-scale gene expression analysis, is in fact, a flourishing technology with potential applications in several fields of Biology and Medicine as indicated by the large number of peer-reviewed articles (n=35502) containing the words "gene" and "microarray" found in Pubmed upto June 2011.

Microarray profiling of gene expression is a powerful tool for discovery, but the ability to manage and compare the resulting data can be problematic. Biological, experimental, and technical variations between studies of the same phenotype/phenomena create substantial differences in results. Some of these issues will be discussed in detail.

a) The success of the microarrays experience greatly depends on whether the hypothesis and rationale have been appropriately formulated through a clearly delineated question. It influences the study design as a whole, from sample collection, to experimental design, and finally, the strategies for data analysis (Smith & Rosa, 2007).

b) While most of the early studies used primary tissues involved in the disease, such as tumor biopsies, more recently a number of gene expression profiling studies have focused on peripheral blood to identify systemic markers of disease. However, gene expression patterns in peripheral blood cells greatly depend on inter-individual variations and technical aspects such as blood sampling techniques, cell and RNA isolation as well as storage temperature or delays in processing. However although significant inter-individual variations in gene expression patterns in peripheral blood cells can be seen, these differences are often much less than the differences between blood samples from healthy donors and from patients. These observations and the accessibility of peripheral blood, strongly suggests that gene expression analysis of peripheral blood is probably the best source for the assessment of systemic differences or changes in gene expression associated with disease or drug response. (Debey *et al.*, 2004).

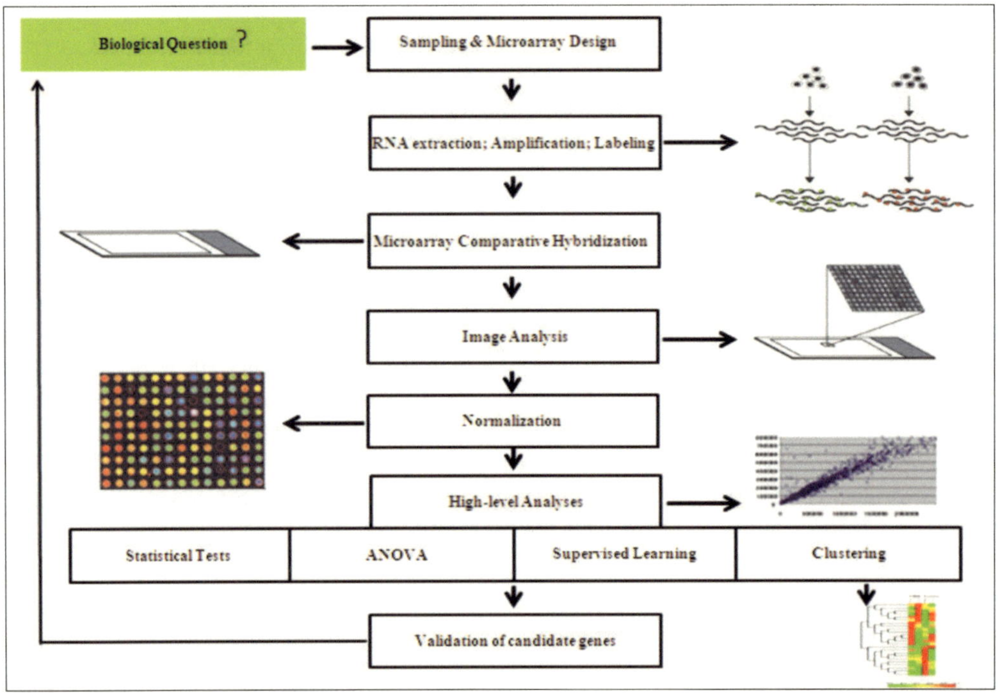

Fig. 1. Design, experimental and data analysis steps in a typical microarray gene expression experiment. Adapted from Repsilber *et al.*, 2005.

c) Appropriate experimental design is another critical step for the success of a microarray experiment. It's important to control and exclude as many biases as possible (Ransohoff, 2007). Integrity and purity of RNA extracted, cDNA labeling and hybridization procedures may affect reproducibility, thus these steps need to be standardized and optimized. However, several key issues regarding appropriate replication remains in discussion: the minimum sample size, the necessity of running multiple arrays with the same samples or the potential benefits and risks associated with pooling samples (Smith & Rosa, 2007). Increasing the sample size will lower the false discovery and false negative rates but it represents an expensive option (Pawitan *et al.*, 2005). Given the well-established reproducible commercially available platforms, technical replication is not required currently. Finally, pooling samples can reduce the variation between arrays but potential outliers may get masked or may compromise the entire pool (Smith & Rosa, 2007). To guaranty an improvement of data quality, replication studies in independent patient series must be performed, but these analyses are often lacking (Ionnidis *et al.*, 2009).

d) Data analysis currently represents a major challenge for researchers. A closer look at the literature reveals many conflicting results. A consensus regarding strategies in data analysis is required. Over the last few years a number of papers have reviewed in detail how to analyze typical microarray data experiments (Allison *et al.*, 2006; Reimers, 2010), to interpret them (Michiels *et al.*, 2007) and to report the results (Dupuy & Simon, 2007). The multidimensionality of microarrays and possible solutions to deal with this issue are well discussed in a recent review (Michiels *et al.*, 2011).

e) Confirmation and validation studies are another crucial step. For confirmation studies the initial results must be reproduced using another assay technology, usually qPCR. Validation studies require an independent study in a new sample cohort to confirm that the gene signatures defined previously replicate satisfactorily in a similar clinical setting. It may be performed by the same research team or ideally by others. These aditional steps reduce false positives and the potential for biases (Michiels *et al.*, 2007, 2011).

Establishing a consensus to optimize each step of the procedure would therefore generate more reproducibility in results from different studies. Evidence-based guidelines to perform meta-analysis of array data are in progress (Ramasamy *et al.*, 2008) but establishing consensus in experimental design and protocols is still the most likely method to minimize variation. Clinical trials to confirm the gene signature's clinical utility on diagnosis and treatment decisions are mandatory, after the identification of reliable biomarkers.

1.3 Microarray applications in rheumatology/spondyloarthritis

Several microarrays studies have been published looking at spondyloarthritis (SpA). A number of early studies used different tissue sources and smaller microarrays with whole-genome arrays prohibitively expensive (Reviewed in Thomas & Brown MA, 2010a, 2010b). The first study in 2002 identified genes more highly expressed in peripheral blood mononuclear cells (PBMC) of patients with SpA, rheumatoid arthritis (RA) and psoriatic arthritis (PsA), in comparison to normal subjects (Gu *et al.*, 2002a). A 588-gene microarray was used as a screening tool and the results were validated by reverse transcription-polymerase chain reaction (RT-PCR). A total of 16 genes were identified encoding differentiation markers, cytokines, cytokine/chemokine receptors and signalling and adhesion molecules. An increased expression of C-X-C chemokine receptor type 4 (*CXCR4*) and its ligand Stromal cell-derived factor-1 (SDF-1), in synovial fluid cells, were seen in all three arthritis groups. The conclusion was that the CXCR4/SDF-1 is a potential pro-inflammatory axis for SpA, PsA and RA. However no genes were identified that could discriminate between the different diseases.

In another study gene expression profiles of synovial fluid mononuclear cells (SFMC) from SpA and RA patients were compared with PBMC of healthy controls to evaluate the unfolded protein response (UPR) hypothesis and identify which cytokines/chemokines were being expressed and which cell fractions were involved. An 1176-gene microarray was used and the results were validated by RT-PCR. There was an increase in transcripts encoding Monocyte chemotactic protein-1 (MCP-1), proteasome subunit C2 and Binding immunoglobulin protein (BiP), which suggest the existence of an UPR. BiP was higher in SpA SFMC compared to RA SFMC and macrophages were potentially identified as the cell type involved (Gu *et al.*, 2002b).

A third study identified a gene expression profile in gut biopsies that could differentiate SpA patients with sub-clinical gut inflammation from SpA patients without gut disease.

2625 differentially expressed sequence tags were initially identified through macroarrays in colon biopsies from Crohn's and SpA patients which were then used to construct a microarray which was used to screen a further sample cohort. Ninety five expressed sequence tags clustered patients with Crohn's and those with SpA and chronic gut inflammation (Laukens *et al.*, 2006).

This chapter, Lessons from Genomic Profiling in AS will be focused on studies using peripheral blood and microarray platforms covering the whole genome. The results seem to be quite heterogeneous reflecting the different methodologies involved, as commented above. Several aspects, summarized in Figure 1, may introduce variability and bias in the results, specifically;

a. Patient selection: numbers of patients, the criteria used to classify and include the patients, different degrees of activity/severity of the disease and patients receiving different therapies are examples of heterogeneity that might influence the final results.
b. Cell Source used for analysis: PBMC vs. whole blood or a specific cell subset.
c. Differences in microarray platform technology and data analysis tools.
d. Differences in methodology used regarding validation of candidate biomarkers.

Based on seven papers published since 2007, several pathways relevant to potential SpA pathological processes have been identified. Moreover, potential biomarkers with applications to diagnosis and treatment response prediction in clinical practice were also flagged. Table 2, summarizes the similarities and methodological differences between the studies and reinforces the caution that should be observed when translating these findings to clinical practice. All the knowledge obtained must be interpreted as hypotheses which need validation in future studies.

	Subjects	Criteria	Samples	Microarray	Validation
Smith *et al.* 2008	6AS+2uSPA 9HC	mNYC ESSG, Amor	Macrophage	Affymetrix	qPCR
Haroon *et al.* 2010	16AS	mNYC	PBMC	Affymetrix	qPCR
Sharma *et al.* 2009	11uSPA+7uSPA 25HC	Likelihood Score	Whole blood	Affymetrix	Microarrays (2nd set)
Duan *et al.* 2010	18AS+18HC 35AS+18HC	mNYC	PBMC	Illumina	qPCR
Gu *et al.* 2009	21AS+28uSPA 23AS+18uSPA 26HC+12RA+5LBP	Calin	PBMC	Illumina	qPCR
Assassi *et al.* 2011	16AS + 14HC+ SLE+SSC 27AS+27HC	mNYC	Whole bood	Illumina	qPCR
Santos *et al.* 2011	18AS+18HC 78AS+78HC	mNYC	Whole blood	Illumina	qPCR

AS: Ankylosing spondylitis; **SPA:** Spondyloarthritis; **HC:** Healthy controls; **RA:** Rheumatoid arthritis; **LBP:** Lumbar back pain; **SLE:** Systemic lupus erythematosus; **mNYC**: modified New York criteria; **ESSG:** European Spondyloarthropathy Study Group; **PBMC:** Peripheral blood mononuclear cells; **qPCR**: Quantitative reverse transcription polymerase chain reaction.

Table 2. Comparison between published microarrays studies in SpA.

2. Lessons from genomic profiling in AS

2.1 The link between an abnormal innate immune response and AS

One of the most intriguing aspects regarding AS pathogenesis is the possible link between pathogens and disease onset. There are several pieces of evidence that an abnormal host response against pathogens is implicated in AS and/or SpA pathogenesis. Sixty percent of patients with SpA without diagnosed Crohn's disease evidenced endoscopic or histological signs of gut inflammation (Mielants *et al.*, 1995). Moreover, studies showing HLA-B27 transgenic rats do not develop inflammatory intestinal or peripheral joint disease in a germ-free environment support a role of commensal gut flora in the shared pathogenesis of gut and joint manifestations (Taurog *et al.*, 1994).

Pattern recognition receptors (PRRs) in innate immune cells play a pivotal role in the first line of the host defense system. These receptors are transmembrane receptors such as Toll-like receptors (TLRs) or C-type lectin receptors (CLRs) and cytosolic receptors RIG-I-like receptors (RLRs) and NOD-like receptors (NLRs) (Jeong & Lee, 2011). Interestingly, expression changes in genes involved in innate immune response such as *TLRs* (Assassi *et al.*, 2011), *NLRP2* (Sharma *et al.*, 2009) and *CLEC4D* (Pimentel-Santos *et al.*, 2011) were consistently observed in several different studies using microarray technology.

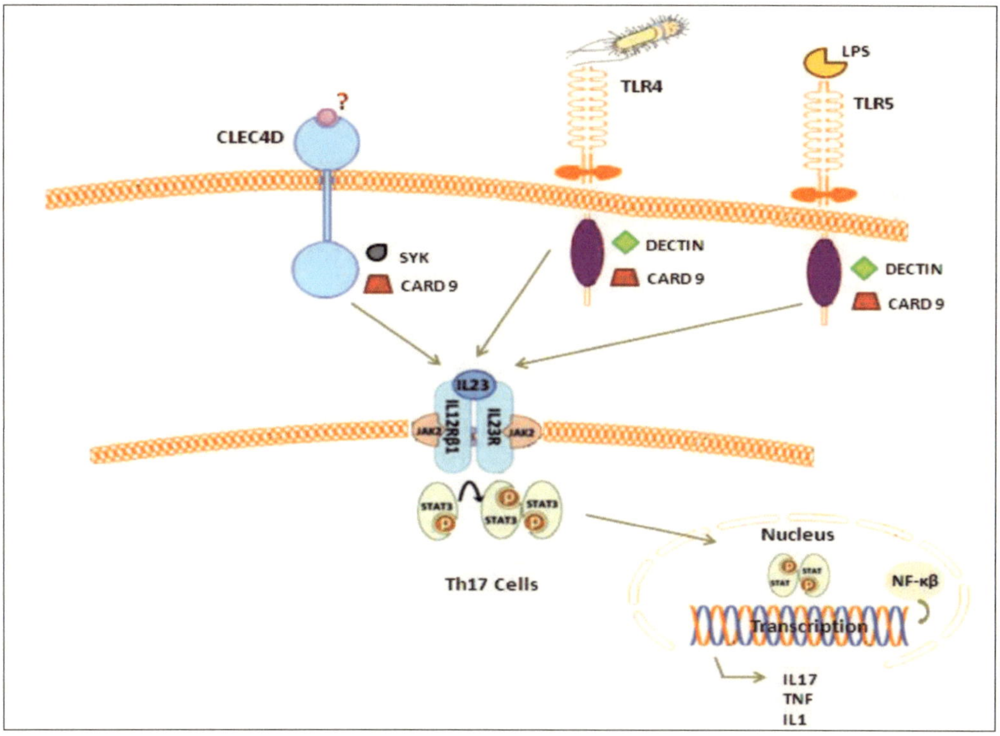

Fig. 2. Possible functional interactions between innate immune receptors and AS candidate genes (Adapted from Thomas & Brown, 2010a).

TLRs are characterized by an extracellular leucine-rich repeat (LRR) domain, a transmembrane domain and a cytoplasmic Toll/IL-1R (TIR) domain. As many as 13 TLR family members have been identified in mammalian systems with TLRs 1 to 10 expressed in humans. They can be divided into 2 groups according to cellular localization and respective ligands. TLRs 1, 2, 4, 5, and 6, are expressed on the cell surface and recognize microbial components in the outer membrane of bacteria. TLRs 3, 7, 8 and 9 are found in intracellular vesicles and recognize microbial nucleic acids (Sirisinha, 2011). TLRs are expressed in various immune (monocytes, macrophages, dendritic cells, B cells) and non-immune (epithelial cells, endothelial cells, fibroblasts) cells. *TLR4* was overexpressed in SpA patients in peripheral whole blood cells, assessed by microarray (Assassi *et al.*, 2011; Pimentel-Santos *et al.*, 2011), in PBMCs, measured by flow cytometry (De Rycke *et al.*, 2005) and in lymphocytes, monocytes and neutrophils by qPCR (Yang *et al.*, 2007). The main ligand for TLR4 is lipopolysaccharide (LPS) in the outer membrane of Gram-negative bacteria, however, it also recognizes other exogenous pathogens such as mannan from *Candida albicans*, glycoinositolphospholipid from *Trypanosoma*, and the envelope proteins from mouse mammary tumor virus (MMTV) and respiratory syncytial virus (RSV). It also recognizes some endogenous molecules, including heat-shock proteins (HSP60, HSP70, and HSP gp96), fibrinogen, oligosaccharides of hyaluronic acid, extracellular domain A of fibronectin, heparan sulfate, myeloid-related proteins (Mrp8 and Mrp14), oxidized LDL, saturated fatty acid and amyloid-β (Jeong & Lee, 2011). Microarray analysis also showed overexpression of TLR5 in peripheral whole blood cells from SpA patients (Assassi S *et al.*, 2011; Pimentel-Santos *et al.*, 2011). Flagellin, a primary component of Gram negative bacteria flagella, is the main ligand for TLR5 (Hayashi *et al.*, 2001), which is mainly expressed on the luminar surface of epithelial cells in the mucosal tissues and respiratory tract (Gewirtz *et al.*, 2001).

The wide responsiveness of TLRs to a wide variety of external and internal signals, and the link that these receptors establish between the innate and adaptative immune systems, reinforces the theory that TLRs are strongly implicated in the development of chronic inflammatory diseases. However, mechanistic studies are needed in order to clarify the role of specific receptor subtypes in AS development.

Members of the NOD-like receptor (NLR) family consist of a central nucleotide-binding and oligomerization (NACHT) domain, which is commonly flanked by C-terminal leucine-rich repeat (LRRs) domain and N-terminal caspase recruitment (CARD) or pyrin (PYD) domains (Schroder & Tschopp, 2010). So far, 20 NLR family members have been identified in humans. Two main subgroups have been described. One, including NODs (NOD 1-5 and CIITA), detects pathogen-associated molecular patterns (PAMPs) existing in Gram-negative bacteria cell walls and elicit responses that are distinct from those of the TLRs. The other NLR subgroup involves a large family of molecular complexes known as the "inflammasomes", the NLRPs (NLRP1-14) and the IPAF subfamily, consisting of IPAF and NAIP (Fitzgerald, 2010; Schroder & Tschopp, 2010). The inflammasomes are macromolecular cytosolic complexes composed of several proteins, some of which are found in all inflammasomes (pro-caspase-1, Apoptosis-associated Speck-like Protein Containing a Caspase Recruitment Domain-ASC), and others which are present depending on the inflammasome type (cardinal, pro-caspase-5, domain with function to find-FIIND). These complexes are involved in the innate immune response recognizing both endogenous signals (adenosine triphosphate, urate, and calcium pyrophosphate crystals) as well as external pathogen-derived products (bacterial RNA, bacterial toxins) (Drenth & van der Meer, 2006).

As such, the reduced expression of Nod-like receptor family, pyrin domain containing 2 *(NLRP2)* in AS was a very interesting observation (Sharma *et al.*, 2009). NLRP2, as with other NLRs, induces an inhibition of the NF*k*B signaling pathway, leading to regulation of IL1β, a relevant cytokine in the disease process. The downregulation of *NLRP2* may therefore lead to upregulation of IL-1β. Supporting this, polymorphisms in *NLR* genes have also been implicated in Behçet's disease and Crohn's disease which share some clinical features with AS (Cummings *et al.*, 2010; Kappen *et al.*, 2009). Another interesting point is the association of *CARD9* with Crohn's disease and AS (Pointon *et al.*, 2010) which has a pivotal role in NOD2 signaling.

Another family of receptors of particular interest are the C-type lectins which display a distinct protein domain, the carbohydrate recognition domain (CRD). Based on the organization of their CRDs, 17 distinct groups have been defined (Drickamer & Fadden, 2002; Zelensky & Gready, 2005). While some recognize DAMPs which facilitate adhesion between cells, adhesion of cells to extracellular matrix and other non-enzymatic functions, others may act as PRRs (Graham & Brown, 2009) after PAMP recognition. Upon ligand biding, C-type lectin receptors can induce a variety of cellular responses, and can be functionally divided into those that inhibit or those that induce cellular activation. In general, inhibitory receptors contain a consensus immunoreceptor tyrosine-based inhibitory motif (ITIM) in their cytoplasmic domains, while activation receptors either contain an immunoreceptor tyrosine-based activation motif (ITAM), or associate with signalling adaptor molecules. Depending on whether signalling is through ITAM or ITIM , either activation of Src homology 2 (SH2) domain-containing protein tyrosine kinases (SyK, ZAP 10) or SH2 containing-phosphatases (SHP-1, SHP-2) are recruited, thereby up or downmodulating cellular activation, respectively (Majeed *et al.*, 2001; Long, 1999).

Genes encoding for each family are distinctly clustered in the telomeric Natural Killer-gene complex (NKC), on chromosome 12. The Dectin-1 cluster of receptors, includes Dectin-1, lectin-like oxidized low-density lipoprotein receptor-1 (LOX-1), C-type lectin-like receptor-1 (CLEC-1), CLEC-2, CLEC12B, CLEC9A and myeloid inhibitory C-type lectin-like receptor (MICL). The Dectin-2 cluster of receptors, includes Dectin-2, DCIR, DCAR, BDCA-2, Mincle and CLEC4D (Graham & Brown, 2009).

Dectin-1, is expressed in dendritic cells, monocytes, macrophages, neutrophils and weakly in a subset of T cells, B cells and eosinophils. It recognizes fungal β-glucan, working as an activating receptor uniquely possessing an ITAM in the cytoplasmic domain. The induction of phagocytosis, production of reactive oxygen species and cytokine production is mediated by NF-kB and spleen tyrosine kinase (Syk). In addition, some of these effects require cooperation with MyD88-mediated TLR signaling (Kanazawa, 2007).

Dectin-2 and Mincle are expressed in macrophages, dendritic cells and weakly in Langerhans cells and monocytes. The receptors recognize several pathogens (*Candida albicans, Saccharomyces cerevisiae, Mycoplasma tuberculosis, Histoplasma capsulatum*) but also endogenous ligands. Both have characteristic short cytoplasmic domains and are associated with FcRγ domains. Their activation, inducing the production of proinflammatory cytokines, is mediated by Syk- and CARD9-dependent pathways but independently of MyD88-mediated TLR signaling (Graham & Brown GD, 2009).

CLEC4D has been found to be expressed in a monocyte/macrophage restricted manner, and although no ligand or biological function has as yet been described, the receptor has been shown to be upregulated at the transcript level in a number of disease settings, similarly to two other members of the family, Mincle and Dectin-2. They are able to recognize and promote pathogen clearance and induce inflammatory signals. This process seems to follow the Syk and CARD9 pathway which was recently implicated in a mouse model of SpA (Ruutu *et al.*, 2010). The upregulation of *CLEC4D*, observed for the first time in an expression profiling study of AS patients (Pimentel-Santos *et al.*, 2011), supports the importance of innate immune mechanisms in AS pathology. However, further studies are required to confirm this hypothesis.

2.2 Proinflammatory *vs.* immunosuppressive signatures

Transcriptional profiling studies have demonstrated that transcripts involved in the inflammatory response were differentially expressed in AS patients and controls, but reports on the nature of these changes seem to vary. A proinflammatory profile in peripheral blood monocyte cells (PBMCs), from undifferentiated spondyloarthritis (uSpA) and AS, is indicated by an increased expression of *RGS1, NR4A2, HBEGF* and *SOCS3,* in both groups (Gu *et al.*, 2009). However, other reports suggest decreased immune responsiveness such as a "reverse *IFNγ* signature" (Smith *et al.*, 2008), and immunosuppressive phenotypes (Duan *et al.*, 2010, Pimentel-Santos *et al.*, 2011). The main reason for these differences in the transcriptomic profiles, between the first study and the 3 later studies, is unknown but differences in patients and methodologies may contribute.

IFNγ dysregulation in AS is supported by previous studies of cytokines expression. A lower frequency of IFNγ positive T cells has been reported in AS patients (Rudwaleit *et al.*, 2001) and gut biopsy samples show a reduced TH1 profile in lymphocytes from SpA patients (Van Damme *et al.*, 2001). Moreover, IFNγ is expressed at lower levels in synovium from SpA compared to rheumatoid arthritis patients (Canete *et al.*, 2000). This knowledge may contribute to understanding AS pathogenesis as decresead IFNγ production by macrophages could impair the host's ability to clear pathogenic organisms. Recent studies support this theory (Rothfuchs *et al.*, 2001; Inman *et al.*, 2006), and may implicate arthritogenic organisms in AS susceptibility. In addition, IFNγ reduction, can contribute to activation of the IL-23/IL-17 axis a major axis in AS pathogenesis.

Complementary to the report in macrophages from peripheral blood of AS patients (Smith *et al.*, 2008), two different studies, from PBMCs and whole blood, have shown an immunosuppressive phenotype (Duan *et al.*, 2010, Pimentel-Santos *et al.*, 2011). The first one validated three downregulated genes, Nuclear receptor subfamily 4, group A, member 2 (*NR4A2*), Tumor necrosis factor, alpha-induced protein 3 *(TNFAIP3)* and CD69 molecule *(CD69)*. NR4A2 has been associated with T-cell subset communication and the macrophage inflammatory response. TNFAIP3 serves as negative feedback system for the TNFα induced by NFkB, acting as an anti-inflammatory molecule to control prolonged inflammation. CD69 is an early leukocyte activation molecule expressed at sites of active inflammation. Of further interest were the results of Ingenuity Pathways Analysis using the differentially expressed geneset showing altered activity of the JAK/STAT signaling pathway in AS patients (Duan *et al.*, 2010). Both *STAT3* and *JAK2* have been shown to be genetically associated with IBD and AS (Barrett *et al.*, 2008; Danoy *et al.*, 2010; The Australo-Anglo-American-Spondyloarthritis-Consortium (TASC), 2011), and represent key downstream molecules of the IL-23/IL-17 pathway (Ma *et al.*, 2008).

In the second study downregulation of several pro-inflammatory genes were described highlighting another aspect of AS pathogenesis (Pimentel-Santos *et al.*, 2011). Protein tyrosine phosphatase, non-receptor type 1 *(PTPN1)* and Dedicator of cytokinesis 10 *(DOCK10)*, which are both involved in mediating IL4 actions (Paul & Ohara., 1987) were downregulated. Protein tyrosine phosphatase 1B (PTP1B), the *PTPN1* protein product, is a ubiquitously expressed enzyme shown to negatively regulate multiple tyrosine phosphorylation-dependent signalling pathways, including the downstream processes involved in C-type lectin receptor activation (Majeed *et al.*, 2001; Long, 1999) and IL4 signalling (Lu *et al.*, 2008). Dock10 is also regulated by IL4 in B cells (Yelo *et al.*, 2008). This is of particular interest as IL4 may play a role in AS pathogenesis. Interleukin 4 (IL4), has a variety of stimulatory and inhibitory actions on B and T cells (O'Garra *et al.*, 1988; Jelinek & Lipsky 1988; Rousset *et al.*, 1988). Recent studies have also indicated a potential role for IL4 producing CD8+ T cells in the pathogenesis of AS. Although CD8+ T cells are predominately associated with the production of 'TH1' cytokines, such as IFNγ, there is now good evidence that some subsets of these cells can also produce 'TH2' cytokines such as IL4, IL5 and IL10 (Baek *et al.*, 2008). The potential functions associated with IL4-producing CD8+ T cells are as yet unclear but the subtype CD8+/TCR αβ+ T cells, with a regulatory phenotype and function (expressing CD25+, CTLA4+, Foxp3+, but negative for IFNγ and perforin), were previously described in peripheral blood of AS patients (Jarvis *et al.*, 2005). These results were confirmed in a recent study suggesting an altered pattern of CD8+ T cell differentiation in AS and in HLAB27+ healthy individuals. This predisposition to generate IL4+CD8+ T cells may play a role in pathogenesis of SpA (Zhang *et al.*, 2009). Further supporting this theory, *RUNX3* was identified as a candidate gene in a GWAS (Australo-Anglo-American Spondyloarthritis Consortium (TASC), 2010). The association of *RUNX3* with AS provides additional evidence of a role for CD8+ T cells in the disease. It's expression in immature lymphocytes is triggered by IL7R signalling, leading to suppression of CD4 and upregulation of CD8 expression (Park *et al.*, 2010).

Although there are some differences between the different expression profiling studies, their findings do contribute to a greater understanding of the pathogenesis of AS, particularly in the delineation of the roles of the innate and adaptive immune responses.

2.3 Bone ossification and resorption processes

Bone formation and bone loss take place at sites closely located to each other presenting an "apparent paradox", which is reflected in the changes in bone and cartilage metabolism occurring in the AS disease process (Carter & Lories, 2011). Ossification is the hallmark of AS and has been linked to aberrant activation of bone morphogenic protein (BMP) and wingless (WNT) signaling. Bone resorption, driven by the impact of inflammation on the bone remodeling cycle, occurs simultaneously, with up to 56% of patients developing systemic osteopenia and some of them systemic osteoporosis (Lange *et al.*, 2005).

Biomarkers, reflecting structural damage and disease activity, constitute a high priority for the understanding of the pathogenesis of AS and for the new therapy discovery. Two microarray-based studies have contributed to the improvement of knowledge in this field. A bone remodeling signature was described associated with an overexpression of *BMP6,* Proprotein convertase subtilisin/kexin type 6 *(PCSK6),* Kringle containing transmembrane protein 1 *(KREMEN1)* and Catenin (cadherin-associated protein) alpha-like 1 *(CTNNAL1)* genes in SpA patients (Sharma *et al.*, 2009).

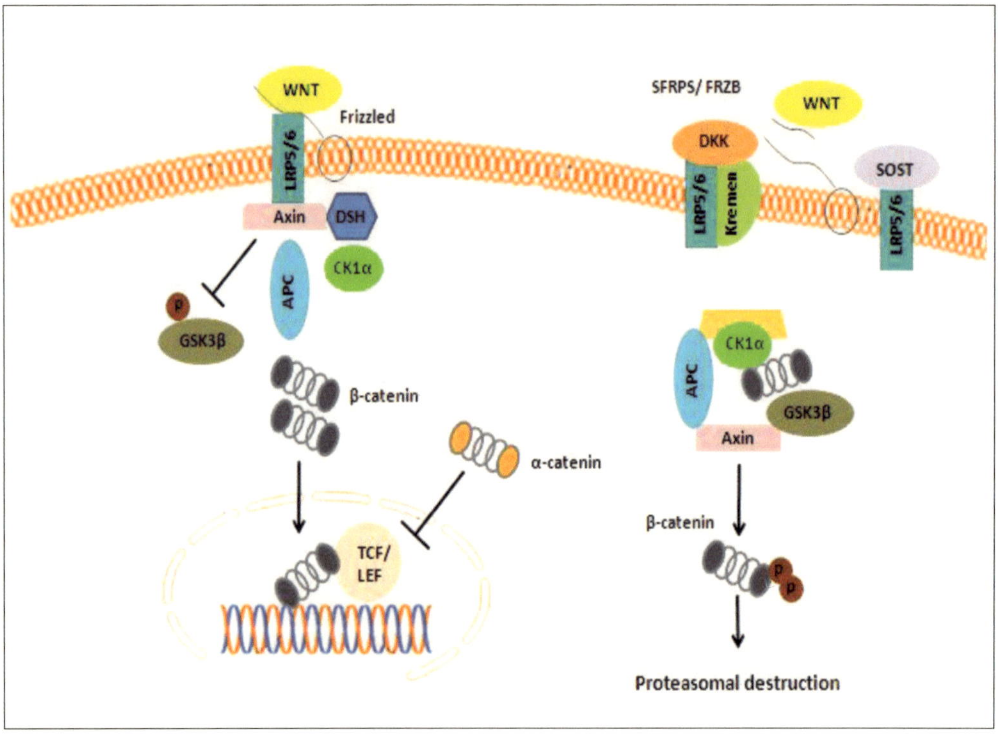

Fig. 3. The canonical WNT signaling pathway (adapted from Carter & Lories, 2011).

KREMEN1 and *CTNNAL1* are negative regulators of WNT/catenin pathway via dickkopf homolog 1 (DKK1), or by direct inhibition of β-catenin, respectively. Although four different intracellular pathways can be triggered upon WNT receptor interaction, the WNT/β-catenin or "canonical" pathway is of particular interest in bone and cartilage biology. This pathway involves the interaction of WNT ligands with frizzled (FZD) receptors and low-density lipoprotein receptor-related protein 4, 5 or 6 (LRP 4, 5 or 6) co-receptors. In the absence of a WNT-FZD-LRP 4/5/6 interaction, cytoplasmic β-catenin is captured within a destruction complex comprising adenomatous polyposis coli (APC), axin, glycogen synthase kinase 3β (GSK-3β), and casein kinase 1α (CK1 α). The kinases phosphorylate β-catenin, which leads to ubiquitinylation and subsequent destruction in a proteasome complex. When WNT does complex with FZD and LRP 4/5/6, axin binds to the cytoplasmic tail of LRP5 or 6, thereby phosphorylating and inhibiting GSK-3β (Gordon & Nusse, 2006). This process enables cytoplasmic β-catenin accumulation which then translocates to the nucleus, where it interacts with transcription factor (TCF)/lymphoid enhancer factor (LEF) family members and modulates WNT target gene expression (Gordon & Nusse, 2006). Several proteins that are not involved in β-catenin stability can also regulate β-catenin signaling. One example is the direct association of α-catenin with β-catenin in the nucleus which interferes with protein-DNA interactions required for TCF-mediated transcription (Giannini *et al.*, 2000). In addition, different endogenous antagonists inhibit WNT signalling; DKK1 and sclerostin (SOST). DKK1 acts by direct binding to and inhibiting the WNT co-receptor LRP6. The related DKK2, however, can function either as LRP6 agonist or antagonist, depending on the cellular context, suggesting that its activity is modulated by unknown co-factors. In this context, the transmembrane proteins KREMEN1 and -2 were recently identified as additional DKK receptors, which bind to both DKK1 and DKK2 with high affinity (Mao & Niehrs, 2003). It was shown that DKK1 was able to simultaneously bind to LRP5/6 and KREMEN and that the ternary complex was rapidly endocytosed, thus preventing the WNT-LRP interaction. The interaction with KREMEN seems to be not essential but it plays a role in facilitating DKK-mediated antagonism if the level of LRP5/6 is high (Wang *et al.*, 2008). The upregulation of *KREMEN1* and *CTNNAL1* genes by these mechanisms can compromise bone formation. In contrast, upregulation of *BMP6* and its regulator *PCSK6* can contribute to the AS ossification process. BMPs, members of the transforming growth factor-β (TGF β) superfamily, play a crucial role in embryonic development, cell lineage determination, and osteoblastic differentiation and function. Enthesitis, a distinctive feature of SpA, is associated with heterotopic cartilage and bone formation (enthesophyte) (Benjamin & McGonagle, 2001). Different BMPs are expressed in distinct stages of ankylosing enthesitis shown in the DBA/1 mouse model. BMP2 is found in proliferating cells and entheseal cells committing their differentiation fate to chondrogenesis. BMP7 is recognized in prehypertrophic chondrocytes and BMP6 in hypertrophic chondrocytes (Lories *et al.*, 2005). Several regulators of endochondral bone formation with different effects in different stages were described (Kronenberg, 2003). It is therefore possible that the presence of progenitor cells at the entheseal site promotes bone formation in SpA patients. Activation of the BMP signaling pathway (phosphorylated Smad1/5) was found in cells at the sites of entheseal inflammation in patients with AS (Lories *et al.*, 2005).

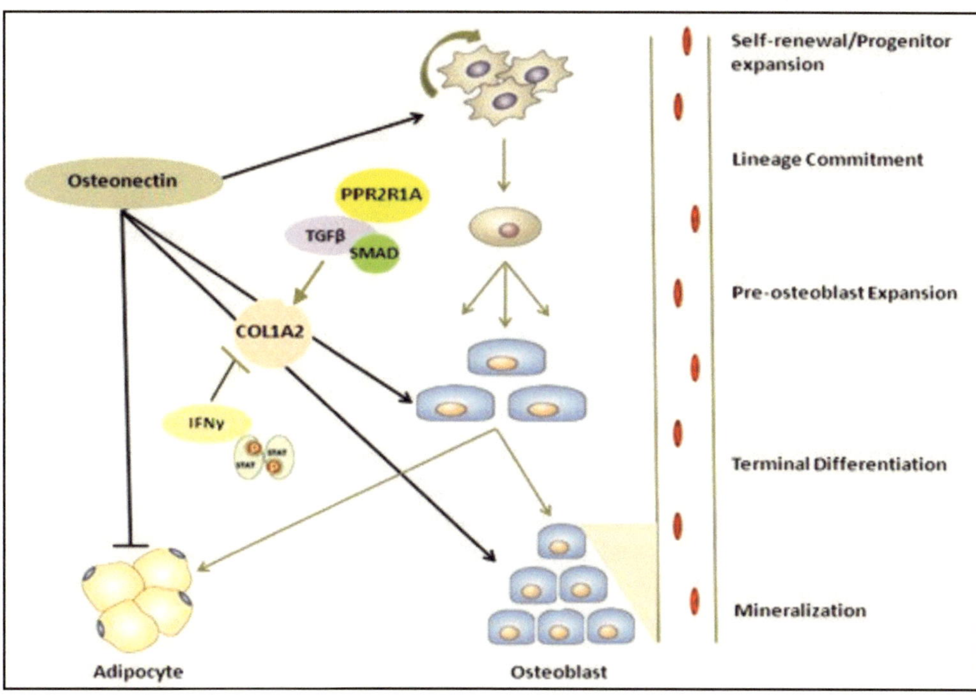

Fig. 4. Model representing the effects of SPARC on marrow mesenchymal progenitors (adapated from Delany & Hankenson, 2009).

Another bone remodeling signature was identified in association with a downregulation of *SPOCK2, EP300* and *PPP2R1A* in AS, which are possible mediators in the ossification process (Pimentel-Santos *et al.*, 2011).

SPOCK2, also known as Sparc/osteonectin, is a non-collagenous bone protein. It is a member of the matricellular class of glycoproteins which includes periostin, tenascin C, osteopontin, bone sialoprotein, thrombospondin-1 and thrombospondin-2 (Alford & Hankenson, 2006). It has been hypothesized to play a role in the regulation, production, assembly and maintenance of the matrix turnover in cartilage (Hausser *et al.*, 2004; Gruber *et al.*, 2005). In this process TGFβ and IFNγ exert antagonistic effects, and play important roles in the physiologic regulation of extracellular matrix turnover. In fact, *TGFβ* positively regulates collagen type 1 (COL1A2) through the Smad signal transduction pathway, whereas *IFNγ* inhibits COL1A2 through Stat1. Additionally, protein phosphatase 2, regulatory subunit A (*PPP2R1A),* also downregulated in AS (Pimentel-Santos *et al.*, 2011), is thought to mediate *TGFβ* regulation through Smad (Heikkinen *et al.*, 2010). Animal models using SPARC-null mice have provided excellent information on the function of this protein in bone. SPARC-null mice develop profound low-turnover osteopenia (bone loss), associated with decreased numbers of osteoblasts and osteoclasts, and a markedly decreased bone-formation rate (Delany *et al.*, 2000; Boskey, 2003). Moreover SPARC-null mice have decreased trabecular bone volume due to decreased trabecular number (Machado dos Reis *et al.*, 2008) and an increase in extra-skeletal adipose deposits (Mansergh *et al.*, 2007). *In vitro* studies showed accumulation of SPARC during early osteoblastic differentiation, likely in association with collagen matrix, which decreases as the cells acquire more osteoblastic characteristics. This expression pattern seems appropriate because SPARC regulates collagen fibril assembly, and matrix is abundantly deposited in the earlier stages of differentiating cultures. SPARC has a positive effect on maintaining and expanding the mesenchymal progenitor pool, and promotes osteoblastogenesis/osteoblast function and decreases adipogenesis (Delany & Hankenson, 2009.). Expression of SPARC by osteoclasts has not been reported. Therefore, the mechanisms by which SPARC limits osteoclast formation may involve the direct interaction with osteoclasts or osteoclast precursors through the bone matrix, and/or the effect of SPARC on immune cells, marrow stromal cells, and osteoblasts supporting osteoclast development (Machado do Reis *et al.* 2008). In summary, recent findings supports the idea that SPARC play a critical role in regulating bone remodeling and maintaining bone mass. Thus its dysregulated expression may contribute to the aberrant matrix formation in AS.

Interestingly, the protein produced by *EP300* belongs to the group of nuclear p300/CBP transcriptional coactivators for both Smad3 and Stat1a that integrate signals that positively or negatively regulate *COL1A2* transcription (Ghosh *et al.*, 2001). Transactivated p300, controlled by phosphoinositide-3 kinase (PI3K)/AKT, is also an important transcriptional co-activator of Sox9, which modulates the expression of the major extracellular matrix component, aggrecan (Cheng *et al.*, 2009). Moreover, there is some evidence supporting a p300 interaction with the Wnt pathway as it is a β-catenin transcriptional coactivator. Downregulation of these genes might lead to a loss of matrix integrity thereby accelerating tissue damage. This may be reinforced by a pro-inflammatory status associated with downregulation of *EP300* (Ahmad *et al.*, 2007).

2.4 Biomarkers for early diagnostic purposes

Low back pain (LBP) is a very common symptom, responsible for 3% of annual medical visits in the USA (Licciardone, 2008). However only 5% of the chronic back pain seen in general practice designated as "inflammatory", is associated with SpA (Underwood & Dawes, 1995). To classify patients with AS or SpA, various criteria sets can be used. The modified New York Criteria (van der Linden *et al.*, 1984) for AS, the Amor criteria (Amor *et al.*, 1990) and the European Spondyloarthropathy Study Group (ESSG) criteria (Amor *et al.*, 1991), developed in the 1990s, before magnetic resonance imaging (MRI) was available, addressed all SpA subtypes. Recently, it has been proposed to divide SpA patients into subgroups according to clinical presentation. The Assessment of SpondyloArthritis International Society (ASAS) group has developed criteria to classify patients with axial SpA with or without radiographic sacroiliitis, and patients with predominant peripheral SpA (Rudwaleit *et al.*, 2009b; Rudwaleit, 2010). With a sensitivity of 82.9% and a specificity of 84.4% , these axial SpA criteria perform better than the ESSG and Amor criteria, even after adding "sacroiliitis on MRI" to the latter. The peripheral criteria with sensitivity of 77.8% and specificity of 82.8% are also promising for use in clinical practice (Rudwaleit, 2010). The ASAS criteria have been developed as classification criteria but they are likely be useful as diagnostic criteria, especially in patients with non-radiographic axial SpA at an outpatient rheumatology clinic (van den Berg & van der Heijde, 2010). This may help to make an early diagnosis and prevent the current diagnostic delay, described as 5 to 10 years between the first occurrence of symptoms and an AS diagnosis (Feldtkeller *et al.*, 2003; Haibel *et al.*, 2007). It prevents unnecessary diagnostic tests and more importantly makes it possible to commence more effective therapies earlier. This is crucial as at early disease stages, even those without definite radiologic sacroiliitis, can suffer as much pain and have as high a disease activity as patients with established AS (Rudwaleit *et al.*, 2009a). Therefore, it's important to consider all patients with SpA with predominantly axial involvement irrespective of the presence or absence of radiographic changes as belonging to one disease continuum (Rudwaleit, 2005). Despite all these advantages with the new ASAS criteria, one of the major reasons for diagnosis delay is a low awareness of AS among physicians in primary care (Sieper, 2009). In this particular setting, several concerns have been raised regarding the use of ASAS criteria for diagnostic purposes (van den Berg &. van der Heijde, 2010). Thus current diagnosis of AS and SpA still relies on clinical and imaging parameters that may be relatively complex for general use in primary care. Screening parameters for an early referral of AS patients, easy to apply by the non-specialist, sensitive, specific and not too expensive, should be identified. For the rheumatology community this represents a great challenge. Expression studies can identify a small number of genes whose expression profile might serve as cost effective set of surrogate biomarkers for AS.

One study has identified a small number of genes whose expression profile might serve as a cost-effective set of surrogate biomarkers for AS and uSpA (Gu *et al.*, 2009). In this PBMC-based microarray study, all included patients fulfilled Calin criteria for inflammatory back pain and were taking non-steroidal anti-inflammatory drugs (NSAID's) and/or sulfasalazine. They concluded that the overall gene expression was higher in uSpA than in AS patients suggesting that early axial SpA is associated with a more systemic inflammatory process. This may represent an interesting point as biomarkers are more helpfull in the early stage of SpA rather than the late stage. (Gu et al., 2009). Alternatively, it may reflect the less accurate diagnosis involved in uSpA and might be due some uSpA patients being misdiagnosed and actually suffering from a different inflammatory condition. A member of the family of regulators of G protein signaling *(RGS1,)* was identified as the most promising biomarker for uSpA and AS, with this gene more highly expressed in uSpA than in AS. They demonstrated a receiver operating characteristic (ROC) area under the curve (AUC) range between 0.93-0.99. Biomarkers with ROC AUC 0.8-1.0 are usually considered to be useful in clinical practice (Rao, 2003). To evaluate arthritis related factors that might enhance *RGS1* expression, a panel of 25 cytokines and chemokines on a monocyte derived human cell line were used. The 2 strongest activators of *RGS1* expression were TNFα and IL-17. However, in order to be implemented in clinical practice further studies are clearly needed. It requires a multicenter, multi-ethnic validation but also comparison with results obtained through MRI and the new ASAS classification criteria. There are several other concerns. This gene was differentially expressed between AS patients and healthy controls, in another microarray study PBMC based (Duan *et al.*, 2010), but contrary to the first study it was underexpressed. Finally, it wasn't identified as differentially expressed in a recent published study from a well defined population of Portuguese ethnicity background (Pimentel-Santos *et al.*, 2011). These distinct results reinforce the need for larger studies involving different ethnic groups.

2.5 Gene expression changes after anti-TNFα therapy

Biomarkers that allow quantitative assessment of treatment response have great potential in clinical practice. They enable appropriate choice of therapy, drug dosage to maximize effect and minimize toxicity, and monitor disease outcomes representing the foundation of evidence-based medicine (de Vlam, 2010). The introduction of biologic therapies targeting TNFα (infliximab, etanercept, adalimumab, golimumab) has changed clinical practice with several benefits regarding clinical management and prognosis. Additionally, the scientific community is waiting for the market introduction of new biological treatments with new targets in the near future. Identification of markers of treatment response would be of great clinical benefit by facilitating better targeting of these treatments to those most likely to respond, and potentially significantly reduce treatment costs by minimizing use of these expensive agents in patients unlikely to respond.

Until now the Visual Analogue Scale (VAS) pain, VAS general health, BASDAI, inflammatory parameters and composite response criteria are used to evaluate treatment effect in AS. ASAS defined and validated three levels of response: ASAS20, ASAS40, and ASAS partial remission, for patients treated with non-steroidal anti-inflammatory drugs and TNFα blockade (Anderson *et al.*, 2001). The recent introduction of the ASDAS criteria (van der Heijde *et al.*, 2009) seems to be a highly discriminatory instrument for assessing AS disease activity and monitoring changes in disease and is finding good use in clinical practice. However all these criteria aren't predictors of response to therapy and greatly rely on subjective self-evaluation and are not free from disease-unrelated influences, so biomarkers with high sensitivity and specificity for treatment response are highly desirable.

Current markers of response such as younger age, HLA-B27 carriage, elevation of acute phase reactants (CRP), and marked spinal inflammation, as shown by MRI, may be predictors of good response; conversely, older age, structural damage and poor function may be predictors of poor- or non-response (Rudwaleit *et al.*, 2004; Rudwaleit *et al.*, 2008). Data from the British Society of Rheumatology Biologics Register has shown raised inflammatory markers at the start of therapy predicted a greater improvement in disease activity, (Lord *et al.*, 2010). Predictors of improvement in function, measured using the BASFI, have shown a strong association with gender (significantly greater improvement in women) and concurrent DMARDs therapy (Lord et al, 2010). Finally, prevention of damage is another important outcome of therapy. Slow radiographic progression of the disease and the relatively small fraction of patients progressing over a period of 2-3 years makes radiographic evaluation less sensitive for damage evaluation. However, the major predictor of progression is previous existing radiographic damage. While it is clear that anti-TNFα agents have a structural benefit in inflammation-mediated resorptive damage as indicated by changes in bone and cartilage metabolism, an effect on radiographic progression remains to be demonstrated in AS (de Vlam, 2010). A study of the relationship of biomarker levels, disease activity and the spinal inflammation detected by MRI was performed in patients with ankylosing spondylitis (AS) receiving Infliximab over a 24 week period. Early reductions in IL-6 (by week 2) but not CRP or vascular endothelial growth factor (VEGF), were significantly associated with reductions in MRI activity and BASDAI scores by week 24 in the infliximab group (Visvanathan *et al.*, 2008). However the structural changes of this effect are not known.

Gene expression profiling constitutes a widely available and promising technology to identify treatment-associated changes. In two recent studies it was demonstrated that anti-TNF alpha treatment leads to significant alteration of gene expression and protein profiles, supporting the use of systematic gene expression and proteomic analysis to shed new light on pathogenic pathways with importance in the chronic inflammation of AS (Haroon *et al.*, 2010; Grcevic *et al.*, 2010). Anti-TNFα therapy induced a rapid change in the expression profile within 2 weeks in AS patients with down-regulation of lymphotoxins exhibiting inducible expression and competing with herpes simplex virus glycoprotein D for herpesvirus entry mediator, a receptor expressed by T lymphocytes *(LIGHT)*, interferon α receptor 1 (*IFNAR1),* interleukin 17 receptor *(IL17R)* and erythropoietin receptor *(EPOR)* genes. *LIGHT*, a member of the TNF superfamily, was the most significantly down-regulated gene and serum soluble LIGHT levels correlate well with other inflammatory markers such as, CRP and ESR. However, no significant differences between responders and non-responders were observed in either *LIGHT* mRNA expression or LIGHT serum levels. A time gap between changes in inflammatory mediators and improvements in subjective disease severity scoring metrics may explain these findings (Haroon *et al.*, 2010). Although these results are interesting more studies are needed for validation. Another study using peripheral blood expression profiles based on PBMCs cells assessed several bone-regulatory factors as potential discriminators of different forms of arthritis, disease activity and therapy responsiveness (Grcevic *et al.*, 2010). ROC curve analysis suggested higher expression of Runx2 was a potential molecular marker for AS. Although no increased gene expression of *BMP-4* or *LIGHT* in AS patients compared with healthy controls were seen, higher expression was evident in AS patients resistant to conventional therapy. Thus *LIGHT* might be considered an interesting biomarker to consider in future studies.

Another marker which must be considered for a treatment-response marker is the CX3CL1-CC3CR1 complex. In RA, CX3CL1 levels decline in patients showing a clinical response to infliximab treatment. Moreover, patients with active RA who did not show a clinical response to infliximab showed higher basal CX3CL1 levels than those who did (Odai *et al.*, 2009). These results suggest that the CX3CL1-CX3CR1 in patients with active RA may be sensitive to anti-TNFα therapy and confirm that CX3CL1 plays a crucial role in the pathogenesis of RA, although further investigations are required. These results suggest that CX3CL1-CX3CR1 may be also relevant in AS process. This is further supported with the underexpression of this gene in AS patients (Pimentel-Santos *et al.*, 2011).

Gene symbol	Designation	Potential role
BMP6	Bone morphogenic protein 6	Bone remodelling and cartilage matrix turnover
PCSK6	Proprotein convertase subtilisin/kexin type 6	
KREMEN1	Kringle containing transmembrane protein 1	
CTNNAL1	Catenin (cadherin-associated protein) alpha-like 1	
SPOCK2	Sparc/osteonectin	
EP300	Nuclear p300	
PPP2R1A	Protein phosphatase 2, regulatory subunit A	
RGS1	Regulators of G protein signaling 1	Diagnosis of early AS/uSPA
LIGHT	Ligand for herpesvirus entry mediator	Response to anti-TNF alpha treatment
CX3CL1-CX3CR1	Chemokine (C-X3-C motif) ligand 1 - chemokine (C-X3-C motif) receptor 1	

Table 3. Potential clinical applications of microarray findings.

3. Conclusion

All the studies described above have contributed to increased knowledge of the physiopathological processes involved in AS and have identified potential disease relevant biomarkers with significance for clinical practice (see Table 3). The integration of the expression profiling data with information obtained from "omic" approaches such as proteomic and metabolomic analyses as well as with clinical and imaging data, may further elucidate disease processes and therapeutic responses in AS.

4. Acknowledgment

We thank Mafalda Matos for her help in figures and tables production.

5. References

Agostini, L.; Martinon, F.; Burns, K.; McDermott, MF.; Hawkins, PN. & Tschopp, J. (2004). NALP3 forms an IL-1beta-processing inflammasome with increased activity in Muckle-Wells autoinflammatory disorder. *Immunity*, Vol.20, No.3 (March 2004) pp. 319-325, ISSN, 1503-0775.

Ahmad, R.; Qureshi, HY.; El Mabrouk, M.; Sylvester, J.; Ahmad, M. & Zafarullah, M. (2007). Inhibition of interleukin 1-induced matrix metalloproteinase 13 expression in human chondrocytes by interferon gamma. *Annals of Rheumatic Disease,* Vol.66, No.6 (June 2007) pp. 782-789, ISSN, 1717-9173.

Alford, AI. & Hankenson, KD. (2006). Matricellular proteins: Extracellular modulators of bone development, remodeling, and regeneration. *Bone,* Vol.38, No.6 (June 2006) pp. 749–757, ISSN, 1641-2713.

Allison, DB.; Cui, X.; Page, GP. & Sabripour, M. (2006). Microarray data analysis: from disarray to consolidation and consensus. *Nature Reviews Genetics,* Vol.7, No.1 (January 2006) pp. 55-65, ISSN, 1636-9572.

Amor, B.; Dougados, M, & Mijiyawa, M. (1990). Criteria of the classification of spondylarthropathies. Révue du Rhumatism et des Maladies Ostéo-articulaires, Vol.57, No.2, (February 1990), pp.:85-89, ISSN 2181-618.

Amor, B.; Dougados, M.; Listrat, V.; Menkes, C.J.; Dubost, J.J.; Roux, H.; Benhamou, C.; Blotman, F.; Pattin, S.; Paolaggi, J.B.; *et al.* (1991). Evaluation of the Amor criteria for spondylarthropathies and European Spondylarthropathy Study Group (ESSG). A cross-sectional analysis of 2,228 patients. *Annales de Médicine Interne* (Paris), Vol.142, No.2, (1991), pp.85-89, ISSN. 2064-170

Anderson, JJ.; Baron, G.; van der Heijde, D.; Felson, DT. & Dougados, M. (2001). Ankylosing spondylitis assessment group preliminary definition of short-term improvement in ankylosing spondylitis. *Arthritis and Rheumatism,* Vol.44, No.8 (August 2001) pp. 1876–1886, ISSN, 1150-8441.

Assassi, S.; Reveille, JD.; Arnett, FC.; Weisman, MH.; Ward, MM.; Agarwal, SK.; Gourh, P.; Bhula, J.; Sharif, R.; Sampat, K.; Mayes, MD. & Tan, FK. (2011). Whole-blood gene expression profiling in ankylosing spondylitis shows upregulation of toll-like receptor 4 and 5. *The Journal of Rheumatology,* Vol.38, No.1 (January 2011) pp. 87-98, ISSN, 2095-2467.

Australo-Anglo-American Spondyloarthritis Consortium (TASC); Reveille, J.D., Sims, A.M., Danoy, P.; Evans, D.M.; Leo, P.; Pointon, J.J.; Jin, R.; Zhou, X.; Bradbury, L.A.; Appleton, L.H.; Davis, J.C.; Diekman, L.; Doan, T.; Dowling, A.; Duan, R.; Duncan, E.L.; Farrar, C.; Hadler, J.; Harvey, D., Karaderi, T.; Mogg, R.; Pomeroy, E.; Pryce, K.; Taylor, J., Savage, L., Deloukas, P.; Kumanduri, V.; Peltonen, L.; Ring, S.M.; Whittaker, P.; Glazov, E.; Thomas, G.P.; Maksymowych, W.P., Inman, R.D., Ward, M.M.; Stone, M.A.; Weisman, M.H.; Wordsworth, B.P. & Brown, M.A. (20109. Genome-wide association study of ankylosing spondylitis identifies non-MHC susceptibility loci. *Nature Genetics,* Vol.42, No.2, (February 2010), pp.123-127, ISSN 2006-2062

Baek, HJ.; Zhang, L.; Jarvis, LB. & Gaston, JS. (2008). Increased IL-4+ CD8+ T cells in peripheral blood and autoreactive CD8+ T cell lines of patients with inflammatory arthritis. (2008). *Rheumatology (Oxford),* Vol.47, No.6 (June 2008) pp. 795-803, ISSN, 1839-0584.

Barrett, JC.; Hansoul, S.; Nicolae, DL.; Cho, JH.; Duerr, R.; Rioux, JD.; Brant, SR.; Silverberg, MS.; Taylor, KD.; Barmada, MM.; Bitton, A.; Dassopoulos, T.; Datta, LW.; Green, T.; Griffiths, AM.; Kistner, EO.; Murtha, MT.; Regueiro, MD.; Rotter, JI.; Schumm, LP.;

Steinhart, AH.; Targan, SR.; Xavier, RJ.; NIDDK IBD Genetics Consortium.; Libioulle, C.; Sandor, C.; Lathrop, M.; Belaiche, J.; Dewit, O.; Gut, I.; Heath, S.; Laukens, D.; Mni, M.; Rutgeerts, P.; Van Gossum, A.; Zelenika, D.; Franchimont, D.; Hugot, JP.; de Vos, M.; Vermeire, S.; Louis, E.; Belgian-French IBD Consortium.; Wellcome Trust Case Control Consortium.; Cardon, LR.; Anderson, CA.; Drummond, H.; Nimmo, E.; Ahmad, T.; Prescott, NJ.; Onnie, CM.; Fisher, SA.; Marchini, J.; Ghori, J.; Bumpstead, S.; Gwilliam, R.; Tremelling, M.; Deloukas, P.; Mansfield, J.; Jewell, D.; Satsangi, J.; Mathew, CG.; Parkes, M.; Georges, M. & Daly, MJ. (2008). Genome-wide association defines more then 30 distinct susceptibility *loci* for crohn's disease. *Nature Genetics,* Vol.40, No.8 (August 2008) pp. 955-962, ISSN, 1858-7394.

Belcher, CE.; Drenkow, J.; Kehoe, B.; Gingeras, TR.; McNamara, N.; Lemjabbar, H.; Basbaum, C. & Relman, DA. (2000). The transcriptional responses of respiratory epithelial cells to Bordetella pertussis reveal host defensive and pathogen counter-defensive strategies. *Proceedings of the National Academy of Science of United States of America,* Vol.97, No.25 (December 2000) pp. 13847-13852, ISSN, 1108-7813.

Benjamin, M. & McGonagle, D. (2001). The anatomical basis for disease localisation in seronegative spondyloarthropathy at entheses and related sites. *Journal of Anatomy,* Vol.199, No.5 (November 2001) pp. 503-526, ISSN, 1176-0883.

Boonen, A.; Braun, J.; van der Horst Bruinsma, IE.; Huang, F.; Maksymowych, W.; Kostanjsek, N.; Cieza, A.; Stucki, G. & van der Heijde, D. (2010). ASAS/WHO ICF core sets for ankylosing spondylitis (AS): how to classify the impact of AS on functioning and health. *Annals of Rheumatic Disease,* Vol.69, No.1 (January 2010) pp. 102-107, ISSN, 1928-2309.

Boskey, AL.; Moore, DJ.; Amling, M.; Canalis, E. & Delany, AM. (2003). Infrared analysis of the mineral and matrix in bones of osteonectin-null mice and their wildtype controls. *Journal of Bone and Mineral Research,* Vol.18, No.6 (June 2003) pp. 1005-1011, ISSN, 1281-7752.

Braun, J.; Bollow, M.; Remlinger, G.; Eggens, U.; Rudwaleit, M.; Distler, A. & Sieper, J. (1998). Prevalence of spondylarthropathies in HLA-B27 positive and negative blood donors. *Arthritis and Rheumatism,* Vol.41, No.1 (January 1998) pp. 58-67, ISSN, 9433-870.

Canete, JD.; Martinez, SE.; Farres, J.; Sanmarti, R.; Blay, M.; Gomez, A.; Salvador, G. & Muñoz-Gómez, J. (2000). Differential Th1/Th2 cytokine patterns in chronic arthritis: interferon gamma is highly expressed in synovium of rheumatoid arthritis compared with seronegative spondyloarthropathies. *Annals of Rheumatic Disease,* Vol.59, No.4 (April 2000) pp. 263–268, ISSN, 1073-3472.

Carter, S. & Lories, RJ. (2011). Osteoporosis: A Paradox in Ankylosing Spondylitis. *Current Osteoporosis Reports.* (June 2011) [Epub ahead of print], ISSN, 2164-7573.

Cheng, CC.; Uchiyama, Y.; Hiyama, A.; Gajghate, S.; Shapiro, IM. & Risbud, MV. (2009). PI3K/AKT regulates aggrecan gene expression by modulating Sox9 expression and activity in nucleus pulposus cells of the intervertebral disc. *Journal of Cellular Physiology,* Vol.221, No.3 (December 2009) pp. 668-676, ISSN, 1971-1351.

Cummings, JR.; Cooney, RM.; Clarke, G.; Beckly, J.; Geremia, A.; Pathan, S.; Hancock, L.; Guo, C.; Cardon, LR. & Jewell, DP. (2010). The genetics of NOD-like receptors in Crohn's disease. *Tissue Antigens,* Vol.76, No.1 (July 2010) pp. 48-56, ISSN, 2040-3135

Danoy, P.; Pryce, K.; Hadler, J.; Bradbury, L.A.; Farrar, C.; Pointon, J.; Australo-Anglo-American Spondyloarthritis Consortium; Ward, M.; Weisman, M.; Reveille, J.D.; Wordsworth, B.P.; Stone, M.A.; Spondyloarthritis Research Consortium of Canada; Maksymowych, W.P.; Rahman, P.; Gladman, D.; Inman, R.D. & Brown, M.A. (2010). Association of variants at 1q32 and STAT3 with ankylosing spondylitis suggests genetic overlap with Crohn's disease. *PLoS Genetics,* Vol.6, No.12, (December 2010), e1001195, ISSN 2115-2001

De Rycke, L.; Vandooren, B.; Kruithof, E.; De Keyser, F.; Veys. EM. & Baeten D. (2005) Tumor necrosis factor alpha blockade treatment down-modulates the increased systemic and local expression of Toll-like receptor 2 and Toll-like receptor 4 in spondylarthropathy. *Arthritis and Rheumatism,* Vol.52, No.7 (July 2005) pp. 2146-2158.

De Vlam, K. (2010). Soluble and Tissue Biomarkers in Ankylosing Spondylitis. *Best Practice & Research Clinical Rheumatology,* Vol.24, No.5 (October 2010) pp. 671–682, ISSN, 2103-5087.

Debey, S.; Schoenbeck, U.; Hellmich, M.; Gathof, BS.; Pillai, R.; Zander, T. & Schultz, JL. (2004). Comparison of different isolation techniques prior gene expression profiling of blood derived cells: impact on physiological responses, on overall expression and the role of different cell types. *The Pharmacogenomics Journal,* Vol.4, No.3 (2004) pp. 193-207, ISSN, 1503-7859.

Delany, AM.; Amling, M.; Priemel, M.; Howe, C.; Baron, R. & Canalis, E. (2000). Osteopenia and decreased bone formation in osteonectin-deficient mice. *The journal of clinical investigation,* Vol.105, No.9 (May 2000) pp. 1325, ISSN, 1079-2008.

Delany, AM. & Hankenson, KD. (2009). Thrombospondin-2 and SPARC/osteonectin are critical regulators of bone remodeling. *Journal of cell communication and signalling,* Vol.3, No.3-4 (December 2009) pp. 227–238, ISSN, 1986-2642.

Diehn, M.; Alizadeh, AA.; Rando, OJ.; Liu, CL.; Stankunas, K.; Botstein, D.; Crabtree, GR. & Brown, PO. (2002). Genomic expression programs and the integration of the CD28 costimulatory signal in T cell activation. *Proceedings of the National Academy of Science of United States of America,* Vol.99, No.18 (September 2002) pp. 11796-11801, ISSN, 1219-5013.

Drenth, JPH. & van der Meer, JWM. (2006). The inflammasome: a linebacker of innate defense. *The New England Journal of Medicine,* Vol.355, No.7 (August 2006) pp. 730-732, ISSN, 1691-4711.

Drickamer, K. & Fadden, A.J. (2002). Genomic analysis of C-type lectins. *Biochemical Society Symposium,* Vol.59, No.69, (2002) pp 59-72, ISSN 1265-5774

Duan, R.; Leo, P.; Bradbury, L.; Brown, MA. & Thomas, G. (2010). Gene expression profiling reveals a downregulation in immune-associated genes in patients with AS. *Annals of Rheumatic* Disease, Vol.69, No.9 (September 2010) pp. 1724-1729, ISSN, 1964-3760.

Dupuy, A. & Simon, RM. (2007). Critical review of published microarray studies for cancer outcome and guidelines on statistical analysis and reporting. *Journal of the National Cancer Institute,* Vol.99, No.2 (January 2007) pp. 147-157, ISSN, 1722-7998.

Feldtkeller, E.; Khan, MA.; van der Heijde, D.; van der Linden, S. & Braun, J. (2003). Age at disease onset and diagnosis delay in HLA-B27 negative vs. Positive patients with ankylosing spondylitis. *Rheumatology International,* Vol.23, No.2 (March 2003) pp. 61-66, ISSN, 1263-4937.

Fitzgerald, K.A. (2010). NLR-containing inflamasomes: Central mediators of host defense and inflammation. *European Journal of Immunology,* Vol.40, No.3 (March 2010) pp. 595-598, ISSN, 2020-1007.

Gewirtz, AT.; Navas, TA.; Lyons, S.; Godowski, PJ. & Madara, JL. (2001). Cutting edge: bacterial flagellin activates basolaterally expressed TLR5 to induce epithelial proinflammatory gene expression. *Journal of Immunology,* Vol.167, No.4 (August 2001) pp. 1882-1885, ISSN, 1148-9966.

Ghosh, AK.; Yuan, W.; Mori, Y.; Chen, Sj. & Varga, J. (2001). Antagonistic regulation of type I collagen gene expression by interferon-gamma and transforming growth factor-beta. Integration at the level of p300/CBP transcriptional coactivators. *The Journal of Biological Chemistry,* Vol.276, No.14 (April 2001) pp. 11041-11048, ISSN, 1113-4049.

Giannini, AL.; Vivanco, MM. & Kypta RM. (2000). Alpha-Catenin Inhibits β-Catenin Signaling by Preventing Formation of a β-Catenin T-cell Factor DNA Complex. *The Journal of Biological Chemistry,* Vol.275, No.29 (July 2000) pp. 21883–21888, ISSN, 1089-6949.

Gordon, M.D. & Nusse, R. (2006). Wnt signaling: multiple pathways, multiple receptors, and multiple transcription factors. The Journal of Biological Chemistry, Vol.281, No.32, (August 2006), 22429-22433, ISSN, 1679-3760

Graham, LM. & Brown, GD. (2009). The Dectin-2 family of C-type lectins in immunity and homeostasis. *Cytokine.* Vol.48, No.1-2 (November 2009) pp. 148–155, ISSN, 1966-5392.

Grcevic, D.; Jajic, Z.; Kovacic, N.; Lukic, I.K.; Velagic, V.; Grubisic, F.; Ivcevic, S. & Marusic, A. (2010). Peripheral blood expression profiles of bone morphogenetic proteins, tumor necrosis factor-superfamily molecules, and transcription factor Runx2 could be used as markers of the form of arthritis, disease activity, and therapeutic responsiveness. *The Journal of Rheumatology,* Vol. 37, No.2,(February 2010), pp. 246-56, ISSN, 2000-8919

Gruber, HE.; Sage, EH.; Norton, HJ.; Funk, S.; Ingram, J. & Hanley EN, Jr. (2005). Targeted deletion of the SPARC gene accelerates disc degeneration in the aging mouse. The *Journal of Histochemistry Cytochemistry,* Vol.53, No.9 (September 2005) pp. 1131-1138, ISSN, 1587-9573.

Gu, J.; Marker-Hermann, E.; Baeten, D.; Tsai, WC.; Gladman, D.; Xiong, M.; Deister, H.; Kuipers, JG.; Huang, F.; Song, YW.; Maksymowych, W.; Kalsi, J.; Bannai, M.; Seta, N.; Rihl, M.; Crofford, LJ.; Veys, E.; De Keyser, F. & Yu, DT. (2002a). A 588-gene microarray analysis of the peripheral blood mononuclear cells of spondyloarthropathy patients. *Rheumatology* (Oxford), Vol.41, No.7 (July 2002) pp. 759-766, ISSN, 1209-6225.

Gu, J.; Rihl, M.; Märker-Hermann, E.; Baeten, D.; Kuipers, JG.; Song, YW.; Maksymowych, WP.; Burgos-Vargas, R.; Veys, EM.; De Keyser, F.; Deister, H.; Xiong, M.; Huang, F.; Tsai, WC. & Yu, DT. (2002b). Clues to pathogenesis of spondyloarthropathy derived from synovial fluid mononuclear cell gene expression profiles. The *Journal of Rheumatology*, Vol.29, No.10 (October 2002) pp. 2159-2164, ISSN, 1237-5327.

Gu, J.; Wei, YL.; Wei, JC.; Huang, F.; Jan, MS.; Centola, M.; Frank, MB. & Yu, D. (2009). Identification of RGS1 as a candidate biomarker for undifferentiated spondylarthritis by genome-wide expression profiling and real-time polymerase chain reaction. *Arthritis and Rheumatism*, Vol.60, No.11 (November 2009) pp. 3269-3279, ISSN, 1987-7080.

Guillemin, K.; Salama, NR.; Tompkins, LS. & Falkow, S. (2002). Cag pathogenecity island-specific responses of gastric epithelial cells to Helicobacter pylori infection. *Proceedings of the National Academy of Science of United States of America*, Vol.99, No.23 (November 2002) pp. 15136-15141, ISSN, 1241-1577.

Haibel, H.; Brandt, HC.; Song, IH.; Brandt, A.; Listing, J.; Rudwaleit, M. & Sieper, J. (2007). No efficacy of subcutaneous methotrexate in active ankylosing spondylitis: a 16-week open-label trial. *Annals of Rheumatic* Disease, Vol.66, No.3 (March 2007) pp. 419-421, ISSN, 1690-1959.

Hamilton, L.; Gilbert, A.; Skerrett, J.; Dickinson, S. & Gaffney, K. (2011). Services for people with ankylosing spondylitis in the UK--a survey of rheumatologists and patients. *Rheumatology (Oxford)*, (March 2011) [Epub ahead of print], ISSN, 2142-1687.

Hardiman, G. (2004). Microarrays platforms-comparisons and contrasts. *Pharmacogenomics*, Vol.5, No.5 (July 2004) pp. 487-502, ISSN, 1521-2585.

Haroon, N.; Tsui, FWL.; O'Shea, FD.; Chiu, B.; Tsui, HW.; Zhang, H.; Marshall, WK. & Inman, RD. (2010). From gene expression to serum proteins: biomarker discovery in Ankylosing Spondylitis. *Annals of the Rheumatic Diseases*, Vol.69, No.1 (January 2010) pp. 297-300, ISSN, 1910-3635.

Hausser, HJ.; Decking, R. & Brenner, RE. (2004). Testican-1, an inhibitor of pro-MMP-2 activation, is expressed in cartilage. *Osteoarthritis Cartilage*, Vol.12, No.11 (November 2004) pp. 870-877, ISSN, 1550-1402.

Hayashi, F.; Smith, KD.; Ozinsky, A.; Hawn, TR.; Yi, EC.; Goodlett, DR.; Eng, JK.; Akira, S.; Underhill, DM. & Aderem, A . (2001). The innate immune response to bacterial flagellin is mediated by Toll-like receptor 5. *Nature*, Vol.410, No.6832 (April 2001) pp. 1099-103, ISSN, 1132-3673.

Heikkinen, PT.; Nummela, M.; Leivonen, SK.; Westermarck, J.; Hill, CS.; Kähäri, VM. & Jaakkola, PM. (2010). Hypoxia-activated Smad3-specific dephosphorylation by PP2A. *The Journal of Biological Chemistry*, Vol.285, No.6 (February 2010) pp. 3740-3749, ISSN, 1995-1945.

Hsu, YM.; Zhang, Y.; You, Y.; Wang, D.; Li, H.; Duramad, O.; Qin, XF.; Dong, C. & Lin, X. (2007). The adaptor protein CARD9 is required for innate immune responses to intracellular pathogens. *Nature Immunology*, Vol.8, No.2 (February 2007) pp. 198-205, ISSN, 1718-7069.

Inman, RD. & Chiu, B. (2006). Early cytokine profiles in the joint define pathogen clearance and severity of arthritis in Chlamydia-induced arthritis in rats. *Arthritis and Rheumatism,* Vol.54, No.2 (February 2006) pp. 499–507, ISSN, 1644-7224.

Ioannidis, JP.; Allison, DB.; Ball, CA.; Coulibaly, I.; Cui, X.; Culhane, AC.; Falchi, M.; Furlanello, C.; Game, L.; Jurman, G.; Mangion, J.; Mehta, T.; Nitzberg, M.; Page, GP.; Petretto, E. & van Noort, V. (2009). Repeatability of published microarray gene expression analyses. *Nature Genetics,* Vol.41, No.2 (February 2009) pp. 149-155, ISSN, 1917-4838.

Jarvis, LB.; Matyszak, MK.; Duggleby, RC.; Goodall, JC.; Hall, FC. & Gaston, JS. (2005). Autoreactive human peripheral blood CD8+ T cells with a regulatory phenotype and function. *European Journal of Immunology,* Vol.35, No.10 (October 2005) pp. 2896-2908, ISSN, 1618-0249.

Jelinek, DF. & Lipsky, PE. (1988). Inhibitory influence of IL-4 on human B cell responsiveness. *Journal of Immunology,* Vol.141, No.1 (July 1988) pp. 164-173, ISSN, 2837-507.

Jeong, E. & Lee, JY. (2011). Intrinsic and Extrinsic Regulation of Innate Immune Receptors. *Yonsei Medical Journal,* Vol.52, No.3 (May 2011) pp. 379-392, ISSN, 2148-8180.

Kanazawa, N. (2007). Dendritic cell immunoreceptors: C-type lectin receptors for pattern-recognition and signaling on antigen-presenting cells. *Journal of Dermatological Science,* Vol.45, No.2 (February 2007) pp. 77-86, ISSN, 1704-6204.

Kandpal, R.; Saviola, B. & Felton, J. (2009). The era of 'omics unlimited. *Biotechniques,* Vol.46, No.5 (April 2009) pp. 351-2, 354-5, ISSN, 1948-0630.

Kappen, JH.; Wallace, GR.; Stolk, L.; Rivadeneira, F.; Uitterlinden, AG.; van Daele, PL.; Laman, JD.; Kuijpers, RW.; Baarsma, GS.; Stanford, MR.; Fortune, F.; Madanat, W.; van Hagen, PM. & van Laar, JA. (2009). Low prevalence of NOD2 SNPs in Behçet's disease suggests protective association in Caucasians. *Rheumatology (Oxford),* Vol.48, No.11 (November 2009) pp. 1375-1377, ISSN, 1974-8964.

Kronenberg, HM. (2003). Developmental regulation of the growth plate. *Nature,* Vol.423, No.6937 (May 2003) pp. 332-336, ISSN, 1274-8651.

Lange, U.; Kluge, A.; Strunk, J.; Teichmann, J. & Bachmann, G. (2005). Ankylosing spondylitis and bone mineral density--what is the ideal tool for measurement? *Rheumatol International,* Vol.26, No.2 (December 2005) pp.115-120, ISSN, 1553-8574

Laukens, D.; Peeters, H.; Cruyssen, B.V.; Boonefaes, T.; Elewaut, D.; De Keyser, F.; Mielants, H.; Cuvelier, C.; Veys, E.M.; Knecht, K.; Van Hummelen, P.; Remaut, E.; Steidler, L.; De Vos, M. & Rottiers, P.(2006). Altered gut transcriptome in spondyloarthropathy. *Annals of the Rheumatic Diseases,* Vol. 65, No.10, (October 2006), pp. 1293-1300, ISSN 1647-6712

Li, X.; Quigg, RJ.; Zhou, J.; Gu, W.; Nagesh Rao, P. & Reed, EF. (2008). Clinical Utility of Microarrays: Current Status, Existing Challenges and Future Outlook. *Current Genomics,* Vol.9, No.7 (November 2008) pp. 466-474, ISSN, 1950-6735.

Licciardone, JC. (2008). The epidemiology and medical management of low back pain during ambulatory medical care visits in the United States. *Osteopathic Medicine and Primary Care,* Vol.2 (November 2008) pp.11, ISSN, 1902-5636.

Long, EO. (1999). Regulation of immune responses through inhibitory receptors. *Annual Review of Immunology,* Vol.17 (1999) pp. 875–904, ISSN, 1035-8776.

Lord, PAC.; Farragher, TM.; Lunt, M.; Watson, KD.; Symmons, DPM.; HYrich, KL. & BSR Biologics Register. (2010). Predictors of response to anti-TNF therapy in ankylosing spondylitis: results from the British Society for Rheumatology Biologic register. *Rheumatology* (Oxford), Vol.49, No.3 (March 2010) pp.563-570, ISSN, 2003-2223.

Lories, RJ.; Derese, I. & Luyten, FP. (2005). Modulation of bone morphogenetic protein signaling inhibits the onset and progression of ankylosing enthesitis. *The Journal of Clinical Investigation,* Vol.115, No.6 (June 2005) pp. 1571-1579, ISSN, 1590-2307.

Lu, X.; Malumbres, R.; Shields, B.; Jiang, X.; Sarosiek, KA.; Natkunam, Y.; Tiganis, T. & Lossos, IS. (2008). PTP1B is a negative regulator of interleukin 4-induced STAT6 signaling. *Blood,* Vol.112, No.10 (November 2008) pp. 4098-4108, ISSN, 1871-6132.

Ma, CS.; Chew, GYJ.; Simpson, N.; Priyadarshi, A.; Wong, M.; Grimbacher, B.; Fulcher, DA.; Tangye, SG. & Cook, MC. (2008). Deficiency of the Th17 cells in Hyper IgE syndrome due to mutation in STAT3. *The Journal of Experimental Medicine,* Vol.205, No.7 (July 2008) pp. 1551-1557, ISSN, 1859-1410.

Machado do Reis, L.; Kessler, CB.; Adams, DJ.; Lorenzo, J.; Jorgetti, V. & Delany, AM. (2008). Accentuated osteoclastic response to parathyroid hormone undermines bone mass acquisition in osteonectin-null mice. *Bone,* Vol.43, No.2 (August 2008) pp. 264–273, ISSN, 1849-9553.

Majeed, M.; Caveggion, E.; Lowell, CA. & Berton, G. (2001). Role of Src kinases and Syk in Fcgamma receptormediated phagocytosis and phagosome-lysosome fusion. *Journal of Leukocyte Biology,* Vol.70, No.5 (November 2001) pp. 801–811, ISSN, 1169-8501.

Mansergh, FC.; Wells, T.; Elford, C.; Evans, SL.; Perry, MJ.; Evans, MJ. & Evans, BA. (2007). Osteopenia in Sparc (osteonectin)-deficient mice: characterization of phenotypic determinants of femoral strength and changes in gene expression. *Physiological Genomics,* Vol.32, No.1 (December 2007) pp. 64-73, ISSN, 1787-8319.

Mao, B. & Niehrs, C. (2003). Kremen2 modulates Dickkopf2 activity during Wnt/LRP6 signaling. *Gene,* Vol.302, No.(1-2) (January 2003) pp. 179-183, ISSN, 1252-7209.

Michiels, S.; Koscielny, S. & Hill, C. (2007). Interpretation of microarray data in cancer. *British Journal of Cancer,* Vol.96, No.8 (April 2007) pp. 1155-1158, ISSN, 1734-2085.

Michiels, S.; Kramarb, A. & Koscielny, S. (2011). Multidimensionality of microarrays: Statistical challenges and (im)possible solutions. *Molecular Oncology,* Vol.5, No.2 (April 2011) pp.190-196, ISSN, 2134-9780.

Mielants, H.; Veys, EM.; Cuvelier, C.; De Vos, M.; Goemaere, S.; De Clercq, L.; Schatteman, L. & Elewaut, D. (1995). The evolution of spondyloarthropathies in relation to gut histology. II. Histological aspects. *The Journal of Rheumatology,* Vol.22, No.12 (December 1995) pp. 2273-2278, ISSN, 8835-561.

Odai, T.; Matsunawa, M.; Takahashi, R.; Wakabayshi, K.; Isozaki, T.; Yajima, N.; Miwa, Y. & Kasama, T. (2009). Correlation of CX3CL1 and CX3CR1 Levels with Response to Infliximab Therapy in Patients with Rheumatoid Arthritis. *The Journal of Rheumatology,* Vol.36, No.6 (June 2009) pp. 1158-1165, ISSN, 1936-9458.

O'Garra, A.; Umland, S.; De France, T. & Christiansen, J. (1988). 'B-cell factors' are pleiotropic. *Immunology Today,* Vol.9, No.2 (February 1999) pp. 45-54, ISSN, 3151-436.

Park, J.H.; Adoro, S.; Guinter, T; Erman, B.; Alag, A.S.; Catalfamo, M.; Kimura, M.Y.; Cui, Y.; Lucas, P.J.; Gress, R.E.; Kubo, M.; Hennighausen, L.; Feigenbaum, L.& Singer, A. (2010). Signaling by intrathymic cytokines, not T cell antigen receptors, specifies CD8 lineage choice and promotes the differentiation of cytotoxic-lineage T cells. *Nature Immunology,* Vol.11, No.3, (Mars 2010), pp. 257-264, ISSN 2011-8929

Paul, WE. & Ohara, J. (1987). B-cell stimulatory factor-1/interleukin 4. *Annual Review of Immunology,* Vol.5, (1987) pp. 429-459, ISSN, 3297-106.

Pawitan, Y.; Michiels, S.; Koscielny, S.; Gusnanto, A. & Ploner, A. (2005). False discovery rate, sensitivity and sample size for microarray studies. *Bioinformatics,* Vol.21, No.13 (July 2005) pp. 3017-3024, ISSN, 1584-0707.

Pimentel-Santos, FM.; Ligeiro, D.; Matos, M.; Mourão, AF.; Costa, J.; Santos, H.; Barcelos, A.; Godinho, F.; Pinto, P.; Cruz, M.; Fonseca, JE.; Guedes-Pinto, H.; Branco, JC.; Brown, MA. & Thomas, GP. (2011). Whole blood transcriptional profiling in ankylosing spondylitis identifies novel candidate genes that might contribute to the inflammatory and tissue-destructive disease aspects. *Arthritis Research & Therapy,* Vol.13, No.2 (April 2011) R57 [Epub ahead of print], ISSN, 2147-0430.

Pointon, JJ.; Harvey, D.; Karaderi, T.; Appleton, LH.; Farrar, C.; Stone, MA.; Sturrock, RD.; Brown, MA. & Wordsworth, BP. (2010). Elucidating the chromosome 9 association with AS; CARD9 is a candidate gene. *Genes and Immunity,* Vol.11, No.6 (September 2010) pp. 490-496, ISSN, 2046-3747

Raetz, E.A. & Moos, P.J. (2004).. Impact of microarray technology in clinical oncology. *Cancer Investigation,* Vol. 22, No. 2, (2004), pp. 312-320, ISSN 1519-9613

Ramasamy, A.; Mondry, A.; Holmes, C.C. & Altman, D.G. (2008). Key issues in conducting a meta-analysis of gene expression microarray datasets. *PLoS Medicin,* Vol.5, No.9, (September 2008), e184, ISSN, 1876-7902

Ransohoff, D.F. (2007). How to improve reliability and efficiency of research about molecular markers: roles of phases, guidelines, and study design. *Journal of Clinical Epidemiology,* Vol.60, No.12, (December 2007), pp. 1205-1219, ISSN 1799-807

Rao, G. (2003). What is an ROC curve? *The Journal of Family Practice,* Vol. 52, No. 9, (September 2003), pp. 695, ISSN 1296-7540

Reimers, M. (2010). Making informed choices about microarray data analysis. *PLoS Computational Biology,* Vol.6, No.5, (May 2010), e1000786, ISSN 2052-3743

Repsilber, D.; Mansmann, U.; Brunner, E.& Ziegler, A. (2005). Tutorial on Microarray Gene Expression Experiments. *Methods of Information in Medicine* (2005), Vol.44, No.3, pp. 392-399, ISSN 1611-3762

Rothfuchs, A.G.; Gigliotti, D.; Palmblad, K.; Andersson, U.; Wigzell, H.& Rottenberg, M.E. (2001). IFN-alpha betadependent, IFN-gamma secretion by bone marrow-derived macrophages controls an intracellular bacterial infection. *Journal of Immunology,* Vol.167, No.11, (December 2001), pp. 6453–6461, ISSN .1171-4812

Rousset, F.; Malefijt, R.W.; Slierendregt, B.; Aubry, J.P., Bonnefoy, J.Y.; Defrance, T.; Banchereau, J.& de Vries, J.E.(1988). Regulation of Fc receptor for IgE (CD23) and class II MHC antigen expression on Burkitt's lymphoma cell lines by human IL-4 and IFN-gamma. *Journal of Immunology,* (April 1988), Vol.140, No.8, pp. 2625-2632, ISSN 2965-726

Rudwaleit. M.; Siegert, S.; Yin, Z.; Eick, J.; Thiel, A.; Radbruch, A.; Sieper, J.& Braun, J. (2001).. Low T cell production of TNFα and IFN γ in ankylosing spondylitis: its relation to HLA-B27 and influence of the TNF-308 gene polymorphism. *Annals of the Rheumatic Diseases,* Vol.60, No.1, (January 2001), pp.36–42, ISSN 1111-4280

Rudwaleit, M.; Listing, J.; Brandt, J.; Braun, J.& Sieper, J. (2004). Prediction of a major clinical response (BASDAI 50) to tumour necrosis factor alpha blockers in ankylosing spondylitis. *Annals of the Rheumatic Diseases,* Vol.63, No.6, (June 2004), pp. 665-670, ISSN 1503-7444

Rudwaleit, M.; Khan, M.A. & Sieper, J. (2005). The challenge of diagnosis and classification in early ankylosing spondylitis: do we need new criteria? *Arthritis and Rheumatism,* Vol.52, No.4, (April 2005), pp.1000-1008, ISSN 1581-8678

Rudwaleit, M.; Schwarzlose, S.; Hilgert, E.S.; Listing, J.; Braun, J. & Sieper, J. (2008). MRI in predicting a major clinical response to anti-TNF-treatment in ankylosing spondylitis. *Annals of the Rheumatic Diseases,* Vol. 67, No.9, (September 2008), pp.1276-1281, ISSN 1800-6539

Rudwaleit, M.; Haibel, H.; Baraliakos, X.; Listing, J.; Märker-Hermann, E.; Zeidler, H.; Braun, J.& Sieper, J. (2009a). The early disease stage in axial spondylarthritis results from the German Spondyloarthritis Inception Cohort. *Arthritis and Rheumatism,* Vol.60, No.3, (Mars 2009), pp. 717-727, ISSN. 1924-8087

Rudwaleit, M.; Landewe, R.; van der Heijde, D.; Listing, J.; Brandt, J.; Braun, J.; Burgos-Vargas, R.; Collantes-Estevez, E.; Davis, J.; Dijkmans, B.; Dougados, M.; Emery, P.; van der Horst-Bruinsma, I.E.; Inman, R.; Khan, M.A.; Leirisalo-Repo, M.; van der Linden, S.; Maksymowych, W.P.; Mielants, H.; Olivieri, I.; Sturrock, R.; de Vlam, K.& Sieper, J. (2009b). The development of Assessment of SpondyloArthritis international Society classification criteria for axial spondyloarthritis (part I): classification of paper patients by expert opinion including uncertainty appraisal. *Annals of the Rheumatic Diseases,* Vol.68, No.6, (June 2009), pp.770-776, ISSN 1929-7345

Rudwaleit, M.(2010). New approaches to diagnosis and classification of axial and peripheral spondyloarthritis. *Current Opinion in Rheumatology.* Vol.22, No.4, (July 2010), pp. 375-380, ISSN 2047-3175

Ruutu, M.; Yadav, B.; Thomas, G.; Steck, R.; Strutton, G.; Tran, A.; Velasco, J.; Deglia Esposti, M., Zinkernagel, M.; Brown, M.& Thomas, R. (2010) Fungal beta-glucan triggers spondyloarthropathy and Crohn's disease in SKG mice. *Arthritis and Rheumatism,* Vol.62, Suppl.10, (2010), pp.1446.

Schroder, K.& Tschopp, J. (2010). The inflammasomes. *Cell,* Vol.140, No.6, (Mars 2010), pp.821-832, ISSN 2030-3873

Shaffer, A.L.; Yu, X.; He, Y.; Boldrick, J.; Chan, E.P. & Staudt, L.M. (2000). BCL-6 repress genes that function in lymphocyte differentiation, inflammation, and cell cycle control. *Immunity,* Vol.13, No.2, (August 2000), pp.199-212, ISSN 1098-1963

Shalon, D.; Smith, S.J. & Brown, P.O. (1996). A DNA microarray system for analyzing complex DNA samples using two-color fluorescent probe hybridization. *Genome Research,* Vol.6, No.7, (July 1996), pp. 639-645, ISSN 8796-352

Sharma, S.M.; Choi, D.; Planck, S.R.; Harrington, C.A.; Austin, C.R.; Lewis, J.A.; Diebel, T.N.; Martin, T.M.; Smith, J.R. & Rosenbaum, J.T. (2009). Insights in to the pathogenesis of axial spondyloarthropathy based on gene expression profiles. *Arthritis Research & Therapy,* Vol.11, No.6, (November 2009), R168, ISSN 1990-0269

Sieper, J. (2009). Developments in the scientific and clinical understanding of the Spondyloarthritides. *Arthritis Research & Therapy,* Vol.11, No.1, (January 2009), R208, ISSN 1923-2062

Simon, R.; Lam, A.; Li, M.C.; Ngan, M.; Menenzes, S. & Zhao, Y. (2007). Analysis of Gene Expression Data Using BRB-Array Tools. *Cancer Informatics,* Vol.3, (February 2007), pp.11-17, ISSN 1945-5231

Sirisinha, S. (2011). Insight into the mechanisms regulating immune homeostasis in health and disease. *Asian Pacific Journal of Allergy and Immunology*, Vol.29, No.1, (Mars 2011); pp.1-14, ISSN 2156-0483

Smith, G.W.& Rosa, G.J.M. (2007). Interpretation of microarray data: Trudging out of the abyss towards elucidation of biological significance. *Journal of Animal Science,* Vol.85, Suppl.13, (Mars 2007), E20–23, ISSN 1732-2122

Smith, J.A.; Barnes, M.D.; Hong, D.; DeLay, M.L.; Inman, R.D.& Colbert, R.A. (2008). Gene expression analysis of macrophages derived from ankylosing spondylitis patients reveals interferon-gamma dysregulation. *Arthritis and Rheumatism,* Vol.58, No.6, (June 2008), pp.1640-1649, ISSN 1851-2784

Southern, E.M. (1975). Detection of specific sequences among DNA fragments separated by gel electrophoresis. *Journal of Molecular Biology,* Vol.98, No.3, (November 1975) pp.503-517, ISSN 1195-397

Taurog, J.D.; Richardson, J.A., Croft, J.T.; Simmons, W.A.; Zhou, M.; Fernandez-Sueiro, J.L.; Balish, E. & Hammer, R.E. (1994). The germfree state prevents development of gut and joint inflammatory disease in HLA-B27 transgenic rats. *Journal of Experimental Medicine,* Vol.180, No.6, (December 1994), pp.2359-2364, ISSN 7964-509

The Australo-Anglo-American Spondyloarthritis Consortium (TASC); the Wellcome Trust Case Control Consortium 2 (WTCCC2); Evans. D.M.; Spencer, C.C.; Pointon, J.J.; Su, Z.; Harvey, D.; Kochan, G.; Opperman, U.; Dilthey, A; Pirinen, M.; Stone, M.A.; Appleton, L.; Moutsianis, L.; Leslie, S.; Wordsworth, T.; Kenna, T.J.; Karaderi, T.; Thomas, G.P.; Ward, M.M.; Weisman, M.H.; Farrar, C.; Bradbury, L.A.; Danoy, P.; Inman, R.D.; Maksymowych, W.; Gladman, D.; Rahman, P.; Spondyloarthritis Research Consortium of Canada (SPARCC); Morgan, A.; Marzo-Ortega, H.; Bowness, P.; Gaffney, K.; Gaston, J.S.; Smith, M.; Bruges-Armas, J.; Couto, A.R.; Sorrentino, R.; Paladini, F.; Ferreira, M.A.; Xu, H.; Liu, Y.; Jiang, L.; Lopez-Larrea, C.; Díaz-Peña, R.; López-Vázquez, A.; Zayats, T.; Band, G.; Bellenguez, C.; Blackburn, H.; Blackwell, J.M.; Bramon, E.; Bumpstead, S.J.; Casas, J.P.; Corvin, A.; Craddock, N.; Deloukas, P.; Dronov, S.; Duncanson, A; Edkins, S.; Freeman, C.; Gillman, M.; Gray, E.; Gwilliam, R.; Hammond, N.; Hunt, S.E.; Jankowski, J.; Jayakumar, A.; Langford, C.; Liddle, J.; Markus, H.S.; Mathew, C.G.; McCann, O.T.;

McCarthy, M.I.; Palmer, C.N.; Peltonen, L.; Plomin, R.; Potter, S.C.; Rautanen, A.; Ravindrarajah, R.; Ricketts, M.; Samani, N.; Sawcer, S.J.; Strange, A.; Trembath, R.C.; Viswanathan, A.C.; Waller, M.; Weston, P.; Whittaker, P.; Widaa, S.; Wood, N.W.; McVean, G.; Reveille, J.D.; Wordsworth, B.P.; Brown, M.A. & Donnelly, P. (2011). Interaction between ERAP1 and HLA-B27 in ankylosing spondylitis implicates peptide handling in the mechanism for HLA-B27 in disease susceptibility. *Nature Genetics,* (July 2011) [Epub ahead of print], ISSN 2174-3469

Thomas, G.P. & Brown, M.A. (2010a). Genetics and genomics of ankylosing spondylitis. *Immunological Reviews,* Vol 233, No.1, (January 2010), pp.162-180, ISSN 2019-2999

Thomas, G.P. & Brown, M.A. (2010b). Genomics of ankylosing spondylitis. *Discovery Medicine,* Vol.10, No.52, (September 2010), pp. 263-271, ISSN 2087-5348

Underwood, M.R. & Dawes, P. (1995). Inflammatory back pain in primary care. *British Journal of Rheumatology.* Vol.34, No.11, (November 1995), pp. 1074–1077, ISSN 8542-211

van Damme, N.; De Vos, M.; Baeten, D.; Demetter, P.; Mielants, H.; Verbruggen, G.; Cuvelier, C.; Veys, E.M.& De Keyser, F. (2001). Flow cytometric analysis of gut mucosal lymphocytes supports an impaired Th1 cytokine profile in spondyloarthropathy. *Annals of Rheumatic Diseases,* Vol.60, No.5, (May 2001), pp.495–499, ISSN 1130-2872

van den Berg, R.; van der Heijde, D. (2010). How should we diagnose spondyloarthritis according to the ASAS classification criteria. A guide for practicing physicians. *Polskie Archiwum Medycyny Wewnetrznej,* Vol.120, No.11, (November 2010), pp.452-457, ISSN 2110-2381

van der Heijde, D.; Lie, E.; Kvien, T.K.; Sieper, J.; Van den Bosch, F.; Listing, J.; Braun, J.; Landewé, R. & Assessment of SpondyloArthritis international Society (ASAS). (2009). ASDAS, a highly discriminatory ASAS-endorsed disease activity score in patients with ankylosing spondylitis. *Annals of the Rheumatic Diseases,* Vol.68, No.12, (December 2009), pp.1811-1818, ISSN 1906-0001

van der Linden, S.; Valkenburg, H.A. & Cats, A. (1984). Evaluation of diagnostic criteria for ankylosing spondylitis. A proposal for modification of the New York criteria. *Arthritis and Rheumatism,* Vol.27, No.4, (April 1984), pp.361–368, ISSN 6231-933

Visvanathan, S.; Wagner, C.; Marini, J.C.; Baker, D.; Gathany, T.; Han, J.; van der Heijde, D.& Braun, J. (2008). Inflammatory biomarkers, disease activity and spinal disease measures in patients with ankylosing spondylitis after treatment with infliximab. *Annals of the Rheumatic Diseases,* Vol.67, No.4, (April, 2008), pp.511-517, ISSN 1764-4552

Wang, K.; Zhang, Y.; Li, X.; Chen, L.; Wang, H.; Wu, J.; Zheng, J. & Wu, D. (2008). Characterization of the Kremen-binding Site on Dkk1 and Elucidation of the Role of Kremen in Dkk-mediated Wnt Antagonism. *The Journal of Biological Chemistry,* Vol.83, No.34, (August 2008), pp.23371–23375, ISSN 1850-2762

Workman, C.; Jensen, L.J.; Jarmer, H.; Berka, R.; Gautier, L.; Nielser, H.B.; Saxild, H.H.; Nielsen, C.; Brunak, S.& Knudsen, S. (2002). A new non-linear normalization method for reducing variability in DNA microarray experiments. *Genome Biology,* Vol. 3, No.9, (August 2002), research0048, ISSN 1222-5587

Yang, Z.X.; Liang, Y.; Zhu, Y.; Li, C.; Zhang, L.Z.; Zeng, X.M. & Zhong, R.Q. (2007). Increased expression of Toll-like receptor 4 in peripheral blood leucocytes and serum levels of some cytokines in patients with ankylosing spondylitis. *Clinical and Experimental Immunology,* Vol.149, No.1, (July 2007), pp.48-55, ISSN 1745-9079

Yelo, E.; Bernardo, M.V.; Gimeno, L.; Alcaraz-García, M.J.; Majado, M.J. & Parrado, A. (2008). Dock10, a novel CZH protein selectively induced by interleukin-4 in human B lymphocytes. *Molecular Immunology* Vol.45, No.12, (July 2008), pp.3411-3418, ISSN 1849-9258

Zelensky, N.A. & Gready, J.E. (2005). The C-type lectin-like domain superfamily. *The FEBS Journal,* Vol.272, No.24, (December 2005), pp. 6179-6217, ISSN 1742-4658

Zhang, L, Jarvis, L.B.; Baek, H.J. & Gaston, J.S. (2009). Regulatory IL4+CD8+ T cells in patients with ankylosing spondylitis and healthy controls. *Annals of the Rheumatic Diseases,* Vol.68, No.8 (August 2009), pp.1345-1351, ISSN 1864-7857